Substance Abuse

Recent Titles in the
CONTEMPORARY WORLD ISSUES
Series

Books in the **Contemporary World Issues** series address vital issues in today's society such as genetic engineering, pollution, and biodiversity. Written by professional writers, scholars, and nonacademic experts, these books are authoritative, clearly written, up-to-date, and objective. They provide a good starting point for research by high school and college students, scholars, and general readers as well as by legislators, businesspeople, activists, and others.

Each book, carefully organized and easy to use, contains an overview of the subject, a detailed chronology, biographical sketches, facts and data and/or documents and other primary source material, a forum of authoritative perspective essays, annotated lists of print and nonprint resources, and an index.

Readers of books in the Contemporary World Issues series will find the information they need in order to have a better understanding of the social, political, environmental, and economic issues facing the world today.

Substance Abuse

A REFERENCE HANDBOOK

Second Edition

David E. Newton

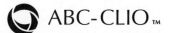

ABC-CLIO™

An Imprint of ABC-CLIO, LLC

Santa Barbara, California • Denver, Colorado

Library of Congress Cataloging-in-Publication Data

Names: Newton, David E., author.
Title: Substance abuse : a reference handbook / David E. Newton.
Description: Second edition. | Santa Barbara, California :
    ABC-CLIO, an Imprint of ABC-CLIO, LLC, [2017] |
    Series: Contemporary world issues | Includes bibliographical
    references and index.
Identifiers: LCCN 2017012076 (print) | LCCN 2016056067
    (ebook) | ISBN 9781440854774 (acid-free paper) |
    ISBN 9781440854781 (ebook)
Subjects: LCSH: Substance abuse—Handbooks, manuals, etc.
Classification: LCC HV4998 .N488 2017 (ebook) |
    LCC HV4998 (print) | DDC 362.29—dc23
LC record available at https://lccn.loc.gov/2017012076

ISBN: 978-1-4408-5477-4
EISBN: 978-1-4408-5478-1

21 20 19 18 17   1 2 3 4 5

This book is also available as an eBook.

ABC-CLIO
An Imprint of ABC-CLIO, LLC

ABC-CLIO, LLC
130 Cremona Drive, P.O. Box 1911
Santa Barbara, California 93116–1911
www.abc-clio.com

This book is printed on acid-free paper ∞

Manufactured in the United States of America

For Ed and Marnie Semeyn,
Still the tops!

The story of substance abuse and efforts to exert control over the misuse of drugs remains one of the most fascinating tales in American culture. For nearly a century, the American legal system has treated the misuse of marijuana, cocaine, heroin, LSD, amphetamines, and other psychoactive substance as a critical social problem requiring legal remedies in the vast majority of cases. During the 1970s, when American culture itself appeared to be threatened by the widespread use of such substances, President Richard M. Nixon declared a "war on drugs" that has, for the most part, continued to the present day. In light of the apparent failure of that "war" to resolve the nation's drug problems, more and more legislators, addiction experts, psychologists and sociologists, and other interested parties are calling for a new approach to the nation's "drug problem." That approach is based on the assumption that substance abuse and addiction are primarily physiological problems that should be dealt with by means other than legal remedies, as are other health and medical problems. So, the first two decades of the twenty-first century have seen some movement away from the crime-based approach to substance abuse to a more medical-centered view of the problem.

In the brief period between the two editions of this book, evidence of this evolution has become more and more apparent. As the second edition goes to press, for example, the U.S. Congress has just passed the first meaningful legislation on substance abuse in decades, legislation that, for the first time, takes a long-term view on the problem and its resolution. Thus, while some features of the first edition still seem as fresh as if they were written yesterday, a new tone—one that often seems subsumed by elements of new hope and optimism—can also be found within these pages.

The format of the new edition is largely the same, although there have been some revisions in the content and arrangement of chapters.

Substance Abuse

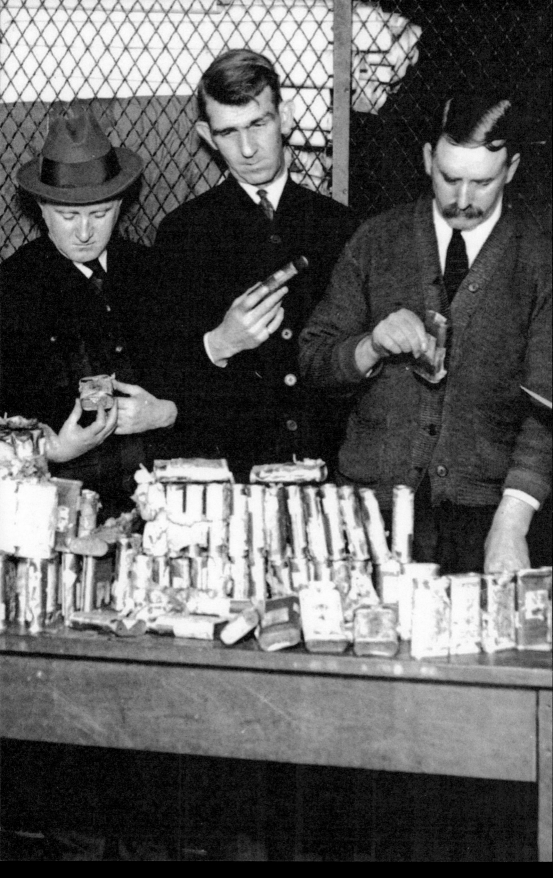

Introduction

The nation was startled by the news at the end of 2015. The U.S. National Center for Health Statistics (NCHS) issued a report that the death rate among Americans had *increased* in the previous year, a trend that had not been seen in over a decade. Although progress in combating deaths from cancer, heart attacks, and other traditional disease-killers had continued to decrease for the most part, death rates began to move upward for a few specific conditions, including Alzheimer's disease, suicide, and substance abuse. NCHS reported, for example, that the death rate for drug overdoses had increased by 137 percent between 2000 and 2015, a trend that reflected more than anything the growing epidemic of opioid abuse and addiction (Rudd et al. 2016). Ironically, the group most at risk for the increase in death rates was relatively well-to-do middle-class white males, a category of Americans that had been experiencing a drop in death rates for many decades. The country was shocked and baffled at the new trend. Had substance abuse become the new killer "disease" capable of sweeping through the nation in coming decades?

A Brief History of Substance Use and Abuse

The use of natural and synthetic products that alter one's consciousness has been part of human culture as far back as records

---

Smoking opium valued at $25,000 was seized on a ship in Brooklyn, New York, by members of the Surveyors' Searching Squad of New York on March 9, 1925. The opium was hidden in a coal bunker. (AP Photo)

3

exist. In some instances, it even predates any written or picto-
rial accounts that humans left behind. In 1992, for example,
Jan Lietava, of Comenius University in Bratislava, reported on
the discovery of a number of natural herbs with mind-altering properties, including ephedra, at a Neanderthal burial site
in the Shanidar region of Iraq dating to at least 50,000 BCE.
Lietava wrote that the substances found at the site had "marked
medical activity" (Lietava 1992). The discovery is thought to be
the earliest evidence of drug use by humans.

Most other drugs with which humans are familiar today
have long histories also. The first references to the cultivation
of the cannabis plant, from which marijuana is produced, date
to at least 10,000 BCE. The precise use of these plants is not
clear, however, as the plant is used not only for the production
of marijuana but also for the manufacture of hemp, a valuable
fiber used to make cloth. The earliest evidence of a cannabis
product, in fact, is a piece of cord attached to pottery dating to
about 10,000 BCE in China. The first reliable evidence that the
plant was also used to make a product that could be smoked
dates to somewhat later, about the first or second century CE,
also in China. Myths dating to the period claim that the Chinese deity Shen Nung tested hundreds of natural products,
including marijuana, to determine their medical and pharmacological properties (Iversen 2000, 18–19). These myths
form the basis for a very early Chinese pharmacopeia, which
describes the hallucinogenic properties of marijuana, which is
called *ma*, a Chinese pun for "chaotic" (Iversen 2000, 19).

The use of marijuana as an intoxicant also has a long history
in Indian culture, where its first mention dates to about 2000–
1400 BCE in the classic work *Atharvaveda* (*Science of Charms*).
According to legend, the Indian god Shiva became embroiled
in a family argument that so angered him he wandered off
into the fields, where he lay down and fell asleep under a leafy
cannabis plant. When he awoke, he tasted a leaf of the plant
and found that it so refreshed him that it became his favorite
food. Thus was born the tradition of making and consuming a

concoction of the cannabis plant known as *bhang* in honor of the Lord Shiva at many religious ceremonies, a tradition that continues today (Booth 2003, 24; see also Cannabis: India 1500 BC; Grierson [1894]).

The history of opium and other opiates (derivatives or chemical relatives of opium) is similar to that of marijuana and other psychoactive substances. Although there is some evidence that the poppy was cultivated and used by the Neanderthals, the first concrete, written evidence of its use dates to about 3500 BCE in lower Mesopotamia. Tablets found at the Sumerian spiritual center at Nippur describe the collection and treatment of poppy seeds, presumably for the preparation of opium. The Sumerians gave the name of *hul gil*, or "joy plant," to the poppy, almost certainly reflecting the sensations it produced when eaten (Kritikos and Papadaki 1967). Thereafter, the plant and the drug are mentioned commonly in almost every civilization of antiquity, where they were used for medical and, apparently, psychoactive reasons, probably in association with religious ceremonies. Interestingly, opium was almost universally ingested by mouth rather than by smoking. In fact, the first mention of the drug's use by smoking is not found until about 1500, when the Portuguese introduced the practice, then thought by the residents of all other nations as being a "barbaric and subversive" custom (Childress 2000, 155).

Although marijuana and opium were apparently not known in the New World, the Western Hemisphere had its own psychoactive drugs of choice, one of which was mescaline, derived from the peyote cactus (*Lophophora williamsii*). As in the Old World, this drug was apparently popular thousands of years ago, although it became known to Europeans only with the Spanish conquests of South America in the sixteenth century. One of the early chroniclers of the history of peyote was a Spanish priest, Bernardino de Sahagun, who estimated from extant documents that the drug had been in use for at least 1,800 years before the Spanish arrived in the New World. De Sahagun's estimate is problematic, however, partly because the conquistadors so aggressively destroyed all historical documents of the natives on which they could lay their hands. Later ethnologists and archaeologists think his estimates are conservative, and that the drug was used at least a thousand years earlier. One writer has placed the first use of peyote in the New World of at least 8,000 years ago (Spinella 2001, 344). In any case, it was still being widely used for both religious and recreational purposes when the Spaniards arrived, and the conquerors' efforts to abolish this practice were largely unsuccessful.

One of the most thorough and detailed observers of native practices in the region, Danish ethnologist Carl Lumholtz, described peyote ceremonies he observed during an extended trip to Mexico:

> The plant, when taken, exhilarates the human system and allays all feeling of hunger and thirst. It also produces colour-visions. . . . Although an Indian feels as if drunk after eating a quantity of hikuli [native name for peyote], and the trees dance before his eyes, he maintains the balance of his body even better than under normal circumstances. (Lumholtz 1902, 364)

The other psychoactive plant native to the New World is the coca plant, *Erythroxylum coca*. Recent studies have shown that the plant was being used at least 3,000 years ago. Two of 11 mummies from a burial area in northern Chile contained small quantities of the drug, whose age was determined by carbon-14 dating. Historically, archaeologists had previously set 600 CE as the earliest date for which good evidence of the use of coca has been set. That evidence consists of mummies that had been buried with a supply of coca leaves and whose cheeks were deformed by a bulge characteristic of those who chew leaves of the plant (Peterson 1977, 17). As with peyote, the Spaniards attempted to abolish the practice of coca use but were entirely unsuccessful. As they discovered, coca provides the chewer with energy and stamina, qualities of considerable benefit especially to those who lived in the thin air of the high Andes, and also of use for the exhausting manual labor in mining and other occupations to which the natives were assigned by the conquistadors.

The use of psychoactive substances has often been the subject of dispute within nations and regions. Indeed, Chapter 2 of this book discusses in some detail some of the issues surrounding the use of such substances in the United States and the rest of the world today. An example of the historical controversies about the use of psychoactive substances is the Opium Wars of the mid-nineteenth century between China and Great Britain. Although opium had been known in China and used for medical purposes for hundreds of years, by 1800 it had been banned for recreational use. Coincidentally, however, Great Britain had just come into control of the world's largest source of opium with its conquest of the Indian subcontinent. That situation was a tinderbox, with the British eagerly searching for a market for the massive amounts of opium they now controlled and the Chinese determined not to permit the importation of the drug to their country.

The British took advantage of this opportunity in 1836, when they bribed officials at the port of Canton to allow them to bring opium into the country. Before long, the drug was widely available throughout China, and the number of people addicted to its use rose to an estimated two million (Chrastina 2009). The Chinese government finally decided to take vigorous action against the smuggling of opium into their country by the British in 1839. Emperor Tao-kuang appointed a trusted bureaucrat named Lin Tse-hsü to lead an anti-opium campaign across the country. Lin was especially aggressive against British merchants in China who trafficked in opium and against merchant ships who were attempting to deliver the drug at the port of Canton. As the year progressed, skirmishes between the Chinese and British increased in number and severity, and war between the two nations broke out in mid-1840. The result of the conflict was a foregone conclusion, with the British then having one of the largest and strongest military establishments in the world. In 1842, the Chinese sued for peace, which was confirmed by the Treaty of Nanjing, signed on August 29 of that year. The treaty called for China to open five ports to foreign trade, to pay significant reparations to Great Britain, and to cede Hong Kong to the British. The treaty settled matters temporarily, but discord between the two nations continued, and war broke out again in 1856. As before, the British prevailed, and the war ended with the Treaty of Beijing in 1860. Again, the Chinese were required to open more ports to foreign trade (ten this time) and to pay very large reparations to Great Britain and its ally, France. (For an excellent overview of the Opium Wars, see Beeching 1975.)

Controversies over the use of psychoactive substances have extended to every material that might fit that description. Even a substance that hardly attracts opprobrium today—coffee—has been the subject of controversy at a number of times in the past. In 1511, for example, the governor of Mecca banned all coffeehouses within his district. His action was based on the belief that coffee is an intoxicant and therefore forbidden by Islamic law. To his misfortune, the governor was later overruled by his superior, the sultan of Cairo, and paid with his own life.

After a coffee craze swept through Europe in the seventeenth century, similar concerns about its use arose in a number of locations. In 1600, for example, a number of Christian clerics asked Pope Clement VIII to ban coffee because it came from the land of the infidels (the Islamic world) and it would cause drinkers to lose their souls. After tasting the new drink, however, Clement had a somewhat different take on the issue. He could not believe, he said, that such a delicious drink could be evil. Instead, he decided to "fool the devil" by baptizing coffee and allowing its free use among all Christians (Grierson 2009).

The pope's decision did not, however, resolve the controversy over the use of coffee in many parts of Europe. The disputes that arose illustrate that fact that such controversies may or may not arise solely out of the medical or health effects of a substance. In some cases, for example, objections to the rapid spread of coffeehouses were raised by tavern owners, who probably cared little one way or another about the psychoactive effects of coffee, and a great deal more about the competition coffeehouses posed to their businesses. Like earlier Christian leaders, they argued that coffee was a product of unbelievers, and that good Christian men should drink only the brew that had been prepared traditionally by monks: beer.

Other efforts to close coffeehouses did focus on their supposed health risks. Perhaps the most famous of these efforts was the "Women's Petition against Coffee," published in 1674 in London. In this petition, a group of women asked the authorities to close coffeehouse because the drink was harming their sexual lives with their husbands. They complained of the "Grand INCONVENIENCIES accruing to their SEX from the Excessive Use of that Drying, Enfeebling LIQUOR" (Clarkson and Gloning 2003). (Some critics have observed that women's greatest complaint about coffeehouses, to the contrary, was that they were not permitted to enter such establishments [Grierson 2009].) The Women's Petition drew a comparable response from men, or at least a man purporting to represent the male position on coffeehouses. The "Men's Answer to the Women's Petition against Coffee" was a long harangue that insisted that the coffeehouse is "the citizen's academy, where he learns more wit than ever his granmum taught him [and that] . . . 'Tis Coffee that . . . keeps us sober." He continues: "[Let] all our wives that hereafter shall presume to petition against it, be confined to lie alone all night, and in the day time drink nothing but bonny clabber" (Clarkson and Gloning 2005). If there is any lesson to be learned from this contretemps, and the longer history of coffee itself, it is that virtually any substance with some effect on a person's mental or physical condition is likely to be the subject of controversy at some point in history.

The aforementioned review provides only a modest introduction to the earliest history of drug use in the Old and New

Worlds. Similar stories could be told for other naturally occurring psychoactive plants and their products, such as tobacco, alcohol, caffeine, and psilocybin, as well as a host of synthetic products developed in the last century, such as amphetamine, the barbiturates, lysergic acid diethylamide (LSD), and MDMA (3,4-methylenedioxymethamphetamine). Those stories would require a series of books much larger than this work, however, although salient points in that history will be discussed in this and following chapters. (For more on the history of psychoactive substances, see also Austin 1978; Merlin 2003; Rudgley 1999.)

Speaking of Drugs

Any discussion of substance abuse makes use of a number of terms whose definitions are essential to a clear understanding of the subject. Some of the most important of these terms are the following.

Drug is probably the most fundamental term used in talking about substance abuse, but it is also the term with the greatest variety of meanings. According to *Merriam-Webster's Dictionary*, for example, the two major definitions of the term refer to its medical use and its recreational use. In the former instance, the term *drug* is defined as:

(1) a substance recognized in an official pharmacopoeia or formulary (2) a substance intended for use in the diagnosis, cure, mitigation, treatment, or prevention of disease (3) a substance other than food intended to affect the structure or function of the body (4) a substance intended for use as a component of a medicine but not a device or a component, part, or accessory of a device." In the latter instance, the term is defined as "something and often an illegal substance that causes addiction, habituation, or a marked change in consciousness. (*Merriam-Webster* 2016) (The terms *pharmacopoeia* and *formulary* refer to books or

lists of drugs, usually prepared and issued by recognized authorities such as medical groups or governmental agencies.)

Legal and *illegal* are terms that describe substances that are or are not permitted by law to be manufactured, transported, sold, and consumed. The term *legal drugs* refers both to prescribed drugs, that is, drugs that can be obtained only with a medical professional's prescription, and over-the-counter (OTC) drugs, which are freely available to any consumer without a prescription. A number of substances that produce psychoactive effects are also legal in the United States. These substances include amyl nitrite, betel nuts, caffeine, catnip, henbane, hops, a variety of inhalants, kava kava, ketamine, mandrake, nitrous oxide, nutmeg, and tobacco. Illegal drugs cannot be obtained legally except by clearly specified medical applications. Legal and illegal drugs are also known as *licit* and *illicit* drugs, respectively.

Substance abuse is a term now more widely used than the formerly popular *drug abuse*. The term has become more common at least partly because it can be used for a wider variety of materials that are not in and of themselves illegal, such as alcohol, tobacco, and caffeine, which may also be abused in much the same way as illegal drugs, such as marijuana, cocaine, and heroin.

The term *substance abuse* itself is somewhat vague, since it can refer to a variety of conditions ranging from relatively harmless to life-threatening. In his book *Illegal Drugs*, Paul Gahlinger describes four levels of drug abuse (Gahlinger 2004, 90). The first level he calls "experimental use," because it involves the first exposure people have to drugs. They "try out" a glass of beer, a cigarette, or a lid of marijuana. For some people, that is as deeply as one becomes involved in "substance abuse." They do not enjoy the experience or decide not to go any further. (Although, as Gahlinger points out, even this level of drug abuse is an illegal act for substances such as marijuana and cocaine, although not for alcohol and tobacco.) The next level of drug use is one that Gahlinger labels "recreational use."

It refers to cases in which a person takes a drink, has a cigarette, or uses an illegal drug from time to time "just for the fun of it." The person's life is not disrupted in any way by this occasional, low-key use of a substance. Gahlinger calls the next level of drug use "circumstantial use," because it includes those occasions when substance use develops into a certain pattern: a person uses a drug to deal with a personal problem, because of the feelings the drug produces, or just to be sociable with others. Again, drug use at this level is not necessarily harmful, but it may be the gateway to the fourth level, "compulsive use," or, as most people would describe the situation, an addiction.

Professional caregivers, such as physicians, psychologists, psychiatrists, and counselors, encounter this whole range of substance abuse behaviors, but usually provide a more detailed and sophisticated definition of the conditions they see. The standard reference in the field of psychiatry, for example, is the *Diagnostic and Statistical Manual of Mental Disorders,* fifth edition, often referred to simply as DSM-5. DSM-5, released in 2013, differs substantially in the way it defines substance abuse disorders from its predecessor, DSM-IV. DSM-5 recognizes substance abuse disorders for nine categories of drugs: alcohol; caffeine; cannabis; hallucinogens; inhalants; opioids; sedatives, hypnotics, and anxiolytics; stimulants; and tobacco. It also defines four levels of impairment resulting from a substance abuse: impaired control (over use of the substance), social impairment (involving interruption of one's normal daily activities), risky use (that results, for example, in a person's placing himself or herself into physical danger), and pharmacological indicators (involving development of tolerance or withdrawal symptoms) (Gorski 2013; Horvath 2016).

Narcotics is a term that was traditionally used for opioids, drugs that are derivatives of or similar to opium. The word *narcotics* comes from the Greek term "narko-sis," which means "to make numb." Today, the term is used more generally for any substance that causes numbness or stupor, induces sleep, and relieves pain.

Psychoactive is an adjective used for any substance that acts on the central nervous system (CNS) and alters one's consciousness or mental functioning. The word *psychotropic* is sometimes used as a synonym for "psychoactive." A number of other terms with the prefix *psycho-* are also used to describe certain specific types of psychoactive drugs. Psychotomimetic drugs, for examples, are compounds that produce symptoms similar to ("mimic") those of a psychosis. Psychedelic drugs are those that produce altered sense of consciousness or distorted sensory perceptions.

One large class of psychoactive drugs are the *hallucinogens*, which, as their name suggests, cause hallucinations, or perceptions of images and events for which there is no real stimulus. Psychoactive drugs have been used throughout history for a number of purposes: as medicines, as recreational drugs, and as a means for achieving spiritual experiences in religious ceremonies. Drugs used for the last of these purposes are sometimes called *entheogen* substances, from the Greek words for "to create," "the divine," and "within."

Generic is a term used to describe a particular form of a drug, or the name given to such a drug. Most drugs have at least two names, and often, they have three. The first name is its *systematic*, or scientific, name. For example, the systematic name for the compound that we commonly call aspirin is sodium acetylsalicylic acid. The systematic names for compounds are derived from rules established by the International Union of Pure and Applied Chemistry (IUPAC) and have the advantage of unambiguously identifying every different compound in the world. Such names are essential for researchers because they prevent any confusion whatsoever as to the substance about which a person is talking. The practical difficulty with IUPAC names is that they can be long and quite beyond the understanding of the ordinary person. The systematic name for the drug known as Ecstasy, for example, is (RS)-1-(benzo[d][1,3]dioxol-5-yl)-N-methylpropan-2-amine.

The generic name for a compound does not necessarily follow rules like those established by IUPAC. It is a simpler, shorter name to which one can more easily refer. The compound officially known as (±)-1-phenylpropan-2-amine, for example, is more commonly known by the generic name of *amphetamine*. Proprietary formulations of drugs always carry a specific brand name also that associates that formulation with the company that makes the drug. Some brand names for amphetamine (sometimes mixed with other compounds) are Dexedrine, Adderall, Biphetamine, Desoxyn, and Vyvanse.

Finally, illegal drugs almost always have a number of street names, nicknames by which they are known among substance abusers, professionals, and the general public. The list of street names is very long indeed. Table 1.1 shows only a sample of some of these names and the drugs for which they are used.

A much more detailed list of street names can be found on the Internet at White House Office of National Drug Control Policy, "Street Terms," http://www.whitehousedrugpolicy.gov/streetterms/Default.asp.

Classifying Drugs

In many cases (as in the last part of this chapter), it may be useful to discuss the specific characteristics of individual drugs, such as cocaine, heroin, and PCP. In other cases, it is helpful to focus on the common properties of large classes of drugs. Drugs can be classified in a number of ways: on the basis of their chemical structures, as to their medical uses, by the mental and physical effects they produce, and on the basis of their legal status. A chemical system of classification organizes drugs according to their chemical structures. One might speak, for example, about the amphetamines, which are all derivatives of the specific compound, amphetamine; barbiturates, which are all derivatives of barbituric acid; and the benzodiazepines, which are all derivatives of the chemical compound by that name. Figure 1.1 shows three members of the barbiturate family with its parent compound, barbituric acid.

Table 1.1   Some Street Names for Illegal Drugs

Generic Name	Street Names
Amphetamine	Black Dex, Bennies, Black and White, Black Bombers, Bumblebees, Dexies, Fives, Footballs, French Blue, Horse Heads, Jolly Beans, Lid Poppers, Lightning, Oranges, Pep Pills, Rhythm, Rippers, Snap, Sparkle Plenty, Sweets, Thrusters, Uppers
Cocaine	All-American Drug, Aunt Nora, Bazulco, Bernie, Big C, Bolivian Marching Powder, Burese, C, Carrie Nation, Cecil, Charlie, Chloe, Double Bubble, Dream, Flake, Florida Snow, Happy Trails, Henry VIII, Merck, Monster, Powder Diamonds, Scorpion, Snow White
Heroin	Al Capone, Antifreeze, Aunt Hazel, Big H, Big Harry, Blow, Bozo, Brown Sugar, Dead-on-Arrival, Dr. Feelgood, Galloping Horse, Good and Plenty, Him, Joy Flakes, Old Steve, Rambo, Rawhide, Smack
Marijuana	Acapulco Red, Black, Boo, Canadian Black, Crying Weed, Don Juan, Flower Tops, Giggle Weed, Grass, Indian Hemp, Jane, Kentucky Blue, Locoweed, Magic Smoke, Muggles, Pot, Rainy Day Woman
MDMA	Adam, Batmans, Bermuda Triangles, Care Bears, E, Ecstasy, Four Leaf Clover, Hug Drug, Igloo, Lover's Special, Orange Bandits, Pink Panthers, Smurfs, Tom and Jerries, Tweety Birds, Wafers
Methamphetamine	Beannies, Black, Boo, Blue Devils, Chicken Feed, Clear, Cris, Hot Ice, Mercedes, Meth, Motocycle Crack, Pink, Po Coke, Scootie, Sketch, Speckled Birds, Spoosh, Tick Tick, Wash
PCP	Angel Dust, Black Dust, Busy Bee, Crazy Coke, Crystal Joint, Dipper, Elephant Tranquilizer, Green Tea, Heaven & Hell, K, Lemon 714, Soma, Super, Tic Tac, Wack
Peyote	Half moon, Hikori, Hikuli, Hyatari, Nubs, Seni, Tops

Another common system of classification is based on the effects produced by drugs. The most common categories included in such a system are depressants, stimulants, and hallucinogens. The first group of substances, the depressants, gets their name from the fact that they depress the CNS, reducing pain, relieving anxiety, inducing sleep, and, in general, calming a person down. Some common depressants are opium and

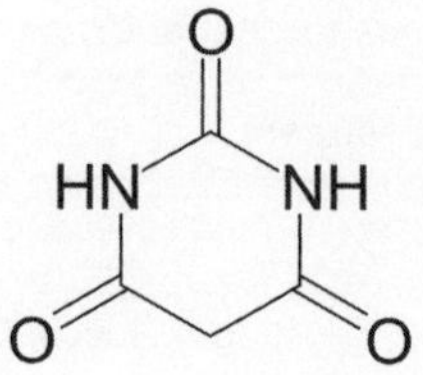

Figure 1.1a   Barbituric Acid

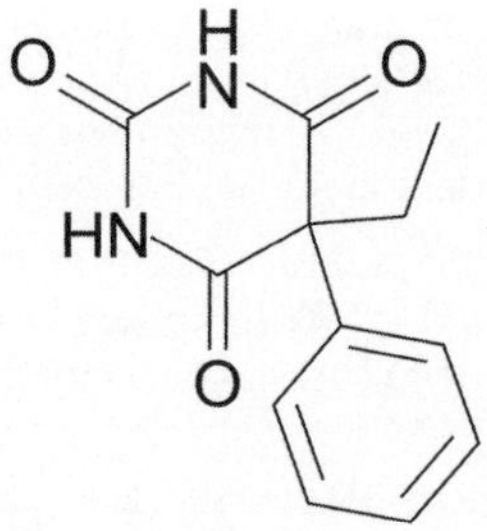

Figure 1.1b   Phenobarbital

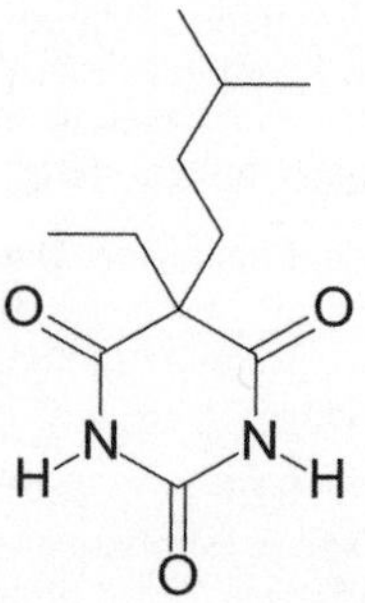

Figure 1.1c   Amobarbital

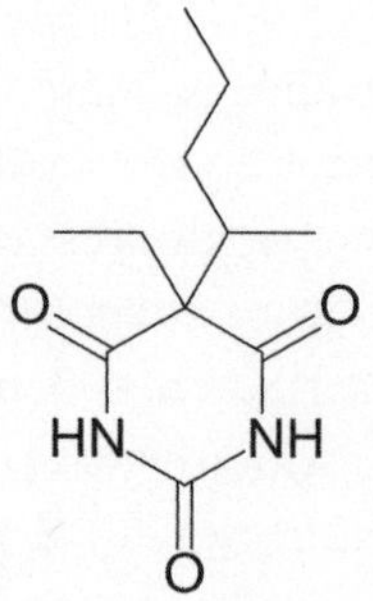

Figure 1.1d   Pentobarbital

its relatives, cannabis, alcohol, the barbiturates, the benzodiazepines, muscle relaxants, antihistamines, and antipsychotics.
Depressants are commonly referred to as "downers" because
they reduce the activity of the CNS.

Stimulants have just the opposite effect. They increase the
activity of the CNS, promoting physical and mental activity.
Stimulants are used medically to treat a number of conditions
that are characterized by depression, such as sleepiness, lethargy, and fatigue; to improve attentiveness and concentration;
to promote weight loss by decreasing appetite; and to treat
attention deficit hyperactivity disorder and clinical depression.
Because of their effects, compounds in this category are sometimes called "uppers." Some common stimulants are amphetamine and its chemical analogs, caffeine, cocaine, Ecstasy
(methylenedioxymethamphetamine), and nicotine. (In chemistry, analogs [or analogues] are chemical compounds similar in
structure and function to other chemical compounds.)

Hallucinogens differ from stimulants and depressants in
one important way. The latter classes of drugs amplify normal
mental sensations, increasing those sensations in the case of
stimulants and decreasing them in the case of depressants. Hallucinogens, by contrast, produce qualitatively different mental
states, such as the perception of objects and events that do not,
in fact, actually exist. The experiences produced by hallucinogens are, in some respects, similar to other kinds of so-called
out-of-body experiences, such as those experienced during
dreaming, meditation, and trances. Ironically, the one effect
that is not produced by hallucinogens is hallucination, an experience in which a person completely accepts as real an event or
object that has no basis whatsoever in reality. To someone who
has taken a hallucinogen, by contrast, there is almost always
some realization that the bizarre experiences he or she is having
do have at least some basis in reality.

Hallucinogens can be subdivided into three groups: psychedelics, dissociatives, and deliriants. The term *psychedelic* comes
from two Greek words, *pysche*, meaning "soul," and *delos*,
meaning "to reveal." The term thus suggests a chemical that

allows a person to look into her or his innermost self to discover his or her authentic person. For this reason, psychedelics
(as well as other hallucinogens) have a very long history of use
in religious and mystical ceremonies since they are thought to
allow a person to go beyond the simple (and limited?) reality
of everyday life. Dissociatives are chemicals that disrupt normal nerve transmissions in the brain so that one loses touch,
to a greater or lesser extent, with the physical world. He or
she literally "disassociates" from that world with the result, as
with psychedelics, that one can focus on one's innermost soul
without the distraction of physical reality. Deliriants are a form
of dissociative that have even more extreme effects on an individual. A person who takes a dissociative may be aware of the
mental changes he or she is experiencing, while someone who
has taken a deliriant is probably not aware of these changes.
Of all hallucinogens, deliriants are most likely to produce true
hallucinations.

Some categories of drugs in addition to stimulants, depressants, and hallucinogens are antipsychotics, used to treat psy-
choses because of their calming effects; antidepressants, used to
treat depression and similar mood disorders; inhalants, abused
by some individuals as a way of achieving some type of altered
mental states, such as a "high"; and marijuana, which is often
listed as a drug group in and of itself.

Finally, drugs can be categorized on the basis of their legal
status in any particular nation. This method of categorization
is of special interest and concern, of course, because it clarifies
which substances are legal for individuals to use and which are
not. The basis for classifying the legal status of drugs in the
United States was established by the Controlled Substances Act
of 1970. That law created five classes, or "schedules," of drugs
according to their medical use and potential for abuse. Drugs
placed in Schedule I, for example, currently have no approved
legitimate medical use in the United States and a high potential for abuse. Some Schedule I drugs include the stimulant
cathinone, the depressant methaqualone (Quaalude), the

psychedelic MDMA, and most opiates. Schedule II drugs include a number of substances that, while strongly subject to use as recreational drugs, do have some legitimate medical uses. These drugs include the amphetamines, most barbiturates, cocaine, morphine, opium, and phencyclidine (PCP). An excerpt of the law creating the drug schedules and a list of drugs in each schedule are to be found in Chapter 5 of this book.

How Do Drugs Work?

Drugs produce their effects on the body by acting on the brain. Specifically, they alter in one way or another the mechanisms by which nerve messages are sent from one part of the brain to another part of the brain. The transmission of a nerve impulse within the CNS, of which the brain is a major component, is a two-step process, one of which is an electrical mechanism, and one of which is chemical. A nerve impulse passes along a neuron (nerve cell) by means of a constantly changing electrical charge on the membrane of that cell. When that electrical impulse, called an *action potential*, reaches the outermost edge of a cell, known as an *axon*, it initiates the release of chemicals from the axon into the space between that neuron (the presynaptic neuron) and some other adjacent neuron (the postsynaptic neuron), a space known as the *synapse*, or *synaptic gap*. These "message-carrying" chemicals are known as *neurotransmitters*. Some examples of neurotransmitters are acetylcholine, epinephrine (adrenaline), γ-aminobutyric acid (GABA), dopamine, serotonin, and nitrous oxide. After a neurotransmitter has crossed the synaptic gap, it attaches itself to a section of the dendrite on a receiving cell. A *dendrite* is a short projection in a neuron designed for the acceptance of neurotransmitters from another neuron. The point at which a neurotransmitter docks is called a *receptor site*. A specifically designed receptor site exists for each different type of neurotransmitter. Once a neurotransmitter has bonded to a receptor site on a dendrite, it stimulates the dendrite to initiate an electrical impulse, similar to the one that traveled through the first neuron. That electrical impulse then passes through the dendrite and into the neuron cell body, repeating the process of nerve transmission from the presynaptic neuron. Meanwhile, the neurotransmitter is released from the dendrite, travels back across the synaptic gap to the presynaptic neuron, and is available for reuse in transmission of the nerve message. (For a visual representation of this process, see The Brain 2011; The Chemical Synapse 2012 [first half]; Nerve Conduction 2016.)

Most drugs exert their effects on the CNS by altering the action of neurotransmitters at some point in the process described previously. Stimulants, for example, tend to prevent the reuptake of a neurotransmitter at the very end of the process. As a result, neurotransmitters tend to accumulate in the synaptic gap and reinsert themselves into receptor cells on the second neuron, which is, as a result, restimulated over and over again. This repetitious stimulation is responsible for the increased activity observable in the brain after the ingestion of a stimulant.

Other stimulants have other modes of action. Nicotine, for example, causes its effects because its structure is somewhat similar to that of the neurotransmitter acetylcholine. Just as acetylcholine works by stimulating an acetylcholine receptor in a dendrite, so nicotine exerts its influence by stimulating a receptor similar to that for acetylcholine, called the nicotinic receptor. Caffeine operates in yet another way on the nervous system. It exerts its effects by acting as antagonist at a dendrite receptor site for the neuromodulator adenosine. A *neuromodulator* is a substance that affects the rate at which nerve messages pass through the brain. In the case of adenosine, the effect is to slow down this process. Thus, whenever an adenosine molecule locks onto one of its receptor sites in a dendrite, no other neurotransmitter can enter that site, and a nerve message is interrupted. The brain's reaction rate slows down as a result of this event. If caffeine is present in the bloodstream, it may also enter the brain and dock at a receptor site normally reserved for adenosine molecules. A molecule that is able to act in a manner similar to some other molecule to produce a diminished response is said to be an *antagonist* for the second molecule. (By contrast, a molecule that acts like another molecule to produce an augmented response is called an *agonist*.) Thus, caffeine is an antagonist for adenosine. The only difference between the two substances is that caffeine has no effect on the rate at which nerve messages are transmitted. When it docks at an adenosine receptor, it prevents an adenosine molecule from docking there also, preventing a slowdown in the brain's activity. A person who has had a cup of coffee, then, does not experience the "slow down" responses, such as drowsiness, that might typically result from the action of adenosine in the brain.

As one might expect, the action of depressants on the nervous system is quite different from that of stimulants. In most cases, the neurotransmitter most commonly affected is γ-aminobutyric acid, generally known as GABA. GABA is a somewhat unusual neurotransmitter in that it tends to reduce the rate at which nerve transmission takes place. (Most neurotransmitters increase brain activity.) That is, the flow of GABA from the presynaptic neuron to the postsynaptic neuron causes changes in the structure of the latter that tends to reduce the rate at which nerve transmission continues. Depressants tend to enhance this effect. For example, members of the benzodiazepine family, a group of depressants, are able to bind to GABA receptor sites on postsynaptic neurons, increasing the efficiency with which those receptors work. Thus, with benzodiazepine molecules present in the brain, GABA neurotransmitters operate more efficiently and tend to significantly slow down brain activity, resulting in drowsiness and slower mental activity.

Another process by which depressants work takes advantage of the body's natural system for dealing with pain. Neurons contain receptor cells especially adapted to a group of natural opiate neurotransmitters called endorphins, enkephalins, and dynorphin. These neurotransmitters are often called *endog-enous opiates* or *endogenous opioids* because they are opium-like compounds that occur naturally within ("endo-") the body. By contrast, the class of drugs generally known simply as "opiates" are more correctly called *exogenous opiates* (or *exogenous opioids*) because they occur naturally outside of ("exo-") the body (as in plants). Endogenous opiates exert their effect on a receptor in the presynaptic neuron that controls the release of GABA from that neuron. When an opiate neurotransmitter docks at this receptor site, it reduces the release of GABA. Fewer GABA molecules flow through the synaptic gap and stimulate the postsynaptic neuron.

The importance of this change is that the amount of GABA in a neuron affects the amount of a second neurotransmitter, dopamine, also present in the neuron. Specifically, the more GABA, the less dopamine (recall that GABA is an inhibitory neurotransmitter). Thus, with less GABA present in the post-synaptic neuron, the greater the amount of dopamine. The significance of this change is that one of the primary effects of dopamine is the production of feelings of elation and well-being. The effect in an endogenous opiate on the presynaptic neuron, then, is to produce a sense of euphoria. Scientists now believe that this system, beginning with the release of endog-enous opiates from the pituitary gland, has evolved as a way for the body to deal with pain.

The action of depressants (exogenous opiates) is simply to enhance this process. If one ingests heroin, for example, there are simply more opiate molecules in the bloodstream, some of which reach the brain. Once in the brain, the heroin molecules act in a virtually identical fashion to the way endogenous opi-ates work. A person who has taken heroin, then, feels the same sense of pleasure and rapture that comes from the action of endogenous opiates.

The previous discussion might be taken to mean that sci-entists have now essentially solved the puzzle as to how drugs affect the CNS. Such is not the case. In fact, the mechanism(s) by which some drugs affect mental and physical behavior is still largely a mystery. The case of LSD is a case in point. For some time, scientists have known that LSD has a chemical structure similar to that of the neurotransmitter serotonin. Serotonin itself is a bit of a puzzle for neuroscientists because there are so few cells that produce the chemical in the brain (only a few thousand), but its influence is widespread, with each seroto-nergic (serotonin-making) cell activating at least 500,000 other neurons (Frederickson 1998). The presence of LSD molecules in the brain almost certainly means that the substance will dock with serotonin receptor sites, either in the presynaptic or post-synaptic neuron, exerting either an agonistic or an antagonistic effect. Theories have been developed around all of four these possibilities, with a number of variations. Thus far, however, no one theory has been shown to explain the bizarre physical and mental effects that occur as the result of the ingestion of LSD. In fact, it was only in 2016 that researchers at Imperial College London obtained the first high-quality images of brains from people who were "high" on LSD, the first real clue to how the drug may affect the human CNS (Sample 2016).

A Survey of Legal and Illegal Drugs

The rest of this chapter is devoted to a review of some of the most common and most important substances involved in sub-stance abuse problems. Each section deals, where appropriate, with a brief history of the use of the drug in the United States, current and historical patterns of drug consumption, and health effects associated with each substance. Other consider-ations, such as legal, political, social, moral, and other issues for each substance, are discussed in Chapter 2.

Tobacco

Tobacco is a product obtained from the leaves of plants belong-ing to the genus *Nicotiana*, the most widely cultivated of which is the species *Nicotiana tabacum*. When dried and cured, tobacco leaves are used to make a variety of products, including cigarettes, cigars, snuff, chewing tobacco, dipping tobacco, and snus, a moist form of the powder placed under the lip. Tobacco was first grown in the New World, where it was used almost exclusively for religious ceremonies and other special occasions, such as the signing of treaties and the celebration of important life events such as birth and marriages. Tobacco was used for these purposes largely because of its mild hallucinatory effects. Europeans who arrived in the New World in the fifteenth century and later were introduced to the product and began using it for purely recreational purposes. When they returned home, they brought with them samples of tobacco, which soon became widely popular for chewing, smoking, and for use as snuff.

Chemically, tobacco is a very complex substance, with at least 7,000 discrete components having been identified as constituents. The most important of these components is probably nicotine, a toxic stimulant that produces the "high" for which tobacco is used and which also produces the substance dependence that results from tobacco use. The health effects of tobacco use were largely unknown or ignored until the second half of the twentieth century. At that point, a number of scientific studies began to show that tobacco and tobacco smoke contain a number of ingredients with possible health effects, ranging from respiratory disorders, to diseases of the eyes and nose, to heart problems, to cancer. Table 1.2 lists some of the most important constituents of tobacco smoke, with the health risks they pose.

Although the health effects of tobacco use were ignored for most of its history, such is no longer the case. Public health agencies, private groups, and nonprofit organizations now work diligently to advertise the harmful effects of tobacco products on the human body. In its most recent announcements about the health effects of smoking, the Office of Smoking and Health of the U.S. Centers for Disease Control and Prevention (CDC) pointed out that tobacco use is responsible for an estimated 480,000 deaths in the United States every year, about

Table 1.2   Some Constituents of Tobacco Smoke and Their Health Risks

Constituent	Concentration in Smoke[1,2]	Health Risk to Humans
Acrolein	60–140 µg	Toxin
4-Aminobiphenyl	2–5.6 ng	Carcinogen
Ammonia	10–130 µg	Respiratory irritant
Arsenic	40–120 µg	Carcinogen
Benzene	20–70 µg	Carcinogen
Benzo(a)pyrene	20–40 ng	Carcinogen
Cadmium	7–350 ng	Carcinogen
Carbon monoxide	10–23 mg	Toxin
Chromium (VI)	4–70 ng	Carcinogen
Ethylene oxide	7 µg	Carcinogen
Hydrogen cyanide	400–500 µg	Toxin
Hydrogen sulfide	10–90 µg	Respiratory irritant
Maleic hydrazine	1.16 µg	Mutagen
Methanol	100–250 µg	Toxin
2-Naphthylamine	1–334 ng	Carcinogen
Nickel	0–600 ng	Carcinogen
Nicotine	1–3 mg	Toxin
Nitrogen oxides (NO$_x$)	100–600 µg	Respiratory irritant
Polonium-210	0.03–1.0 pCi	Carcinogen
Prussic acid	400–500 µg	Toxin
Pyridine	16–40 µg	Respiratory irritant
Vinyl chloride	11–15 ng	Carcinogen

[1]As measured by a standard cigarette-smoking machine
[2]ng = nanograms
µg = micrograms
mg = milligrams
pCi = picocuries

Source: Adapted from Knut-Olaf Haustein and David Groneberg. *Tobacco or Health?: Physiological and Social Damages Caused by Tobacco Smoking*, 2nd ed. Berlin; New York: Springer, 2009, 35–37, Tables 3.1–3.3.

one out of every five deaths in the nation. That total is greater than the total number of deaths from human immunodeficiency virus (HIV), illegal drug use, alcohol use, motor vehicle injuries, and firearms-related incidents combined (Health

Effects of Cigarette Smoking 2016). The CDC report went on to note that tobacco use is responsible for cancer of a number of organs, including the bladder, blood (leukemia), oral cavity, pharynx, larynx, esophagus, cervix, kidney, lung, pancreas, and stomach. In fact, tobacco use is now implicated in about 90 percent of all cases of lung cancer in men and 80 percent of all cases of lung cancer in women in the United States. In addition, many diseases of the respiratory system are caused by the use of tobacco products, with an estimated 90 percent of all cases of chronic obstructive lung diseases based on the use of tobacco (Health Effects of Cigarette Smoking 2016).

In recent years, health authorities have become increasingly concerned about the effects of tobacco use—especially smoking—even among those individuals who do not use tobacco. Research has shown that the smoke emitted by cigarette use can affect individuals in close proximity to a smoker, and even, in some cases, those who are at some distance from a smoker. Evidence now suggests that approximately 41,000 deaths in the United States annually can be attributed to secondhand smoke, of which about 7,330 are caused by lung cancer and 33,950 by heart disease (Health Effects of Secondhand Smoke 2016). Secondhand smoke, also referred to as *environmental tobacco smoke, involuntary smoke,* or *passive smoke,* is a special problem for children, partly because their immune systems may not be fully developed, and partly because they may be less able to remove themselves from locations in which they are exposed to smokers (as when their parents smoke). According to some estimates, secondhand smoke may be responsible for as many as 150,000 to 300,000 cases of lower respiratory tract infections among children in the United States each year, and an estimated 202,000 children with asthma may have their conditions aggravated by exposure to secondhand smoke (Health Effects of Secondhand Smoke 2016).

The considerable health risks posed by tobacco use have led to increased regulation of the product and more aggressive campaigns to discourage smoking and other tobacco use in the

United States and other parts of the world, a topic discussed in more detail in Chapter 2. The results of these efforts have begun to bear fruit in the United States, where the percentage of smokers has continued to drop over the past 50 years from a maximum of 41.9 percent of the general population (51.2% of men and 33.7% of women) in 1965 to an estimated 16.8 percent of the general population in 2012 (18.8% of men and 14.8% of women) (Health, United States 2013, Table 56, page 192; and Current Cigarette Smoking among Adults in the United States 2016). The only group for which this trend did not hold was high school students, among whom the proportion of smokers rose from 27.5 percent in 1991 (the first year for which data were available) to 36.4 percent in 1997, before falling back to a recent low of 15.7 percent in 2013, in line with patterns for older Americans (Trends in Current Cigarette Smoking among High School Students and Adults, United States, 1965–2014, 2016).

A new factor was introduced into the discussion over tobacco smoking in the early twenty-first century. In 2003, a Chinese pharmacist named Hon Lik invented a new way of smoking tobacco that consists of a metallic tube consisting of four basic parts: an inhaler, which contains a replaceable cartridge that holds a liquid consisting of nicotine, water, and other liquids; an atomizing chamber, in which the liquid is converted to a vapor; a battery, used to bring about the vaporization process; and an LED light to replicate the burning tip of a traditional cigarette. (For a diagram of an e-cigarette, see http://www.e-cig-bargains.com/HowItWorks.jsp.) This type of *electronic cigarette*, *e-cigarette*, or *vaporizer* allows a person to enjoy the experiencing of ingesting nicotine, as with cigarette smoking, but without having to inhale the numerous other unhealthy tobacco components.

E-cigarettes became very popular very quickly in the United States and other parts of the world. Studies found that by 2014, 12.6 percent of all adults in the United States had tried an e-cigarette at least once in their life, with 14.2 percent of all men and 11.2 percent of all women falling into this category. The product was especially popular with younger Americans. In the 2014 survey, 21.6 percent of all individuals between the ages of 18 and 26 had tried an e-cigarette at least once in their life, with 5.1 percent of that group reporting that they now smoke e-cigarettes on a regular basis then. The comparable numbers for adults age 25 to 44 was 4.7 percent; those 45 to 64, 3.5 percent; and adults over the age of 65, 1.4 percent (Schoenborn and Gindi 2015).

One of the most interesting aspects of the e-cigarette phenomenon is that many people had come to believe that e-cigarettes are safer than traditional cigarettes. This point of view is reflected in the fact that 9.7 percent of individuals questioned in this survey who had *never* tried a tobacco cigarette had decided to try an electronic cigarette (Schoenborn and Gindi 2015). In fact, the safety of e-cigarettes has not yet been adequately determined. Some evidence suggests that the devices deliver some of the same risky chemicals present in traditional tobacco smoke, although the total amount of harmful ingredients obtained from e-cigarettes is almost certainly substantially less than that obtained from traditional tobacco cigarettes (E-cigarettes and Lung Health 2016).

Alcohol

The production and use of alcoholic beverages dates to the earliest periods of human civilization. The first evidence of jugs designed to hold alcoholic beverages dates to about 10,000 BCE, while the world's first winery was discovered in modern-day Armenia, dating to about 4000 BCE (Patrick 1952, 12–13; Owen 2011). The production of alcoholic beverages is generally thought to be one of the first chemical processes discovered by humans, at least partly because the fermentation of fruit and vegetable matter, a process that results in the production of alcohol, occurs naturally and commonly. It is not difficult to imagine early humans discovering that the taste and effects of fermented plant products were pleasant enough to prompt them to find ways of making such beverages artificially.

Today, alcoholic beverages of one kind or another are a part of every human culture of which we know. In some cases, they are used for religious or ceremonial purposes, but most commonly, they are enjoyed solely for recreational purposes. In the United States, the annual consumption of alcohol per person has tended to remain at 2.0–2.5 gallons for more than 150 years. In 1850, for example, the average consumption for all alcoholic beverages was 2.10 gallons, the largest proportion of which consisted of hard liquor, such as gin and whiskey (also referred to as *spirits*; 1.88 gal), with much smaller amounts of beer (0.14 gal) and wine (0.08 gal). In 2013, average consumption was 2.34 gallons annually, although the proportions of beverages had changed, with consumption of beer at 1.12 gallons, wine at 0.42 gallons, and hard liquor at 0.80 gal). Except for a number of years that include World War II and the years following Prohibition, when alcoholic beverage consumption fell significantly, Americans' consumption of beer, wine, and hard liquor has remained remarkably constant (Apparent per Capita Ethanol Consumption, United States, 1850–2013 2016).

Alcohol consumption differs widely among individuals and has been classified in a variety of ways by researchers and specialists. For example, the National Institute on Alcohol Abuse and Alcoholism defines four levels of drinking:

- Moderate Drinking: Defined as one drink per day for women and two drinks per day for men, where a "standard drink" is defined as 12 fluid ounces of regular beer, five fluid ounces of wine, or 1.5 fluid ounces of hard liquor;

- Heavy Drinking: Defined as drinking five or more standard drinks on the same occasion on at least five days within one 30-day period;

- Binge Drinking: Defined as a pattern of drinking that brings a person's blood alcohol concentration to 0.08 g/dL (grams per deciliter) within two hours, typically about four standard drinks for women and five standard drinks for men within that period of time.

- At Risk for Developing Alcohol Use Disorder: Defined as having more than three drinks per day or seven drinks per week for women or four drinks in a single day or 14 drinks in a week for men.

(Note that differing standards for men and women are not an act of sexism, but a reflection of differences in the way the two sexes metabolize alcohol [Drinking Levels Defined 2016]).

Over the last decade or so, binge drinking has been of special concern among specialists in alcohol abuse and alcoholism. Newspapers and the Internet often carry stories about high school or college students who "go on a binge" that ends badly for the drinker and/or his or her companions. For example, a Stanford University student and star swimmer was convicted in June 2016 for raping a young woman, at least partly because he was under the influence of binge drinking (Xu 2016).

In fact, binge drinking affects all levels of American society. According to the most recent data available, 60.9 million people reported having engaged in binge drinking in the 30 days preceding the survey, accounting for about one-quarter of Americans over the age of 11. The age group with the highest percentage of binge drinkers (37.7% of the total population in that age group) was those between the ages of 18 and 25, or about 13.2 million young adults. By comparison, the rate of binge drinkers was lower among those over the age of 25 (22.5%) and those in the age group 12 to 17 (6.1%) (Hedden et al. 2015, Figure 26, page 20). Interestingly enough, these numbers for all age groups have remained relatively constant over at least the past decade during which records have been kept.

Whatever the specific numbers, the finding that tens of millions of Americans acknowledge to binge drinking on a regular basis is quite significant. And that fact is associated with a range of personal and social issues that can occur as a result of binge drinking. Studies have shown, for example, that binge drinkers are 14 times as likely as non-binge drinkers to report driving in an impaired state. The condition has now also been associated with a range of physical and mental problems such as unintentional injuries of all kinds; intentional injuries, such as domestic violence and sexual assault; transmission of sexual diseases; alcohol poisoning; unintended pregnancies; high blood pressure and other cardiac disorders; liver disease; neurological damage; and sexual dysfunction (Binge Drinking 2015).

Binge drinking is by no means the only form of alcohol abuse about which there is concern. Alcohol consumption at levels lower than those seen in binge drinking has also been implicated in a number of life-threatening diseases and conditions. Some of the medical and psychiatric problems that are associated with alcohol use include liver disease, pancreatitis, cardiovascular disease, malignant neoplasms, depression, dysthymia, mania, hypomania, panic disorder, phobias, generalized anxiety disorder, personality disorders, schizophrenia, suicide, neurologic deficits, brain damage, hypertension, coronary heart disease, ischemic stroke, and cancers of the esophagus, respiratory system, digestive system, liver, breast and ovaries (Cargiulo 2007, S5). Overall, alcohol consumption is the fourth-leading cause of preventable deaths in the United States, accounting for about 88,000 deaths (62,000 men and 26,000 women) each year (Alcohol Facts and Statistics 2016).

The news about alcohol consumption is not, however, entirely negative. Some researchers have found, for example, that moderate consumption of alcohol may have some health benefits, such as reducing the risk of coronary disease, dementia, and diabetes (Alcohol Facts and Statistics 2016). This evidence appears to be strong enough that the U.S. Department of Health and Human Services and the U.S. Department of Agriculture included a comment in their 2015 Dietary Guidelines for Americans that "moderate alcohol intake can be a component of a healthy dietary pattern" (Scientific Report of the 2015 Dietary Guidelines Advisory Committee 2015, 4; see also Table D2.3, page 43). Given the very serious health problems associated with alcohol consumption, however, most statements like this one are followed by a warning that consumption of alcohol should be restricted to adults, that excessive consumption can pose a serious risk to human health, and that, for some people, even moderate amounts of alcohol can be harmful.

Marijuana

As indicated earlier in this chapter, marijuana and related substances (such as hashish) have been used in some parts of the world for many centuries. The use of the drug in the United States, however, appears to have been relatively limited until the 1960s. Prior to that time, marijuana was largely the drug of choice of certain small, specialized groups, such as jazz musicians (Harrison, Backenheimer, and Inciardi 1995). The first public opinion polls in which Americans were asked about marijuana use apparently date to the late 1960s, when use rate was recorded as being very low. The first such poll, for example, was conducted by Gallup in 1967. The poll found that about 5 percent of Americans said that they had used marijuana at once in their lifetime. Usage was significantly higher among college students, 12 percent of whom reported having smoked marijuana in a similar poll conducted two years later. Those results began to change rapidly, however, possibly as a reflection of more general cultural changes associated with the Vietnam War and other protests occurring during the late 1960s and early 1970s. For example, a Gallup Poll in 1970 found that 43 percent of all college students queried said that they had tried marijuana at least once in their lives, with 28 percent saying that they had used it in the drug in the preceding year (Harrison, Backenheimer, and Inciardi 1995).

Gallup continued to track Americans' use of marijuana for the next four decades; it is the best source of those data prior to the late twentieth century, when the U.S. government also began keeping such records. After its earliest survey on the topic in 1969, Gallup found in 1972 that the fraction of Americans who had admitted to trying marijuana at least once had risen seven points to 11 percent. That trend continued in succeeding polls, reaching 12 percent in 1973, 24 percent in 1977, 33 percent in 1985, 38 percent in 2013, and 44 percent in July 2015 (Illegal Drugs 2016).

Almost certainly the best information about the use of marijuana by high school students became available with the initiation in 1975 of the Monitoring the Future (MTF) study, conducted for the National Institute on Drug Abuse by the Institute for Social Research at the University of Michigan, a study that continues to the present day. MTF researchers have asked a sample of U.S. 12th grades annually about their use of and attitudes toward marijuana and a similar sample of 8th and 10th grades the same questions since 1991. Those studies indicate that the percentage of 12th graders who had used marijuana within the 30-day period preceding the study was 27.1 percent in 1975, before rising to its highest level ever in 1978, 37.1 percent. Marijuana use among 12th graders then dropped off over the next 15 years or so, reaching a low point of 11.9 percent in 1992 before beginning to rise once more. It reached another high of 23.7 percent in 1997 before falling once more, this time to around 20 percent, where it has remained ever since. In 2015, the rate of 30-day marijuana use among 12th graders was 21.3 percent. Data for 8th and 10th graders followed a similar trajectory from 1991 to 2015 (Johnston et al. 2014, Table 5–3, pages 227–228; Johnston et al. 2016, Table 7, page 72).

One of the most controversial issues in the field of substance abuse concerns the health effects of consuming marijuana. Even though literally thousands of studies on the topic have been conducted, experts still disagree as to the precise effects that result from consuming marijuana and the severity of these effects. In its own review of the research, the National Institute on Drug Abuse has listed the following acute and chronic effects of marijuana ingestion:

- impairment of short-term memory;
- impairment of attention, judgment, and other cognitive functions;

- loss of coordination and balance;
- increase in heart rate;
- reduction and memory and learning skills in a medium time range;
- increased risk of cough, bronchitis, emphysema, and cancer of the head, neck, and lungs;
- increased risk of addiction (Marijuana 2016).

Research conducted for well over a century also suggests that ingestion of marijuana may also have some health benefits. Although a number of claims have been made for the use of marijuana in treating many medical conditions, strong scientific evidence is still somewhat more cautious. In one large review of studies on the medical benefits of marijuana, for example, researchers found what they called "moderate-quality evidence" for the use of marijuana to treat chronic pain and spasticity and "low-quality evidence" to support its use for the treatment of nausea and vomiting due to chemotherapy, weight gain in HIV infection, sleep disorders, and Tourette syndrome (Whiting et al. 2015, 2456). A significant number of experts in the field believe that marijuana has a much greater range of uses in treating medical problems, however, and, as of 2016, 25 states, the District of Columbia, and Guam have taken the step of legalizing the use of marijuana for medical purposes (Medical Use 2016; Welsh and Loria 2014).

Cocaine

Cocaine is obtained from various plants belonging to the genus *Erythroxylum*, most commonly the coca plant *E. coca*. Residents of the South American Andes Mountains have used the leaves of the coca plant for religious, recreational, and medical reasons for many hundreds (or thousands) of years. In Bolivia and Peru, for example, people chew coca leaves as a way of dealing with the lassitude that results from living in very thin air at altitudes of 3,000 meters or more. Once the plant was introduced to Europe by early Spanish conquerors, it became widely popular for medical applications and as a recreational drink. One preparation was a coca-infused wine, Vin Mariani, which apparently was a favorite of Pope Leo XIII (Malin 2016). Coca products were also imported to the United States, where they appeared in any number of preparations, ranging from toothache remedies to a popular soft drink to pills, liquids, and even an injectable solution from the drug firm of Parke-Davis (Cocaine 1885, 124–125; Parke-Davis & Co. Cocaine Injection Kit 2016).

By 1900, evidence of the health consequences of cocaine use had become widely known, and legal prohibitions on the drug's use were being instituted. Illegal cocaine was still readily available, however, usually in the form of the salt cocaine hydrochloride, in the form of a white powder that users inhaled or dissolved in water and injected. Reports of serious damage to the nasal passages as a result of cocaine "snorting" appeared as early as 1910, although these studies appear not to have much effect on the use of the drug for recreational purposes (Coca Timeline 2016).

Until the 1970s, powder cocaine was the drug of choice among many substance abusers, especially among well-to-do individuals. Its cost was usually too high for low- or moderate-income persons, accounting for its common name "the champagne of drugs" (Gahlinger 2004, 242). In the mid-1970s, a new form of cocaine became available, so-called *freebase cocaine*. The name comes from the method by which the product is made: cocaine hydrochloride is treated with a base, such as sodium bicarbonate, which neutralizes the acidic cocaine hydrochloride, leaving behind free cocaine. The cocaine is extracted from the reaction mixture with ether, which is then allowed to evaporate, leaving behind pure cocaine crystals, which can then be smoked. (The one serious risk here is smoking crystals that still contain some ether, resulting in a fire when the product is lighted.) Freebase cocaine rapidly became very popular because it was generally purer than powder cocaine and, as a result of being smoked, reached the brain more rapidly.

About a decade after the discovery of freebasing, yet another form of cocaine was developed: crack cocaine. The process for making crack cocaine is essentially the same as that for making freebase cocaine. Powder cocaine is neutralized with sodium bicarbonate, sodium hydroxide, or another base and heated. When the excess water in the mixture has evaporated, pure cocaine and additional by-products remain in the form of a rocklike crystalline substance. The substance gets its name of "crack" from the sound it makes during the chemical reaction by which it is formed. Because it is much safer and cheaper to make than freebase cocaine, crack cocaine soon became very popular among low- and middle-income individuals, resulting in an epidemic that peaked between 1984 and 1990 in the United States.

The number of Americans over the age of 12 who have used cocaine "occasionally" or "chronically" was an estimated 6,000,000 and 3,984,000, respectively, in 1988, the first year in which such data were collected. Those numbers both decreased regularly over succeeding years until they reached an all-time low of 3,216,000 and 2,755,000 respectively in 1999. Since 2002, government agencies have been counting the percentage of cocaine (and other illicit drug) users, rather than raw numbers. Those data suggest that the percentage of 30-day cocaine users dropped only very slowly from 0.9 percent of the U.S. population in 2002 to 0.6 percent in 2013 (National Drug Control Strategy [2013], Table 7; Results from the 2013 National Survey on Drug Use and Health: Summary of National Findings 2014, Figure 2.2; see also Drug Use Trends 2002).

Considerably more detailed information is available about cocaine use among young adults by means of the MTF study. According to the most recent version of that report, 1.9 percent of 12th graders used cocaine at least once in the 30 days preceding the survey. The number increased significantly in the following decade, reaching 6.7 percent in 1985. It then fell off rapidly until it reached 1.3 percent in 1992. Over the last

25 years, it remained close to 2 percent before dropping again to its lowest point in history, 1.1 percent in 2012 (Johnston et al. 2014, Table 5.3, pages 227–228).

Users of cocaine do so because of the heightened feelings of sensation they experience, which may be described as an increased sense of energy and alertness, a feeling of supremacy, an elevated mood, and a sensation of euphoria. These feelings may not be entirely positive, as they can be accompanied by more unpleasant reactions, such as a sense of anxiety or irritability or a sensation of paranoia. As with any drug, however, these short-term feelings are balanced by longer-term physiological and psychological effects such as an increase in heart rate that may lead to cardiovascular problems; irritation of the upper respiratory tract and lungs among those who inhale the drug; constriction of blood vessels in the brain, which may lead to seizures or stroke; disruption of the gastrointestinal system, which can result in perforation of the inner walls of the stomach and intestines; kidney damage that can be serious enough to lead to kidney failure; and impairment of sexual function among both men and women.

Opioids

The terms *opiate* and *opioid* occur commonly in the literature of substance abuse. At one time, the two terms had slightly different meanings. *Opiate* was taken to refer to any compound that was derived from the opium plant, *Papaver somniferum*. The most common and best known of these products are probably morphine, heroin, and codeine. The term *opioid* was originally proposed to describe synthetic analogs of opium compounds, such as oxycodone (Oxycontin), hydrocodone (a component of Vicodin), meperidine (Demerol), hydromorphone (Dilaudid), and fentanyl citrate (Sublimaze). Today, experts in the field have chosen to use the term *opioid* for any analog of opium, natural, synthetic, or semisynthetic (Opiates/Opioids 2016).

Opioids are arguably the most problematic of all abused substances in use today. Throughout history, they have played a dual role of useful medical product and dangerous recreational drug. This pattern arises because of the way opioids act on the brain. They attach to opioid receptors in the CNS, reducing the perception of pain and producing drowsiness and a general sense of relaxation and apathy. Opioids are so successful in this regard that they tend to be the most popular drug for treating levels of pain for which aspirin, acetaminophen, and other painkillers are ineffective. The problem arises when a person ingests opioids to achieve these same sensations—relaxation, a sense of ease, and euphoria—for nonmedical purposes. The brain easily becomes dependent upon and addicted to the effects produced by opioids, leading to harmful and dangerous long-term psychological consequences (How Do Opioids Affect the Brain and Body? 2014; How Does the Opioid System Work? 2007).

Opioid abuse is a problem in the United States and other parts of the world today because the legitimate demand for their use for medical purposes has produced a flood of the products that then easily become available to individuals who use them for recreational, nonmedical purposes. This pattern has led to the so-called *prescription drug epidemic*, in which legal, useful, effective substances are being diverted to individuals who have no medical problem, but often do become dependent upon or addicted to drugs such as oxycodone, hydromorphone, and fentanyl. According to the most recent data available, 4.3 million individuals 12 years of age and older in the United States in 2014 reported using one or more prescription drugs for nonmedical purposes in the 30 days preceding the survey (Hedden et al. 2015, 1).

In some respects, the most difficult aspect of this problem involves finding a way of preventing prescription drug abuse. One obvious approach is simply to cut back on the quantity of opioids prescribed by health care professionals, thus reducing the amount of such drugs available to abusers. But that approach means that people who legitimately need opioids for the treatment of pain or other uses may find it more difficult to obtain the drugs they need. This complex problem is discussed in more detail in Chapter 2 of this book.

Amphetamines

Amphetamine was first synthesized in 1887 by the Romanian chemist Lazăr Edeleanu while conducting research on ephedrine, one of the oldest psychoactive stimulants known to humans. Edeleanu's discovery was largely ignored for four decades before British chemist Gordon Alles, working at the time at the University of California at Los Angeles, repeated Edeleanu's work and decided to explore the effects of amphetamine on humans (using himself as a subject). Alles found that amphetamine worked as a stimulant, much as does ephedrine, but even more effectively. He decided to continue and expand his research, eventually synthesizing and studying the effects of two amphetamine analogs, 3,4-methylenedioxyamphetamine (MDA) and MDMA. Alles soon realized the potential medical benefits of amphetamine and its analogs and sold the process for making the drugs to the pharmaceutical company of Smith, Kline, and French, who first marketed amphetamine for the control of high blood pressure and the symptoms of asthma under the commercial name of Benzedrine in 1932.

The potential use of the amphetamines for recreational use did not escape the attention of many individuals, and the drugs soon became widely popular for this purpose in the mid-twentieth century (Rasmussen 2008). Even national governments realized their potential benefits as stimulants during World War II, when the armed forces of both Allied and Axis nations distributed amphetamines in large quantities to improve the endurance and aggression of their troops (Borin 2003). One problem was that the end of the war did not mean a loss of interest in amphetamines by former members of the armed services, and amphetamine abuse became a major public health problem in the late 1940s and 1950s. Eventually, the U.S. government attempted to solve the problem by banning the over-the-counter sale of amphetamine products in 1953.

Although these efforts at controlling the production and use of amphetamines were moderately successful at first, they were only the beginning of a long war between users of the drugs and drug enforcement agencies, a history that will be told in more detail in Chapter 2 of this book. Suffice to say that the abuse of methamphetamine and its analogs still poses a serious problem of substance abuse in the United States and some other parts of the world. According to the most recent National Survey on Drug Abuse and Health, an estimated 569,000 Americans (about 0.2% of the general population) could be classified as regular users of methamphetamine in 2014, of whom about 45,000 (0.2% of the age group) were between the ages of 12 and 17; 86,000 (0.2%) were between the ages of 18 and 25; and 438,000 (0.2%) were over the age of 25 (Hedden et al. 2015, Figure 10 Table, and pages 9–10).

The immediate results of taking amphetamines result from stimulation of the CNS and include increased heart rate and blood pressure, a sense of euphoria, increased wakefulness and need for physical activity, increased respiration, and decreased appetite. An excessive dose of an amphetamine can lead to irregular heartbeat, respiratory problems, cardiovascular collapse, and death. Some long-term effects of amphetamine use are related to these short-term effects, as overstimulation of the body may result in more serious respiratory and cardiac problems. It may also result in the onset of psychotic episodes that may include anxiety, confusion, insomnia, mood disturbances, violent behavior, feelings of paranoia, visual and auditory hallucinations, and delusions.

Legal Medications

Another category of substances that are being abused today includes medications that are legally sold without prescription, so-called *over-the-counter,* or *OTC,* drugs. A relatively small number of OTC drugs contain ingredients that can have psychoactive effects on an individual if taken in doses not recommended for their legal medical use. Probably the most commonly abused of these drugs are cough and cold medicines, which typically include the compound dextromethorphan (DXM) as an active ingredient. DXM is an ingredient in more than two dozen popular OTC medications including Alka-Seltzer Plus, Cheracol, Contac, Coricidin, Diabetic Tussin, Kids Eeze, Mucinex DM & Cough Products, Robitussin, Sine-Off, Sudafed, Triaminic, Tylenol Cough, Cold, & Flu Products, and a variety of Vicks products. Products containing DXM are also available on the street under names such as candy, drank, dex, robo, skittles, triple c, tussin, and velvet. The practice of using such products is also known commonly as *robotripping*.

According to the most recent data available, 2.0 percent of all eighth graders, 3.70 percent of all 10th graders, and 4.10 percent of all 12th graders in the United States reported using a cough medicine product for nonmedical purposes in the year preceding the study. At all three grade levels, these percentages represented significant decreases from data collected in 2011, 2012, and 2013 (Monitoring the Future Study: Trends in Prevalence of Various Drugs 2015).

DXM has an inhibitory effect on neuroreceptors in the brain. That is, it tends to bind to those receptors and interrupt the flow of normal neural messages through the brain. In this respect, DXM acts in the brain in much the same way as do hallucinogens. This process has the general effect of slowing down mental processes in such a way as to produce a sense that one is removed from his or her body, a dissociative effect. DXM abusers often say that they feel completely relaxed and at ease, with a sense that they are floating through the air, released from their bodies. It is these feelings of euphoria and escape for which abusers are searching when they take DXM products (Cough and Cold Medicine [DXM and Codeine Syrup] 2015).

But the nonmedical use of DXM may also have a number of other side effects that are not as pleasurable as those a user is hoping for. These side effects include nausea, numbness, slurred speech, dizziness, sweating, insomnia, and lethargy. At more advanced stages, a user may also experience more serious effects, such as delusions, hallucinations, hyperexcitability, and hypertension. With prolonged use, liver and brain damage may result, and physical dependence and addiction may occur.

Another OTC product that is sometimes misused or abused, especially by teenagers, is called *bath salts*. The term has only the most tenuous relationship with the legitimate commercial product that many people add to their bath water for the soothing and relaxing feeling it can produce. The "bath salts" described here contain one or more synthetic analogs of cathinone, an alkaloid found in the leaves of the *Catha edulis* (khat) plant. It has physiological effects on the brain similar to those produced by amphetamine and its analogs. The product is sold under a variety of names, of which "bath salts" is only one. It is also marketed as plant food, a jewelry cleaner, or cleaner for a cell phone screen. The package in which the product comes is usually labeled "Not for Human Consumption" to avoid having to deal with regulations for legitimate drugs (DrugFacts: Synthetic Cathinones ["Bath Salts"] 2012). When sold on the Internet, the product may carry trade names such as Bloom, Cloud Nine, Ivory Wave, Lunar Wave, Scarface, Vanilla Sky, or White Lightning.

Bath salt products are typically ingested in a variety of ways, including by inhalation, by injection, or orally. Individuals take bath salts because of the sense of euphoria they provide, along with feelings of greater sociability, increased sex drive, and higher energy levels. These feelings may be accompanied, however, by other side effects that are not as pleasant, such as shortness of breath, abdominal pain, abnormal vision, anxiety, confusion, fever, rash, drowsiness, confusion, and dizziness. More serious side effects include abnormal renal function and renal failure, paranoia, psychosis, abnormal liver function and liver failure, and cardiovascular disorders (Prosser and Nelson 2012, Table 4).

Conclusion

The use of psychoactive substances dates back to the earliest years of human civilization. Those materials have been used for a variety of purposes: religious and ceremonial, medical, and recreational. Because of the variety of uses to which tobacco, alcohol, marijuana, cocaine, opium, and other products can be put, societies have almost always had mixed feelings about their use, encouraging the more positive applications and discouraging (sometimes strongly) their less desirable uses. That tradition continues today. In 2015, the federal government spent about $26 billion trying to prevent, control, monitor, and treat public and personal health problems and social issues arising out of substance abuse, with nearly the same amount ($25 billion) spent by states and local communities on the same problems. Chapter 2 provides an introduction to some of the most important problems and issues related to substance abuse and actions that have been and are being taken to prevent and treat related problems.

References

"Alcohol Facts and Statistics." 2016. National Institute on Alcohol Abuse and Alcoholism. https://www.niaaa .nih.gov/alcohol-health/overview-alcohol-consumption/ alcohol-facts-and-statistics. Accessed on June 18, 2016.

"Apparent per Capita Ethanol Consumption, United States, 1850–2013." 2016. National Institute on Alcohol Abuse and Alcoholism. http://pubs.niaaa.nih.gov/publications/ surveillance102/tab1_13.htm. Accessed on June 17, 2016.

Austin, Gregory A. 1978. *Perspectives on the History of Psychoactive Substance Use*. Research Issues 24, National Institute on Drug Abuse. https://babel.hathitrust.org/cgi/ pt?id=uc1.32106001081378;view=1up;seq=6. Accessed on June 14, 2016.

Beeching, Jack. 1975. *The Chinese Opium Wars.* New York: Harcourt Brace Jovanovich.

"Binge Drinking." 2015. Centers for Disease Control and Prevention. http://www.cdc.gov/alcohol/fact-sheets/binge-drinking.htm. Accessed on June 18, 2016.

Booth, Martin. 2003. *Cannabis: A History.* New York: Thomas Dunne Books/St. Martin's Press.

Borin, Elliott. 2003. "The U.S. Military Needs Its Speed." *Wired.* http://archive.wired.com/medtech/health/news/2003/02/57434. Accessed on June 20, 2016.

"The Brain." 2011. YouTube. https://www.youtube.com/watch?v=p5zFgT4aofA. Accessed on June 15, 2016.

"Cannabis: India 1500 BC." *Inity Weekly.* http://inityweekly.com/mmj-india-1000-bc/. Accessed on June 14, 2016.

Cargiulo, Thomas. 2007. "Understanding the Health Impact of Alcohol Dependence." *American Journal of Health-System Pharmacy.* 64(1): S5–S11.

"The Chemical Synapse." 2012. YouTube. https://www.youtube.com/watch?v=TevNJYyATAM. Accessed on June 17, 2016.

Childress, David Hatcher. 2000. *A Hitchhiker's Guide to Armageddon.* Kempton, IL: Adventures Unlimited Press.

Chrastina, Paul. 2009. "Emperor of China Declares War on Drugs." Opium. http://opioids.com/opium/opiumwar.html. Accessed on June 14, 2016.

Clarkson, Janet, and Thomas Gloning. 2005. "The Women's Petition against Coffee (1674)." http://www.uni-giessen.de/gloning/tx/wom-pet.htm. Accessed on June 14, 2016.

"Coca Timeline." 2016. The Vaults of Erowid. https://www.erowid.org/plants/coca/coca_timeline.php. Accessed on June 19, 2016.

"Cocaine." 1885. *St. Louis Medical and Surgical Journal.* https://books.google.com/books?id=6xNYAAAAMAAJ&

pg=PA124&lpg=PA124&dq=parke+davis+cocaine+injec tion+kit&source=bl&ots=8pQSXBYHPD&sig=Lg4FO C5I4xMyG5uTvkjPvuNM33Y&hl=en&sa=X&ved=0ah UKEwim37u9x7TNAhVM7mMKHTMtBns4ChDoAQ gkMAI#v=onepage&q=parke%20davis%20cocaine%20 injection%20kit&f=false. Accessed on June 19, 2016.

"Cough and Cold Medicine (DXM and Codeine Syrup)." 2015. NIDA for Teens. http://teens.drugabuse.gov/drug-facts/ cough-and-cold-medicine-dxm-and-codeine-syrup. Accessed on June 20, 2016.

"Current Cigarette Smoking among Adults in the United States." 2016. Centers for Disease Control and Prevention. http://www.cdc.gov/tobacco/data_statistics/fact_sheets/ adult_data/cig_smoking/. Accessed on June 17, 2016.

"Drinking Levels Defined." 2016. National Institute on Alcohol Abuse and Alcoholism. https://www.niaaa.nih .gov/alcohol-health/overview-alcohol-consumption/ moderate-binge-drinking. Accessed on June 17, 2016.

"Drug." 2016. *Merriam-Webster*. http://www .merriam-webster.com/dictionary/drug. Accessed on June 15, 2016.

"Drug Use Trends." 2002. Office of National Drug Control Policy. *file:///C:/Users/David/Downloads/20719.pdf.* Accessed on June 19, 2016.

"DrugFacts: Synthetic Cathinones ('Bath Salts')." 2012. National Institute on Drug Abuse. http://www.drugabuse .gov/publications/drugfacts/synthetic-cathinones-bath-salts. Accessed on June 20, 2016.

"E-Cigarettes and Lung Health." 2016. American Lung Association. http://www.lung.org/stop-smoking/ smoking-facts/e-cigarettes-and-lung-health. html?referrer=https://www.google.com/. Accessed on June 20, 2016.

Frederickson, Anne. 1998. "Mechanisms of LSD: A Glimpse into the Serotonergic System." http://serendip.brynmawr .edu/bb/neuro/neuro98/202s98-paper3/Frederickson3. html. Accessed on December 23, 2016.

Gahlinger, Paul. 2004. *Illegal Drugs: A Complete Guide to Their History, Chemistry, Use and Abuse.* New York: Plume.

Gorski, Terry. 2013. "DSM 5 Substance Use Disorders: A Concise Summary." https://terrygorski.com/2013/10/15/ dsm-5-substance-use-disorders-a-concise-summary/. Accessed on June 15, 2016.

Grierson, G. A. [1894.] Indian Hemp Drugs Commission Report. http://www.druglibrary.org/schaffer/library/studies/ inhemp/6app1.htm. Accessed on June 14, 2016.

Grierson, James A. 2009. "The History of Coffee." Mr. Breakfast.com. http://www.mrbreakfast.com/article .asp?articleid=26. Accessed on June 14, 2016.

Harrison, Lana D., Michael Backenheimer, and James A. Inciardi. 1995. "Cannabis Use in the United States: Implications for Policy." In Peter Cohen and Arjan Sas, eds. *Cannabisbeleid in Duitsland, Frankrijk en de Verenigde Staten.* Amsterdam: Centrum voor Drugsonderzoek, Universiteit van Amsterdam, 81–197. Available in English at http://www.cedro-uva.org/lib/harrison.cannabis.01 .html#prev. Accessed on June 18, 2016.

"Health, United States 2013." 2013. Hyattsville, MD: National Center for Health Statistics. http://www.cdc.gov/ nchs/data/hus/hus13.pdf. Accessed on June 17, 2016.

"Health Effects of Cigarette Smoking." 2016. Centers for Disease Control and Prevention. http://www.cdc.gov/ tobacco/data_statistics/fact_sheets/health_effects/effects_ cig_smoking/. Accessed on June 17, 2016.

"Health Effects of Secondhand Smoking." 2016. American Lung Association. http://www.lung.org/stop-smoking/ smoking-facts/health-effects-of-secondhand-smoke.html. Accessed on June 17, 2016.

Hedden, Sarra L., et al. 2015. "Behavioral Health Trends in the United States: Results from the 2014 National Survey on Drug Use and Health. HHS Publication No. SMA 15-4927, NSDUH Series H-50. http://www.samhsa.gov/data/sites/default/files/NSDUH-FRR1-2014/NSDUH-FRR1-2014.pdf. Accessed on June 18, 2016.

Horvath, A. Tom, et al. 2016. "The Diagnostic Criteria for Substance Use Disorders (Addiction)." AMHC. http://www.amhc.org/1408-addictions/article/48502-the-diagnostic-criteria-for-substance-use-disorders-addiction. Accessed on June 15, 2016.

"How Do Opioids Affect the Brain and Body?" 2014. National Institute on Drug Abuse. https://www.drugabuse.gov/publications/research-reports/prescription-drugs/opioids/how-do-opioids-affect-brain-body. Accessed on June 20, 2016.

"How Does the Opioid System Work?" 2007. *News Medical.* http://www.news-medical.net/news/2007/10/15/31153.aspx. Accessed on June 20, 2016.

"Illegal Drugs." 2016. Gallup. http://www.gallup.com/poll/1657/illegal-drugs.aspx. Accessed on June 18, 2016.

Iversen, Leslie L. 2000. *The Science of Marijuana.* New York: Oxford University Press.

Johnston, Lloyd D., et al. 2014. "Monitoring the Future National Survey Results on Drug Use, 1975–2013: Volume I, Secondary School Students." Ann Arbor: Institute for Social Research. The University of Michigan. http://www.monitoringthefuture.org/pubs/monographs/mtf-vol1_2013.pdf. Accessed on June 18, 2016.

Johnston, Lloyd D., et al. 2016. "Monitoring the Future. National Survey Results on Drug Use, 1975–2015: Overview, Key Findings on Adolescent Drug Use." Ann Arbor: Institute for Social Research, The University of Michigan. http://www.monitoringthefuture.org/pubs/monographs/mtf-overview2015.pdf. Accessed on December 23, 2016.

Kritikos, P. G., and S. P. Papadaki. 1967. "The History of the Poppy and of Opium and Their Expansion in Antiquity in the Eastern Mediterranean Area." *Bulletin on Narcotics.* 19(3): 17–38 and 19(4): 5–10.

Lietava, Jan. 1992. "Medicinal Plants in a Middle Paleolithic Grave." *Journal of Ethnopharmacology.* 35(3): 263–266.

Lumholtz, Carl. 1902. *Unknown Mexico.* 2 vols. New York: Charles Scribner & Sons.

Malin, Joshua. 2016. *VinPair.* http://vinepair.com/wine-blog/vin-mariani-bordeaux-wine-coca/. Accessed on June 19, 2016.

"Marijuana." 2016. Drug Facts. National Institute on Drug Abuse. https://www.drugabuse.gov/sites/default/files/marijuanadrugfacts_march_2016.pdf. Accessed on June 18, 2016.

"Medical Use." 2016. NORML. http://norml.org/marijuana/medical. Accessed on June 18, 2016.

Merlin, Mark David. 2003. "Archaeological Evidence for the Tradition of Psychoactive Plant Use in the Old World." *Economic Botany.* 57(3): 295-323. https://www.researchgate.net/publication/225632469_COVER_ARTICLE_Archaeological_Evidence_for_the_Tradition_of_Psychoactive_Plant_Use_in_the_Old_World. Accessed on June 14, 2016.

"Monitoring the Future Study: Trends in Prevalence of Various Drugs." 2015. National Institute on Drug Abuse. http://www.drugabuse.gov/trends-statistics/monitoring-future/monitoring-future-study-trends-in-prevalence-various-drugs. Accessed on June 20, 2016.

"National Drug Control Strategy." [2013.] Office of National Drug Control Policy. https://www.whitehouse.gov/sites/default/files/ondcp/policy-and-research/2013_data_supplement_final2.pdf. Accessed on June 19, 2016.

"Nerve Conduction." 2016. The Brain from Top to Bottom. http://thebrain.mcgill.ca/flash/d/d_01/d_01_m/d_01_m_fon/d_01_m_fon.html. Accessed on June 15, 2016.

"Opiates/Opioids." 2016. The National Alliance of Advocates for Buprenorphine Treatment. http://www.naabt.org/education/opiates_opioids.cfm. Accessed on June 20, 2016.

Owen, James. 2011. "Earliest Known Winery Found in Armenian Cave." National Geographic. http://news.nationalgeographic.com/news/2011/01/110111-oldest-wine-press-making-winery-armenia-science-ucla/. Accessed on June 17, 2016.

"Parke-Davis & Co. Cocaine Injection Kit." 2016. The Herb Museum. http://herbmuseum.ca/content/parke-davis-co-cocaine-injection-kit. Accessed on June 19, 2016.

Patrick, Charles H. 1952. *Alcohol, Culture, and Society*. Durham, NC: Duke University Press.

Prosser, Jane M., and Lewis S. Nelson. 2012. "The Toxicology of Bath Salts: A Review of Synthetic Cathinones." *Journal of Medical Toxicology*. 8(1): 33–42. http://www.ncbi.nlm.nih.gov/pmc/articles/PMC3550219/. Accessed on June 20, 2016.

Peterson, Robert C. 1977. "History of Cocaine." In Robert C. Peterson and Richard C. Stillman, eds. *Cocaine: 1977*. NIDA Research Monograph #13. Rockville, MD: Department of Health, Education, and Welfare.

Rasmussen, Nicolas. 2008. "America's First Amphetamine Epidemic 1929–1971: A Quantitative and Qualitative Retrospective with Implications for the Present." *American Journal of Public Health*. 98(6): 974–985.

"Results from the 2013 National Survey on Drug Use and Health: Summary of National Findings." 2014. Substance Abuse and Mental Health Services Administration. http://www.samhsa.gov/data/sites/default/files/NSDUHresultsPDFWHTML2013/Web/NSDUHresults2013.htm#5.4. Accessed on June 19, 2016.

Rudd, Rose A., et al. 2016. "Increases in Drug and Opioid Overdose Deaths—United States, 2000–2014." *Morbidity and Mortality Weekly*. http://www.cdc.gov/mmwr/preview/mmwrhtml/mm6450a3.htm. Accessed on June 14, 2016.

Rudgley, Richard. 1999. *The Encyclopaedia of Psychoactive Substances*. New York: St. Martin's Press.

Sample, Ian. 2016. "LSD's Impact on the Brain Revealed in Groundbreaking Images." *The Guardian*. https://www.the guardian.com/science/2016/apr/11/lsd-impact-brain-revealed-groundbreaking-images. Accessed on June 17, 2016.

Schoenborn, Charlotte A., and Renee M. Gindi. 2015. "Electronic Cigarette Use among Adults: United States, 2014." National Center for Health Statistics. http://www .cdc.gov/nchs/data/databriefs/db217.pdf. Accessed on June 20, 2016.

"Scientific Report of the 2015 Dietary Guidelines Advisory Committee." 2015. http://health.gov/dietaryguidelines/ 2015-scientific-report/pdfs/scientific-report-of-the-2015-dietary-guidelines-advisory-committee.pdf. Accessed on June 18, 2016.

Spinella, Marcello. 2001 *The Psychopharmacology of Herbal Medicine: Plant Drugs That Alter Mind, Brain, and Behavior*. Cambridge, MA: MIT Press.

"Trends in Current Cigarette Smoking among High School Students and Adults, United States, 1965–2014." 2016. Centers for Disease Control and Prevention. http:// www.cdc.gov/tobacco/data_statistics/tables/trends/cig_ smoking/. Accessed on June 17, 2016.

Welsh, Jennifer, and Kevin Loria. 2014. "23 Health Benefits of Marijuana." *Business Insider*. http://www.businessinsider .com/health-benefits-of-medical-marijuana-2014-4. Accessed on June 18, 2016.

Whiting, Penny F., et al. 2015. "Cannabinoids for Medical Use: A Systematic Review and Meta-analysis." *JAMA*. 313(24): 2456–2473.

Xu, Victor. 2016. "Brock Turner's Statement in Trial and at His Sentencing Hearing." *The Stanford Daily*. http://www .stanforddaily.com/2016/06/10/brock-turners-statement-in-trial-and-at-his-sentencing-hearing/. Accessed on June 18, 2016.

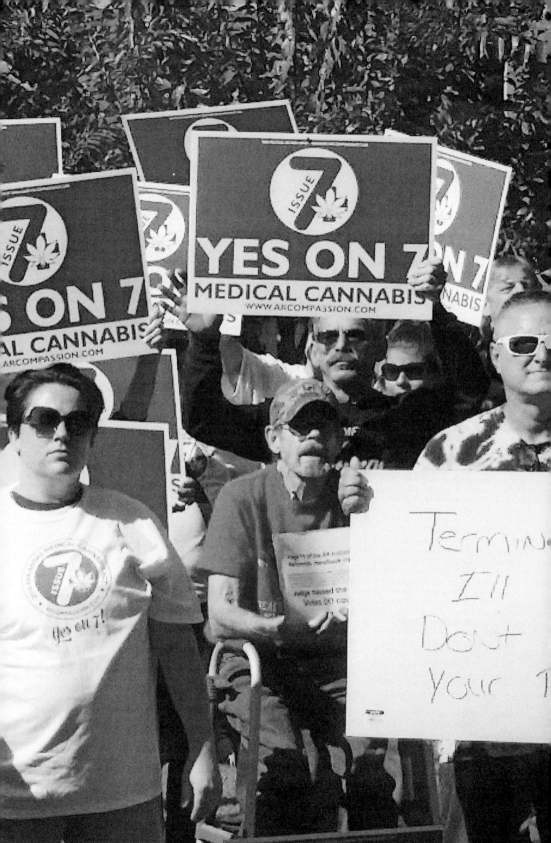

Introduction

We believe that the possession offense [for marijuana] is of little functional benefit to the discouragement policy and carries heavy social costs, not the least of which is disrespect and cynicism among some of the young. Accordingly, even under our policy of discouraging marihuana use, the better method is persuasion rather than prosecution. Additionally, with the sale and use of more hazardous drugs on the increase, and crimes of violence escalating, we do not believe that the criminal justice system can afford the time and the costs of implementing the marihuana possession laws. Since these laws are not mandatory in terms of achieving the discouragement policy, law enforcement should be allowed to do the job it is best able to do: handling supply and distribution. (National Commission on Marihuana and Drug Abuse 1971)

As noted in Chapter 1, the use of psychoactive substances has been the subject of considerable dispute for much of human history in many parts of the world. These disputes are not based on the question as to whether or not individuals should use

Supporters of Arkansas Issue 7, a medical marijuana initiative that would have allowed patients with certain conditions an opportunity to obtain or grow marijuana to ease their symptoms, rally outside the Arkansas Supreme Court building in Little Rock on October 28, 2016. The court invalidated the measure, and it did not appear on the November ballot. (AP Photo/ Kelly P. Kissel) alcohol, tobacco, marijuana, cocaine, heroin, and other psychoactive substances to the point where they become addicted or where their physical and/or mental health begins to deteriorate significantly. Almost no one would dispute that these consequences of substance use are undesirable, and they should be prevented or treated. In the vast majority of instances, the real debate over the use and abuse of psychoactive substances concerns the extent to which they should be legal, if at all. The paragraph with which this chapter opens, for example, comes from a report issued to President Richard M. Nixon in 1971 on the legal status of marijuana. Marijuana had been illegal or closely taxed for almost half a century before this report was issued. Continued aggressive action against drugs such as marijuana, cocaine, and heroin was a key element in President Nixon's domestic program. But the committee reporting to him, the National Commission on Marihuana and Drug Abuse, suggested a new approach to the problem of marijuana use in the United States: decriminalization for possession of small amounts of the drug, and a more vigorous program of prevention to reduce its use. Nixon rejected this and other recommendations made by the committee. As a Schedule I drug, marijuana use continues to be illegal today.

This chapter reviews the ongoing debate about the legal status of alcohol, tobacco, marijuana, and other substances abused by some individuals. First, however, the chapter reviews a discussion of the alternatives posed by the National Commission on Marihuana and Drug Abuse, and by many other expert committees and commissions, professionals in the field of substance abuse, and interested citizens and organizations: the role of prevention and treatment in reducing substance abuse.

Substance Abuse Prevention

No matter how one feels about the legality of alcohol, tobacco, marijuana, and other drugs as substances available for use by the general public, nearly everyone agrees that efforts should be made to prevent people from using these products to a point where their lives are disrupted and to provide treatment for such individuals for the worst effects of substance abuse and addiction. Individuals and agencies at every level—from the federal government to state government to local government to small groups and individuals—have been and are involved in programs of drug prevention. Some groups focus on one part of the problem of substance abuse, targeting alcohol, tobacco, or other drugs for their efforts, while others think that drug prevention programs must include some reference to all substances of abuse.

Literally hundreds of drug abuse prevention programs (also called simply drug education programs) are in existence in the United States today. No brief summary can do justice to the variety of goals, activities, and accomplishments of these programs, but many subscribe to a few general principles. One of the best statements of those principles can be found in a 2003 publication of the National Institute on Drug Abuse (NIDA), *Preventing Drug Use among Children and Adolescents: A Research-Based Guide for Parents, Educators, and Community Leaders* (Robertson, David, and Rao 2003). The authors of that report list 16 general principles that should guide prevention programs, such as the following:

- Prevention programs should enhance protective factors or reduce risk factors;
- Prevention programs should address all forms of substance abuse, including alcohol, tobacco, and other drugs;
- Prevention programs should be designed to address specific characteristics of the target population, such as age, sex, and ethnicity;
- Family-based programs should focus on strengthening family ties, including classes in parenting where necessary;
- Prevention programs are appropriate at every age level, from preschool to adult, and must be tailored to meet the needs of each specific group;

- Programs that involve more than one type of group, such as family and a community organization, tend to be more effective than those that focus on a single type of group;
- Prevention programs should make use of the best information available from research on substance abuse and its prevention; and
- Programs should have a long-term focus, with repetition of key concepts constituting the program. (Adapted from Robertson, David, and Rao 2003, 2–5)

One of the lead federal agencies dealing with drug prevention education is the Center for Substance Abuse Prevention (CSAP) of the Substance Abuse and Mental Health Services Administration (SAMHSA). The mission of CSAP is to work with local communities to develop programs of substance abuse prevention that are appropriate for that community and its specific problems in this area. CSAP uses a five-step approach in achieving this mission, beginning with an assessment of the specific substance abuse issues faced by a community; an analysis of the resources available within that community to develop a program of prevention, planning, and development of such a program; implementation of the program; and an evaluation of its successes and failures (SAMHSA's Center for Substance Abuse Prevention 2016).

A number of for-profit and nonprofit organizations have also been established to assist schools and communities in the development and implementation of substance abuse prevention programs. Perhaps one of the best known of these organizations is D.A.R.E. (Drug Abuse Resistance Education). D.A.R.E. was established in 1983 by Los Angeles police chief Darryl Gates and one of his deputy chiefs, Glenn Levant, as a way of trying to deal with the problem of substance abuse, especially among teenagers, in Los Angeles. D.A.R.E.'s drug prevention program consists of a series of classes run by police

officers who have had at least 80 hours of training in drug prevention programs. The organization claims to have a presence
in 75 percent of all American school districts and in 43 foreign
countries (D.A.R.E. 2016).

An important question about D.A.R.E.—and all other
drug prevention programs—is how effective they are. Does
participation in a D.A.R.E. class, or any other drug prevention program, actually reduce the likelihood that individuals
will become involved in substance abuse? A number of studies
have been conducted to answer this question. One of the best
known of these studies was prepared by the Office of the Surgeon General of the United States in 2000. Among its many
objectives, that report attempted to identify substance abuse
programs that were and were not effective. It classified a number of programs as "model programs," because there was sound
scientific evidence that the programs significantly reduced the
likelihood that participants would become involved in substance abuse: as "promising," because they showed evidence
of achieving this goal; and as "does not work," because available evidence did not support the goal of reducing substance
abuse and, in some cases, actually increased the likelihood that
participants would become involved in substance abuse (*Youth
Violence: A Report of the Surgeon General* 2001, 102–109).
Table 2.1 shows some of the programs that fell into each of
the three categories.

It is interesting that D.A.R.E. was one of only two programs
classified as Does Not Work in the report (the other being a program called "Scared Straight"). Authors of the report acknowledged the widespread popularity of D.A.R.E. but explained
that it was classified as Does Not Work because "numerous well
designed evaluations and meta-analyses . . . consistently show
little or no deterrent effects on substance use. Overall, evidence
on the effects of the traditional DARE curriculum . . . shows
that children who participate are as likely to use drugs as those

Table 2.1   Effectiveness of Selected Drug Prevention Programs

Category	Program
Model	
Violence Prevention	Seattle Social Development Project
	Prenatal and Infancy Home Visitation by Nurses
	Functional Family Therapy
	Multisystemic Therapy
	Multidimensional Treatment Foster Care
Risk Prevention	Life Skills Training
	The Midwestern Prevention Project
Promising	
Violence Prevention	School Transitional Environmental Program
	Montreal Longitudinal Study/Preventive Treatment Program
	Syracuse Family Development Research Program
	Perry Preschool Program
	Striving Together to Achieve Rewarding Tomorrows
	Intensive Protective Supervision Project
Risk Prevention	Promoting Alternative Thinking Strategies
	I Can Problem Solve
	Iowa Strengthening Families Program
	Preparing for the Drug-Free Years
	Linking the Interests of Families and Teachers
	Bullying Prevention Program
	Good Behavior Game
	Parent Child Development Center Programs
	Parent-Child Interaction Training
	Yale Child Welfare Project
	Families and Schools Together
	The Incredible Years Series
	Preventive Intervention
	The Quantum Opportunities Program
Does Not Work	Drug Abuse Resistance Education
	Scared Straight

Source: Youth Violence: A Report of the Surgeon General. 2001. Washington, DC: Department of Health and Human Services. U.S. Public Health Service, 109, Box 5–2.

who do not participate" (*Youth Violence: A Report of the Surgeon General* 2001, 110).

The D.A.R.E. program has been subjected to a number of similar criticisms over the years and has focused on improving its work with young people to reduce substance abuse. In 2014 it announced a new program that it claimed actually worked and attempted to recover some of the good will that it had earned many years earlier (The New D.A.R.E. Program—This One Works 2014).

The question remains, however, how an ordinary person can determine the effectiveness of a drug prevention program. There certainly is no shortage of such programs, many of which are advertised on the Internet. But scientific evidence for the quality of such programs is in short supply, and the average consumer has little to base a decision in the selection of prevention programs to recommend to friends and loved ones. (One modest exception is a review of a small number of such programs provided by SAMHSA on its website at http://nrepp. samhsa.gov/AdvancedSearch.aspx.)

Substance Abuse Treatment

A position on which the vast majority of substance abuse experts can now agree is that people who abuse drugs or become dependent upon or addicted to them require some form of treatment to help them deal with their problem. That treatment is often not available, however, or those who need it do not get the treatment that is available. According to the 2014 National Survey on Drug Use and Health survey, an estimated 22,478,000 Americans over the age of 12 needed some form of treatment for substance abuse in 2014, of whom about 2,606,000 actually received treatment. Corresponding numbers for those in the age group 12 to 17 were 1,284,000 requiring treatment and 109,000 receiving it; 5,845,000 needing treatment in the age group 18 to 25 and 470,000 receiving it; and 15,349,000 in the 26 years and older group needing and 2,028,000 receiving treatment (Results from the 2014 National Survey on Drug Use and Health: Detailed Tables 2015, Table 5.51A).

As is the case with substance abuse prevention programs, a number of organizations and agencies have developed principles upon which programs of substance abuse treatment should be based. The NIDA has provided one such set of guidelines in one of the newsletters in its InfoFacts newsletters. Among the general principles the NIDA suggests are the following:

- Addiction is a complex but treatable disease that affects brain function and behavior.
- No single treatment is right for everyone.
- People need to have quick access to treatment.
- Effective treatment addresses all of the patient's needs, not just his or her drug use.
- Staying in treatment long enough is critical.
- Counseling and other behavioral therapies are the most commonly used forms of treatment.
- Medications are often an important part of treatment, especially when combined with behavioral therapies.
- Treatment plans must be reviewed often and modified to fit the patient's changing needs.
- Treatment should address other possible mental disorders.
- Medically assisted detoxification is only the first stage of treatment.
- Treatment doesn't need to be voluntary to be effective.
- Drug use during treatment must be monitored continuously.
          (quoted from DrugFacts: Treatment
          Approaches for Drug Addiction 2016)

As these guidelines suggest, treatment for substance abuse and addiction usually makes use of two approaches: medication and behavioral therapies. Medications are sometimes the first line of attack for individuals who have actually become addicted to a substance. Such is most often the case with opiate addictions, in which case three medications are generally available for use: methadone, naltrexone, and buprenorphine. A fourth drug, levo-alpha-acetylmethadol (LAAM), is also approved for use, but, because of risky side effects, not as commonly prescribed. Three medications have also been approved by the U.S. Food and Drug Administration (FDA) for the treatment of alcohol dependence and addiction: naltrexone, acamprosate (Campral), and disulfiram (Antabuse). Nicotine dependence and addiction can be treated by a variety of over-the-counter patches, sprays, gums, and lozenges that reduce the need for nicotine, as well as by two FDA-approved drugs: bupropion (Zyban) and varenicline (Chantix). For some types of substances, such as cocaine and marijuana, no medications are available for assisting a person with withdrawal and treatment of a dependence or addiction. After a person has gone through the worst stage of recovery—withdrawal from use of a substance—then personal and group counseling is often helpful in weaning him or her entirely from the substance.

One might reasonably ask which types of treatment work best for each type of substance abuse and addiction for which individuals and under what circumstances. In fact, researchers have conducted many studies on just such issues. Because of the many variables involved, it is not possible to make simple assessments as to any one part of this complex equation. There is, however, an abundance of information about specific types of treatment for specific situations. One of the best resources for that information is a website operated jointly by the NIDA, the National Development and Research Institutes, Inc., the University of California at Los Angeles Integrated Substance Abuse Program, and the Texas Institute of Behavioral Research at Texas Christian University. The website is called Drug Abuse Treatment Outcome Studies (DATOS). Readers interested in learning more about the effectiveness of various types of treatments for individuals of various ages dealing with specific types of substance abuse under specific types of conditions should refer to this website at http://www .datos.org/.

More recent suggestions for successful treatment programs are also available. One book that deals specifically with this issue is *Inside Rehab: The Surprising Truth about Addiction*

Treatment—and How to Get Help That Works, by medical writer Anne M. Fletcher (Viking 2013). Fletcher reports on her visits to 15 treatment programs and interviews with more than 200 clients to explain why most programs work much less effectively than they claim to or could work (see also Brody 2013).

Other Options

As the preceding sections suggest, many specialists in the field of substance abuse are looking for ways for dealing with the problem that goes beyond traditional prevention and treatment options. Two such ideas that have shown promise are drug courts and recovery schools.

Drug courts are facilities that offer modified forms of traditional criminal courts consisting of prosecution, defense, and a judge or jury that meet to hear evidence in a criminal case and then decide on a person's guilt or innocence and any punishment that may be appropriate. In drug courts, all of these elements, along with counselors, social workers, psychologists, mental health experts, and others with specialized knowledge and skills, meet to decide the best response to individuals and cases not well treated in traditional courts. Specialized drug courts have been developed for dealing with adult and young adult substance abusers, veterans, family dependency problems, tribal issues, and DWI (driving while intoxicated).

In general, the goal of drug courts is to find alternatives to sentencing and imprisonment for individuals arrested for substance-related crimes. In most cases, the court team meets to consider an individual's background and involvement in substance abuse and to decide the most appropriate treatment before developing a treatment plan, which may consist of various forms of monitored treatment (counseling, medication, etc.) and preparation for post-release guidance and assistance. Individuals who successfully complete the prescribed course of action may have their records expunged, along with the chance to have a fresh beginning in dealing with their substance abuse issues.

The first drug court was created in Miami-Dade County, Florida, in 1989, in response to the epidemic of crack cocaine abuse then occurring in the area. Over time, the number of drug courts has increased until, at the end of 2014, there were 3,057 such courts in all 50 states, the District of Columbia, Guam, and Puerto Rico (Drug Courts 2016).

Another fairly new approach to substance abuse treatment is recovery schools. A recovery school is an educational program designed for young adults who are recovering from substance abuse. They have been developed because of the high rate of recidivism among such students who leave a (usually successful) treatment program and then return to the educational setting from which they came in the first place. This series of events has a tendency to result in an individual's falling back into old habits and reverting once more to the substance abuse for which he or she had been treated.

The first recovery school was Sobriety High, established in Burnsville, Minnesota, in 1987, with just two students. The school later reached an enrollment of more than 100 before closing down in 2013. As of 2016, there were 25 recovery schools located in eight states, with plans to expand their presence over the next few years (Are Recovery High Schools Really Working? 2016).

Recovery schools may take a number of forms. Some, for example, are located in traditional schools, with some form of physical separation available for recovery students. Others may be housed in freestanding structures separate from traditional schools. Recovery students are expected to complete the state-mandated curriculum required of non-recovery students, but are provided with a variety of support options, such as specialized counseling, guidance, and health services (Vimont 2011). The parent association for recovery schools is the Association of Recovery Schools (https://recoveryschools.org/), from which more detailed information about the topic may be obtained. For an important evaluative study of recovery schools, see Moberg and Finch (2008).

Drug Testing

As noted at the beginning of this chapter, the abuse of psychoactive substances, such as alcohol, tobacco, marijuana, and other drugs, has been a matter of concern in the United States for at least a century. Individuals, private organizations, and government agencies have searched for ways of dealing with this problem, with prevention and treatment programs being viewed as two possible solutions. A number of other ways of dealing with substance abuse have also been developed. One of these methods is drug testing. The 1960s and 1970s saw a dramatic increase in substance abuse in the United States. In some cases, as discussed for the use of marijuana in Chapter 1 of this book, that increase may have represented a general rejection of moral standards by some younger members of society. But increased substance abuse was also directly linked to the Vietnam conflict of the early 1960s to 1975. Many men and women who served in Vietnam sought relief from the horrible conditions they faced there by turning to alcohol and other drugs. By the end of the war, very large numbers of personnel had either used drugs from time to time or had become addicted to them. To track the severity of this problem, the Department of Defense ordered that returning veterans be randomly tested for drug use before being discharged from the service, a program that eventually earned the sobriquet of Operation Golden Flow (Holland 2015).

Drug Testing in the Workplace

For a variety of reasons, President Richard M. Nixon soon overturned the Pentagon's drug testing plan. But the idea of identifying substance abusers in the society as a whole, but especially in the workplace, had already begun to set in. Many studies have been done on the prevalence of drug testing in the workplace over the past four decades, but most seem to suggest that businesses began to see value in screening job applicants (and, less commonly, current employees) for illegal drug use as early as the 1970s. During the 1980s, however, the number of businesses that had adopted such programs increased dramatically, from about 20 percent at the beginning of the decade to more than twice that number at the end of the decade. The longest continuous series of studies on drug testing in the workplace is one conducted by the American Management Association (AMA), which collected data on the topic for more than two decades. AMA surveys show that the percentage of businesses contacted that require preemployment drug testing rose to a peak of 81 percent in 1996. It then began to fall off fairly rapidly until it reached a new low of 62.6 percent in 2004, the last year in which AMA conducted the survey (DePillis 2015). Throughout this period, the number of companies that tested current employees in addition to new hires was consistently much less, usually by a factor of one-half, than those who screened for preemployment purposes.

Proponents of drug testing in the workplace offer a number of arguments in support of their position. First, they point out that workers who are under the influence of illegal substances are more likely to have or cause accidents in the workplace, causing injuries and deaths to coworkers, innocent bystanders, and themselves, and costing the company significant amounts of money in property loss. A number of studies appear to confirm this position. For example:

- About 40 percent of deaths in the workplace and 47 percent of the injuries have been correlated with alcohol use or alcoholism.
- Anywhere from 38 to 50 percent of all workplace accidents involve substance abuse involving alcohol or drugs.

- A 1998 study found that 19 percent of the individuals killed in workplace accidents had alcohol and/or drugs in their bloodstream during a postmortem examination.
- Companies that have adopted drug testing programs have experienced a decrease of more than half (51%) in the number of workplace-related accidents within a two-year period of instituting the program.
- Companies that have instituted drug testing programs have also experienced a decline in workmen's compensation rates of more than 10 percent (Judge 2007, 14).

Proponents of workplace drug testing also pose a number of other arguments in favor of the practice. For example, they point to data that suggest that workers who are drug-free tend to be more productive at their jobs. They also suggest also that the use of illegal substances in the workplace may affect general morale and reduce the ability of coworkers to do their own jobs efficiently. Finally, they believe that testing programs may be an important factor in helping to reduce the problem of substance abuse overall, since workers will have to reduce or discontinue use of illegal substances if they are to be hired for or retain a job (Newton 1999, 31–38).

Opponents of drug testing have their own counterarguments. They point out, in the first place, that drug testing can be a significant intrusion on a person's privacy, which is protected in the United States by the Fourth Amendment to the U.S. Constitution's ban on "unreasonable searches and seizures." Since the vast majority of drug tests are conducted randomly and are not based on some illegal or improper act on the part of the testee, they would appear to violate this constitutional protection. Second, opponents note that drug tests tend to be notoriously unreliable with high percentages of false positives (a positive test when a person has not actually used a drug) and false negatives (a negative test when a person has been using a drug). The authority most often cited in defense of this position is a study conducted by the National Research Council in 1994, which concluded that "[d]espite beliefs to the contrary, the preventive effects of drug-testing programs have never been adequately demonstrated" (Normand, Lempert, and O'Brien 1994, 11).

The debate over the effectiveness of workplace drug testing continues well into the second decade of the twenty-first century. A meta-analysis of 23 studies on the question conducted in 2014 produced mixed results on the question. Researchers concluded that "the effectiveness of testing in improving workplace safety is at best tenuous," but that the quality of the research that had been conducted was, in general, so poor that making firm conclusions was difficult (Pidd and Roche 2014, 154). Still, by the end of 2016, there seemed to be a strong consensus in the general literature that workplace drug testing has not, in its 40-year history, proved its value to industry, to workers, or to the country at large (Engber 2015).

Opponents of workplace drug testing also argue that such programs are not cost-effective. In a 1991 study of the use of drug testing in federal agencies, for example, the cost of identifying a single substance abuser was estimated to be about $77,000 (cited in Zimmer 1999, 14). That number may be a gross underestimate, however, if one assumes (probably correctly) that only one out of ten individuals who tests positive is a serious substance abuser. In such a case, the actual cost of identifying a single individual likely to be a risk in the workplace may range from $700,000 to $1.5 million (Donohoe 2005, 72). Given a number of options for locating potential substance abuser risks in the workplace, some critics say, other options to drug testing should be considered. (An excellent review of the issues involved in workplace drug testing on the Internet is this pair of websites: Olson 2004a and Olson 2004b.)

Finally, opponents of drug testing in the workplace sometimes point to the fact that most testing programs ignore the one drug—alcohol—responsible for by far the greatest proportion of accidents in the workplace.

Arguably the most serious issue about workplace drug testing has arisen because of the actions by some states to legalize the use of marijuana for medical and recreational purposes. Until the early twenty-first century, debates over the pre- and post-hiring testing for marijuana were moderated to some degree because of the fact that the drug was, after all, illegal. It was listed as a Schedule I drug by the federal government. Now, the drug is legal in nearly half of the states, and the question arises as to whether a job candidate or employee can or should be refused employment or fired because of testing positive for marijuana.

For some observers, the answer to that question is simple: Marijuana is an illegal drug; employers can test for it and act on test results. This position was taken perhaps most prominently by the Colorado Supreme Court in 2015 when it ruled in *Coats v. Dish Network* that Brandon Coats, a quadriplegic employee of Dish Network, was fired because he failed a workplace test for marijuana, a drug he takes for the pain associated with his medical condition. The court ruled that the company was within its rights to fire an employee who used an illegal drug (by federal standards), no matter what state law said (*Coats v. Dish* 2015).

Other stakeholders have taken a very different view of the problem. They argue that it is now legal to use marijuana for medical and/or recreational purposes in some states, so actions such as those taken by Dish are simply penalizing private citizens for conducting legal actions in the privacy of their own homes. Dish's action, and that of the vast majority of employers, was not based on a worker's *performance* on his or her job, but on some behavior conducted away from the workplace that may or may not have influenced the quality of his or her work. Since positive results for marijuana smoking can be collected up to ten days following the actual act, it is not clear the extent to which the act of smoking may or may not have affected a person's job performance (Wallace 2015).

As of late 2016, no clear trend had developed as to how this new issue will be resolved. Attendees at an annual conference of the Society for Human Resource Management in 2015 packed a session on the nature of the problem companies were facing, possible actions by employees, and ways in which employers could or should react to those actions (Pratt 2015). Meanwhile, the state of Vermont was holding high-level meetings to determine how the state's new medical marijuana law would affect workplace drug testing policies in the states. A period of controversy and debate can only be expected on this question over the near future (Bielawski 2015; for an excellent overview of this issue, see DuPont 2015).

Drug Testing in Schools

Businesses are by no means the only place where drug testing has become somewhat routine and, at the same time, controversial. The practice is also carried out now in many schools, colleges, and universities, and in professional sports. In fact, the debate over the use of drug testing in schools began just at the nexus of these two issues when a number of school districts in the late 1980s and early 1990s decided to institute mandatory drug tests for students who wished to participate in sports at the schools. Drug testing in schools was initiated among athletic teams for a number of reasons, one being that illicit drug use was sometimes thought to be (correctly or not) especially common among student athletes. In addition, participation in athletics is a voluntary activity, unlike school attendance itself, and so boys and girls can choose whether or not to submit to drug tests. Finally, some school districts felt that student athletes should be presentable as desirable role models for the rest of the student body.

In any case, mandatory drug testing for student athletes was met in some instances by objections from individuals who objected to the practice for one reason or another. The case that eventually drew the most attention nationwide involved a decision by the Vernonia School District in Oregon in 1991 to require student athletes to be tested for a number of illicit drugs. One student, James Acton, objected to the policy and filed suit to have the district's policy declared unconstitutional. That case worked its way through the courts and was eventually decided four years later by the U.S. Supreme Court, which ruled in favor of the school district by a vote of 6 to 3 (*Vernonia School Dist. 47J v. Acton 515 U.S. 646* 1995; an excerpt from that decision also appears in Chapter 5 of this book). That decision served as an important precedent for lower courts, which eventually issued decisions allowing drug testing of students who participate in any extracurricular activity and even of students who drive to school.

Another Supreme Court decision on school drug testing came in 2002 in the case of *Board of Education of Independent School District No. 92 of Pottawatomie County v. Earls* (536 U.S. 822), when the Court ruled by a 5 to 4 vote that schools could require drug tests from students who participate in any extracurricular activity. Writing for the majority, Justice Clarence Thomas made the point that "[g]iven the nationwide epidemic of drug use, and the evidence of increased drug use in Tecumseh schools, it was entirely reasonable for the School District to enact this particular drug testing policy" (*Board of Education of Independent School District No. 92 of Pottawatomie County v. Earls* 2002).

Today, drug testing in schools may take a number of different forms. It may involve student athletes only, participants in other types of extracurricular activities, a random sample of the student body, or all members of the student body on either a voluntary or a required basis. A frequently cited study on this variety of programs found that about 20 percent of all schools (containing about 20% of all students in the country) had one or another of these programs (Yamaguchi, Johnston, and O'Malley 2003, 22–23, Table 2). The most popular program was one in which testing was required only when there was specific cause or reason to suspect illicit drug use, with about

13 percent of all schools (and 13.4% of all students) involved in this type of program. The pattern of drug testing programs in about 170 schools from 1998 to 2002 is shown in Table 2.2 (for more recent, but limited, data, see Ringwalt et al. 2008).

As with workplace drug testing, arguments both in support of and in opposition to drug testing in schools have been presented, and, in many cases, the arguments are similar to those used in the workplace controversy. Most importantly, proponents of testing say, schools should do something to stem the tide of substance abuse in the nation, and carefully controlled testing of all or certain groups of students is one way to do that. Besides, students who do not use drugs have nothing to fear from substance testing. Opponents disagree, pointing out that less invasive methods of drug prevention are available, and students should not have to give up their right of privacy for the purposes of drug testing (see, for example, Anderson 2012).

Research on the effectiveness of school drug testing has produced somewhat conflicting results. A study of seven school districts with 36 high schools that had received grants from

Table 2.2 Drug Testing Programs in U.S. Schools, 1998–2002, Percentage of Schools/Students

Category	1998	1999	2000	2001	2002
Any program	14.4/16.2	19.5/21.1	23.4/24.0	15.9/15.6	20.7/20.1
Athletes	n/a	2.9/4.6	7.0/7.4	5.0/5.7	6.5/6.9
Other extracurricular	n/a	0.6/1.6	2.9/3.1	3.3/2.8	3.0/2.9
Cause/suspicion	n/a	14.4/15.2	15.8/15.7	12.1/11.2	13.0/13.4
School probation	n/a	4.0/3.4	4.1/3.4	2.8/1.4	1.2/1.1
Volunteered	n/a	4.6/5.7	3.5/3.9	3.3/3.0	3.0/2.5
Random	0/0	1.7/1.0	1.2/1.3	0/0	1.2/1.1
Routine	2.5/3.3	3.4/3.4	6.5/5.5	4.4/4.1	3.6/4.2
Mandated	5.6/5.2	2.3/2.0	5.9/4.6	5.5/5.3	4.1/3.3

Source: Yamaguchi, Ryoko, Lloyd D. Johnston, and Patrick M. O'Malley. *Drug Testing in Schools: Policies, Practices, and Association with Student Drug Use.* Occasional Paper No. 2. Ann Arbor: Institute for Social Research. University of Michigan, 2003, 22–23, Table 2.

the U.S. Department of Education for drug prevention programs found that "students subject to MRSDT [the trial program: mandatory-random student drug testing] reported less substance use than comparable students in high schools without MRSDT." The study found no other effects on students in the trial program or any "spillover" effects to students not enrolled in the program (James-Burdumy et al. 2010, xvii). More commonly, research appears to find fewer or no effects on drug use as a result of drug testing programs. At least two large-scale reviews of studies on the effectiveness of school drug testing (Stuart 2010; Sznitman and Romer 2014) have found little or no evidence that those programs changed drug use patterns among students required to take those tests. Perhaps the most significant reflection of this trend was a position paper released by the American Academy of Pediatrics in 2015. That document noted that the organization "opposes widespread implementation of these programs because of the lack of solid evidence for their effectiveness" (Levy, Schizer, and Committee on Substance Abuse 2015, 782). Although the fervor for school testing appears to have cooled to some degree since the late twenty-first century, the debate continues at a reduced level over the practice.

Drug Testing in Amateur and Professional Sports

While interest in drug testing in the workplace and schools appears to have diminished somewhat (in the first instance) or remained about constant (in the second), it has increased quite significantly in one other situation: professional sports. Some modest efforts to limit the use of illegal substances by athletes go as far back as 1970, when the National Collegiate Athletic Association (NCAA) first established a Drug Education Committee to provide information about drug use among college athletes. It took more than 10 years, however, for the NCAA to authorize a study of the use of drugs by college athletes and 16 years before the association actually began testing athletes. That program was initiated for championship and bowl games in the fall of 1986, based on a list of banned sub-stances adopted a year earlier by the NCAA. Today the NCAA bans thousands of drugs that fall into eight major categories: stimulants, anabolic agents, alcohol and beta-blockers, diuret-ics and other masking agents, street drugs, peptide hormones and analogues, anti-estrogens, and beta-2 agonists (2016–2017 NCAA Banned Drugs 2016). Most of these substances have short-term effects and must be taken just prior to an activity or in an effort to mask the use of an illegal substance (masking agents). They are, therefore, relatively easy to detect by stan-dard drug tests.

The exception to that statement is the anabolic agents, also known as anabolic-androgenic steroids (AAS), substances that are chemically similar to the male sex hormone testosterone. AAS are popular among athletes because they produce weight gain, which occurs almost entirely in the form of muscle mass, increasing an individual's strength, speed, and endurance. AAS compounds also have a number of troubling side effects, how-ever, which provide an important argument against their use. These side effects include increased blood pressure and blood cholesterol levels along with increased risk for cardiovascular disease, acne, and liver damage. A number of mental condi-tions have also been associated with steroid use, including aggression and violence (sometimes called "roid rage"), mania, and psychosis.

Anabolic agents are the primary cause of concern among both amateur and professional sports associations because ath-letes value their effects so highly and they are more difficult to detect than are stimulants, masking agents, and other drugs. In many cases, it is difficult to know if an athlete is bigger, stronger, and faster as the result of training or because he or she has been taking AAS drugs. Probably the most dramatic example of this dilemma has been the revelation that many of the best-known and most successful professional baseball play-ers achieved their physical superiority not just by training, but by the use of substances that have long been banned in most sports, although not in professional baseball until 2004 (Newton 2014; Quinn 2015).

Today, nearly all amateur and professional sports organizations have drug testing programs for a number of illegal substances. National Football League regulations, for example, call for a four-game suspension after a first positive test, a six-game suspension after a second positive test, and a one-year suspension after a third positive test. A policy adopted by Major League Baseball in 2005 calls for counseling of a player who tests positive for an illegal substance the first time; a 15-day suspension and maximum fine of $10,000 after a second positive test; a 25-day suspension and a maximum fine of $25,000 after a third positive test; a 50-day suspension and a maximum fine of $50,000 after a fourth positive test; and a one-year suspension and maximum fine of $100,000 after a fifth positive test. Both the National Basketball Association and the National Hockey League have roughly similar drug testing programs (Professional Sports and Their Drug Policies 2016).

Controlling the Use of Drugs

As discussed in Chapter 1, many countries have, at one time or another in their histories, struggled with the question of how to control the use of one psychoactive substance or another within their boundaries. Three approaches have frequently been used in such efforts: education, taxation, and outright prohibition.

Education about Harmful Substances

Educational efforts are based on the assumption that the more people know about the deleterious effects of a substance, the less likely they are to use those substances for recreational purposes. One of the classic examples of this approach to dealing with a psychoactive substance in the United States has been the Women's Christian Temperance Union (WCTU). The WCTU was founded in Cleveland, Ohio, in November 1874 as the outgrowth of an 1873–1874 campaign known as the Woman's Crusade. During this campaign, a number of ordinary housewives decided to rebel against what they saw as the evils of drinking alcohol that they had experienced in their communities firsthand. They organized "sit-ins" and "pray-ins" at local taverns, demanding that the sale of liquor be discontinued. Within the first three months of their campaign, these women had driven more than 250 establishments out of business (Early History 2016).

One of the WCTU's earliest programs was an effort to introduce anti-alcohol education into public schools. In 1879, the organization created a permanent committee, a year later to become the WCTU Department of Scientific Temperance Instruction in Schools and Colleges, for this purpose. WCTU members were encouraged to appear before their local school boards of education to demand that anti-alcohol classes be included in the regular curriculum, and the organization itself began to produce materials to be used in such classes, including a textbook called *Alcohol and Hygiene*. When these efforts proved to be only moderately successful, the organization aimed its sights higher: at state legislatures. It lobbied for the introduction of bills that would require local districts to adopt anti-alcohol curricula, an effort that was first successful in the state of Vermont in 1882. The pressure from WCTU members was so great that Vermont legislators passed the bill by large majorities in both houses (Hanson 2009). This success was replicated elsewhere in the country, and by the end of the century, some form of anti-alcohol education law had been adopted by almost every state, the District of Columbia, and all U.S. possessions (Hanson 2009).

The success of educational efforts like those of the WCTU is difficult to determine. On the one hand, the average annual consumption of alcohol in the United States actually increased in the years in which the WCTU was most successful in passing legislation on anti-alcohol education. That number increased from 1.72 gallons of alcohol per person per year in the decade of 1871–1880 to 2.06 gallons in 1896–1900 to 2.56 in 1911–1915, a 49 percent increase in consumption in about 40 years (Nephew et al. 2002, 18, Table 1). Average alcohol consumption among Americans was not to reach that level again until the 1970s. On the other hand, the efforts of the WCTU have generally been credited with providing the momentum that eventually culminated in the great "noble experiment" to ban alcohol completely in the United States with the Eighteenth Amendment to the U.S. Constitution in 1919. That amendment did not actually ban the consumption of alcoholic beverages; it prohibited the manufacture, sale, and transportation of such beverages within the United States. The educational efforts originally promoted by the WCTU and other temperance organizations thus evolved over time into a very different type of effort to restrict the consumption of alcohol: legal remedies, the strongest of which, of course, was an amendment to the U.S. Constitution.

Many books and untold numbers of scholarly papers have been written about the American prohibition movement, the name given to the effort to stamp out the drinking of alcoholic beverages in the United States between 1919 and 1933 (the year in which the Twenty-First Amendment to the Constitution, rescinding the Eighteenth Amendment, was adopted). Experts in the area have drawn conclusions from across the board, from the experiment having been a great success in terms of reducing the consumption of alcohol among Americans to its having been a nearly total failure, on the basis not only of no change in drinking habits, but also in terms of the explosion of crime engendered by the need to supply drinkers with alcoholic beverages illegally. Of course, statistical data about alcohol consumption during the period of 1919–1933 is unavailable, since alcoholic beverages were illegal at the time. A number of studies suggest, however, that the Eighteenth Amendment had, at best, only limited success in reducing the consumption of alcohol. These studies show that the number of deaths from alcohol-related problems, the age at which males and females began drinking, and the number of arrests for drunkenness and other alcohol-related problems all suggest a significant increase in the amount of alcohol consumption during the period (Schaffer 2016).

Taxation of Drugs

World history is replete with examples of efforts to control the use of psychoactive substances by means of taxation or methods that fall short of actual, total prohibition. Probably the earliest example in American history of such an effort was the whiskey tax of 1791, imposed by the federal government on the producers of that beverage. The tax was imposed by the young U.S. government for a number of reasons, perhaps the most important of which was the dire financial status of the government. Under provisions under which the federal government was established, that government was required to assume all of the debts accumulated by the states in association with the Revolutionary War. The government began operation, then, with a huge debt. The first secretary of the Treasury, Alexander Hamilton, envisioned a modest tax on alcoholic spirits (whiskey, in particular) as being a possible lucrative source of income for paying down this debt. Even before the new government had formed, Hamilton presaged this idea in his earlier writings. In the *Federalist Papers*, for example, he had written that "[t]he single article of ardent spirits, under federal regulation, might be made to furnish a considerable revenue" (Hamilton 1904, 280). Interestingly, Hamilton's interest in a tax on spirits was motivated by more than just a concern about revenue. He concluded the paragraph from which the previous quotation is taken with the observation that "[t]hat article [spirits] would well bear this rate of duty; and if it should tend to diminish the consumption of it, such an effect would be equally favorable to the agriculture, to the economy, to the morals, and to the health of the society. There is, perhaps, nothing so much a subject of national extravagance as these spirits" (Hamilton 1904, 280).

In 1791, then, Hamilton was able to convince the Congress to impose a tax on alcohol, based in part on the size of the manufacturing operation: large companies paid six cents a gallon in tax, while small companies paid nine cents a gallon, a system that was almost guaranteed to produce strong opposition from the latter, most of whom were then located on the western frontier. That opposition eventually boiled over into the so-called Whiskey Rebellion of 1794, with armed uprising breaking out in many of the colonies. That rebellion continued for more than five years and was met with considerable force by federal troops, whose action was necessitated at least in part by the government's desire to establish a strong central government within the new nation. Even though the federal troops prevailed in armed conflict on the field, opposition to the tax was so strong that it was eventually repealed in 1802.

The U.S. government has sometimes taken somewhat circuitous routes—short of outright bans—to the control of psychoactive substances other than alcohol. Such was long the case with cocaine and opiates. During the second half of the nineteenth century, these substances were generally available to the public and unregulated by the government. The Sears, Roebuck catalogs of the late nineteenth century, for example, carried advertisements for "coca wine" that was recommended for the treatment of neuralgia, sleeplessness, and despondency (Pearce 2016). Some catalogs also listed small quantities of cocaine accompanied by a syringe with which to inject the drug, sold for $1.50 (Buxton 2006, 16–17). Perhaps the best-known everyday use of cocaine, however, was as an ingredient in a popular new soft drink invented by Atlanta pharmacist John Pemberton in 1885, Coca-Cola. Originally sold as a patent medicine, the drink soon became widely popular as a refreshing soft drink. As its name clearly announces, the drink originally contained cocaine. By 1903, however, the drug was removed, largely in response to growing concerns about its harmful and addictive effects.

By the turn of the century, pressures for some kind of control over the use of cocaine and opiates began to grow from both national and international sources. The first factor of importance was the annexation by the United States of the Philippine Islands, one of the penalties paid by Spain following its defeat in the Spanish-American War of 1898. Along with the many natural resources provided by the Philippines, the United States inherited a very large population of residents of the island who had become addicted to cocaine. The federal government was forced to develop some program for dealing with these individuals. The decision was finally reached that addiction to cocaine and other drugs, such as opiates, was really an international problem, rather than one restricted to the Philippines. As a consequence, President Theodore Roosevelt called for an international conference, called the International Opium Commission, to be held in Shanghai in February 1909. That meeting was followed by a second international conference, held at The Hague, the Netherlands, in May 1911. The Hague conference adopted the first international treaty for the control of psychoactive substances, calling for all signatories to do whatever they could to "control, or to cause to be controlled, all persons manufacturing, importing, selling, distributing, and exporting morphine, cocaine, and their respective salts, as well as the buildings in which these persons carry such an industry or trade" (International Opium Convention Signed at The Hague January 23, 1912 1912, Article 10, page 197). The treaty provided a powerful impetus for the U.S. government to adopt measures for the control of cocaine and opiates within its own borders.

Domestic issues also contributed to the increasing pressures for regulation of psychoactive substances. By the first decade of the twentieth century, medical studies began to show possible health issues associated with the use of these substances, for example, an increase in respiratory diseases in connection with the use of cocaine. Law enforcement officers also pointed to the legal problems created by addicts needing the money required to support their drug habits. And a number of religious and social leaders grew increasingly concerned about the moral effects of the apparent spread of cocaine and heroin use among Americans. As perhaps to be expected, much of the blame for the nation's growing substance abuse problem fell on minority groups. A committee appointed to study this problem in 1902, for example, singled out Chinese immigrants as a major factor in the substance abuse problem faced by Americans. In its report, the Committee on Acquirement of the Drug Habit noted that opium use was rife among Chinese immigrants and concluded somewhat ominously that "[i]f the Chinaman cannot get along without his dope we can get along without him" (Report of Committee on Acquirement of the Drug Habit 1902, 572). Criticism increasingly fell on the African American community also. A number of legislators, law enforcement personnel, and experts in the field of substance abuse pointed out that cocaine and heroin use was especially common among blacks, often with terrible social consequences. A leading advocate for stricter controls on drugs, Hamilton Wright, the first opium commissioner of the United States, said at the Shanghai convention in 1909 that "cocaine is often the direct incentive to the crime of rape by the Negroes of the South and other sections of the country" (Musto 1987, 43–44). (Somewhat ironically, no credible evidence existed for Wright's claim, or for any of the other similar warnings raised about the special problems that blacks created by their abuse of illegal substances [Courtwright 1995, Chapter 10].)

The confluence of international and domestic pressures led in 1914 to the adoption of the Harrison Act, the first federal legislation designed specifically to control the consumption of cocaine and opiates in the United States. (The act was actually written by Wright, although introduced by Rep. Francis Burton Harrison of New York.) The main provision of the act was the requirement that all individuals who "produce, import, manufacture, compound, deal in, dispense, sell, distribute, or give away opium or coca leaves, their salts, derivatives, or preparations, and for other purposes" register with federal officials and pay a tax on all their proceedings (Harrison Narcotics Tax Act, 1914). The practical effect of the Harrison Act was to make the possession and consumption of cocaine and opiates illegal for any use other than medical applications. As an attempt to solve the nation's substance abuse problems, however, it was a failure, producing almost the opposite result. Individuals who had become dependent on cocaine or an opiate could no longer obtain their drug of choice legally and found it necessary to find ways of getting it on the black market and, in many cases, to commit crimes to get the money they needed for the increasingly expensive product.

Recognizing this disturbing trend, the secretary of the Treasury, William Gibbs McAdoo, appointed a committee to evaluate the effects of the Harrison Act. The committee reported a number of trends as a result of the act's passage, perhaps most significant of which was that (1) the use of cocaine and opiate had actually increased since the adoption of the act and (2) a thriving new community of "dope peddlers" had arisen, bringing drugs illegally into the country from Canada and Mexico (Brecher 1972, Chapter 8). To remedy this situation, the committee recommended more of the same, that is, amendments to the Harrison Act that would increase penalties for illegal use of cocaine and opiates. Within a year of adoption of the new amendments in 1924, signs appeared that stricter enforcement of the Harrison Act was not working either. An editorialist for *The Illinois Medical Journal* wrote in 1926 that "[t]he Harrison Narcotic law should never have been placed upon the Statute books of the United States . . . instead of stopping the [drug] traffic, those who deal in dope now make double their money from the poor unfortunates upon whom they prey" (Brecher 1972, Chapter 8).

The "tax and regulate" approach to controlling cocaine and opiates has also been used with other psychoactive substances. The 1937 Marihuana Tax Act is an example. (Note that the modern spelling of the substance, *marijuana,* is of relatively recent origin, with an "h" instead of a "j" being more common historically.) Marijuana is obtained from the cannabis plant, of which three species are of commercial significance: *Cannabis sativa, C. indica,* and (less commonly) *C. ruderalis.* The plant is an annual dioecious (one type of gamete per plant) flowering herb that grows to a height of about 3 meters (10 feet). It has historically been utilized primarily for two purposes. First, the soft, flexible fibers obtained from its stalk—known as hemp— are used in the manufacture of more than 25,000 industrial products, including paper, cloth, construction materials, medicines, and biofuels (Hemp Facts 1997). Second, the dried flowers and leaves of the plant are smoked to produce a "high" for recreational and religious purposes.

For the first 300 years of American history, hemp was a very popular commercial crop. As early as 1619, the Virginia Assembly passed a law requiring every farmer to grow at least some hemp to be used both for domestic purposes and for exportation and foreign trade. Hemp was also used as legal tender at the time in Maryland, Pennsylvania, and Virginia. The fiber became especially popular during the Civil War when it was used as a substitute for cotton and other natural materials by both sides in the war (Abel 1980, Chapter 8). Largely because of its association with marijuana, hemp largely disappeared as a commercial crop in the United States for many years. Recently, however, a number of states have passed laws allowing the farming of cannabis plants for the production of industrial hemp or the conduct of research on industrial hemp (State Industrial Hemp Statutes 2016).

The use of cannabis products for purely recreational purposes appears to have had its beginning in the United States in the 1910s, when immigrants fleeing the Mexican Revolution arrived in this country, often bringing with them a long-standing recreational habit: the smoking of marijuana. The marijuana used for this purpose comes from cannabis plants botanically different from those used for the production of hemp. The latter have been developed to contain the lowest possible amount of Δ^9-tetrahydrocannabinol (THC), the chemical responsible for the psychoactive effects of ingesting marijuana plant products. By contrast, other types of cannabis plants have been developed with relatively high concentrations of THC which, in general, have stalks that yield poor-quality hemp unsuitable for commercial use. By the early 1930s, the use of marijuana for recreational purposes had become relatively widespread in some parts of the United States, producing a reaction among law enforcement officials, governmental officials, and many private organizations and individuals. In many cases, the objections to the use of marijuana appear to have had their basis in a general fear and dislike of the immigrants who first brought the product to the United States (Abel 1980, Chapter 11). In any case, by 1931, 29 states had outlawed the use of marijuana, and the federal government had begun to consider ways of banning its use nationwide (Abel 1980, Chapter 11).

The first step in this direction occurred in 1937 when the U.S. Congress passed and President Franklin Delano Roosevelt signed the Marihuana Tax Act. Justification for the legislation was based to a considerable extent on some questionable statements about the effects of marijuana on the human personality. In his testimony before Congress as it considered the marijuana bill, for example, Commissioner of Narcotics Harry J. Anslinger said that while the drug first produces feelings of "well-being [and] a happy, jovial mood," that euphoria is soon replaced by much less salubrious emotions, including:

a more-or-less delirious state . . . during which [users] are temporarily, at least, irresponsible and liable to commit violent crimes . . . [and] releases inhibitions of an antisocial nature which dwell within the individual. . . . Then follow errors of sense, false convictions and the predominance of extravagant ideas where all sense of value seems to disappear.

The deleterious, even vicious, qualities of the drug render it highly dangerous to the mind and body upon which it operates to destroy the will, cause one to lose the power of connected thought, producing imaginary delectable situations and gradually weakening the physical powers. Its use frequently leads to insanity. (The Marihuana Tax Act of 1937 2016a)

The bill that was finally passed by Congress did not specifically outlaw the production, sale, or consumption of marijuana, but it did impose a somewhat complex system of taxes and regulations. Anyone involved in any of these activities had to register with the federal government and to pay a tax for each type of activity. For example, anyone who grew or processed a cannabis product had to pay a tax of $24 annually (equivalent to $405 in 2016 dollars). The tax for sale of a cannabis product to anyone who already held a license was $1 per transaction ($17 in 2016 dollars), but $100 ($1,700 in 2016 dollars) to anyone who did not hold such a license (The Marihuana Tax Act of 1937 2016b). Federal authorities did not take long to put the Marihuana Tax Act into effect. On October 1, 1937, they arrested two men in Denver, Colorado, for possession (Moses Baca) and sale (Samuel Caldwell) of marijuana. Judge Foster Symes sentenced Baca to 18 months in jail and Caldwell to four years at hard labor and a $1,000 fine (Uncle Mike 2008).

Assessing the effectiveness of the 1937 legislation is difficult, of course, because marijuana has been, for all practical purposes, illegal since passage of the act. However, substantial evidence is available from arrests for marijuana-related crimes and other sources to suggest that the act was somewhat less than totally successful. A 1998 study found, for example, that the percentage of individuals surveyed who reached the age of 21 in the decades following 1937 and who first used marijuana increased from 0 percent in the 1940s to 2 percent in the 1950s to 6 percent in the 1961–1966 period to 21 percent in the 1967–1971 period to 40 percent in the 1972–1976 period

(Johnson and Gerstein 1998, 29, Table 2). Official government statistics available since 1965 also suggest similar trends, with a gradual increase in the number of marijuana users from that year to a peak in the late 1970s, falling off then to a fluctuating but relatively constant level from that point to the present day (Initiation of Marijuana Use: Trends, Patterns, and Implications 2002, Table 3.3, page 30).

Outright Bans on Substances

The first federal law designed to outlaw the consumption of a psychoactive substance entirely was the Eighteenth Amendment ban on alcohol, certified in 1919 and discussed earlier in this chapter. Similar laws against other psychoactive substances had been enacted much earlier, however, by individual states and municipalities. Probably the first of these laws was the prohibition on the smoking of opium in opium dens, adopted by the city of San Francisco in 1875. That law was very limited, designed to deal almost entirely with Chinese immigrants who brought the habit of opium smoking with them when they immigrated to the United States. All other uses of opium were excluded from the law, and the substance was still widely used by the non-Chinese population for medical and recreational purposes (Gieringer 2000). (Hawaii had passed a similar law in 1856, but had not yet been admitted to the Union as a state [Forbes 1998–2003, 169, #2163].) A number of other California cities, including Oakland, Sacramento, Stockton, and Virginia City, soon followed San Francisco's example. In 1881, the state legislature enacted a similar law applying to all parts of the state (Gieringer 2000).

The first laws prohibiting the consumption of marijuana were enacted in the Rocky Mountain and Southwestern states toward the end of World War I. At the time, a number of Mexicans were fleeing the Mexican Revolution of 1910–1920 and entering the United States. Many of them brought with them the habit of smoking marijuana, a practice largely unknown in the United States at the time. As with the San Francisco law, laws prohibiting the consumption of marijuana usually reflected the dislike and disapproval of foreigners as much as it did opposition to the use of psychoactive substances. Somewhat ironically, however, the first law banning the use of marijuana had a somewhat different motivation. By the mid-1910s, a number of Mormon missionaries returning from assignments to Mexico brought with them the practice of smoking marijuana, a practice that was quickly condemned by the church as opposed to doctrine (as was and is the use of all other kinds of psychoactive substances). In August 1915, the synod of the Mormon church banned the use of marijuana among all church members, and two months later, the Utah state legislature passed similar legislation, as was commonly the case with other church prohibitions at the time in the state (Whitebread 1995).

In the 20 years following adoption of the Utah law, a total of 27 states passed similar legislation, banning the use of marijuana. Although most of those states were west of the Mississippi, some were located in the Northeast, where there were few or no Mexicans. In these states, the justification for the laws was that individuals who had become dependent on alcohol, cocaine, and opiates and who were now deprived of those drugs because of the Eighteenth Amendment and the Harrison Act were likely to turn to marijuana as their new "drug of choice" (Whitebread 1955).

Thus, as has often been the case with the American federalist system for much of the nation's history, individual states made their own decisions as to how they would deal with psychoactive substances, whether they would ban them outright, and, if so, which substances would be prohibited. The federal government itself took a number of piecemeal actions, many (as noted previously) that fell short of outright bans on substances. During the mid-twentieth century, some of the legislation that was adopted to deal with the nation's substance abuse problem were the following:

The Food, Drug, and Cosmetic Act of 1938 was a comprehensive revision of the nation's laws dealing with foods, drugs, and cosmetics. Among its many provisions was the recognition that the definition of a "drug" could include substances that could be used for purposes other than therapeutic applications. It assigned to drug manufacturers the responsibility for deciding whether a product could be sold freely to the general public (over-the-counter use) or required a prescription.

The Opium Poppy Control Act of 1942 banned the growing of opium poppies without a federal license, supposedly to guarantee a dependable supply of opiates for the federal government during World War II.

The Durham-Humphrey Amendment of 1951 established two general categories of drugs: *prescription* (also called *legend*) drugs and *over-the-counter* (OTC) drugs. Legend drugs were defined as substances that were unsafe to use without supervision of a medical professional. They could be purchased only with a prescription from a medical professional and were required to carry the statement: "Caution: Federal law prohibits dispensing without a prescription."

The 1951 Boggs Amendment to the Harrison Narcotic Act was passed by the U.S. Congress in an atmosphere of increasing national concern about the spread of substance abuse, especially among teenagers. The Boggs Amendment was significant in a number of ways, primarily in the dramatic increase in penalties it provided for drug possession and use. It established a minimum mandatory sentence of two years for simple possession of marijuana, cocaine, or heroin, with a maximum sentence of five years; a minimum of 5 years and a maximum of 10 years for a second offense; and a minimum of 10 years and a maximum of 15 years for a third offense. In addition, the Boggs amendment was significant in that it was the first time that marijuana, cocaine, and opiates had been included with each other in a single piece of federal legislation.

The Boggs Amendment was important not only as a piece of federal legislation, but also because it served as a model that the federal government urged states to use for their own state laws. Many states took up the suggestion. Between 1953 and 1956, 26 states passed "mini-Boggs" bills, some of which carried penalties significantly more severe than those in the federal bill. The law in Louisiana, for example, provided for a 5- to 99-year sentence without the possibility of parole, probation, or suspension of sentence for sale or possession of any illegal substance (Bonnie and Whitebread 1974, 210). Similarly, Virginia adopted a mini-Boggs law that made possession of marijuana the most severely punished crime in the state. While first-degree murder earned a mandatory 15-year minimum sentence and rape, a mandatory 10-year sentence, possession of marijuana drew a mandatory minimum of 20 years, and sale of the drug a mandatory minimum of 40 years (Whitebread 1995).

The Narcotic Control Act of 1956 was yet another attempt by the U.S. Congress to solve the nation's drug problem with harsher legislation. Coming on the heels of the widely popular Kefauver hearings on crime in the United States, the Narcotics Control Act of 1956 provided for very stiff penalties on the sale of and trafficking in illegal substances, with a mandatory minimum sentence of five years and a mandatory 10-year sentence for all subsequent violations. In addition, judges were prohibited from suspending sentences or providing probation for convicted offenders (King 1972, Chapter 16).

The Drug Abuse Control Amendments of 1965 was yet another piece of legislation designed to bring under control the spread of illegal drug use in the United States. Among its many provisions was one designed to deal with a new and growing problem, the use of psychoactive substances other than marijuana, cocaine, and heroin. Amateur drug makers had become increasingly skillful in learning how to make products previously available only from drug manufacturers (such as methamphetamines and LSD), as well as analogs of drugs already banned by the federal government. For the federal government, the effort was a bit like trying to grab hold of a balloon. No sooner had some control been achieved over one part of the nation's drug problem when another issue arose elsewhere. Instead of having to deal with three, four, or a handful of illegal substances, the federal government was faced with restricting the use of dozens upon dozens of modifications of these drugs and entirely new drugs invented by imaginative amateur chemists. The Drug Abuse Control Amendments of 1965 attempted to deal with this problem by giving the secretary of health, education, and welfare authority to regulate any substance whatsoever that might have the potential for abuse because of its stimulant, depressant, or hallucinogenic effects. Although penalties against these drugs were less severe than those for marijuana, cocaine, and heroin, they represented the first concerted effort by the federal government to stem the growth of this new arm of the nation's substance abuse problem (King 1972, Chapter 26).

The Controlled Substances Act of 1970 (CSA) was an effort by the federal government to update and revise the various bills previously passed in an effort to control substance abuse in the nation. It was designed to be a comprehensive, overriding statement of federal policy about illegal substance use, along with guiding principles for prosecution and punishment. The act was enacted as Title II of the Comprehensive Drug Abuse Prevention and Control Act of 1970. Arguably the most important part of the CSA was Section 812, in which five "schedules" of drugs were established. The schedules are based on three features of any given substance: (1) its potential for abuse,

(2) its value in accepted medical treatment in the United States, and (3) its safety when used under medical supervision. Thus, substances placed in Schedule I are those that (1) have a high potential for abuse, (2) have no currently accepted use for medical treatments in the United States, and (3) cannot be safely used even under appropriate medical supervision. Examples of Schedule I drugs are heroin, LSD, marijuana, mescaline, peyote, and psilocybin. By contrast, substances listed in Schedule V (1) have minimal potential for abuse, (2) have accepted medical applications in the United States, and (3) are generally regarded as safe to use under medical supervision (although they may have the potential to lead to addiction). Examples of Schedule V drugs are certain cough medications that contain small amounts of codeine and products used to treat diarrhea that contain small amounts of opium. Current information about controlled substances and an up-to-date list of drugs can be found at http://www.dead iversion.usdoj.gov/schedules/index.html.

In its original form, the CSA listed a total of 81 substances in Schedule I, 21 in Schedule II, 17 in Schedule III, 11 in Schedule IV, and five in Schedule V (Controlled Substances Act 2009). As of late 2016, approximately 375 substances are listed among the five Schedules (Controlled Substances 2016).

The Comprehensive Drug Abuse Prevention and Control Act (CDAPCA) also included a perhaps unexpected provision that repealed all mandatory minimum sentences for substance abuse. As noted previously, these sentences were first established in the Boggs Amendment in 1951, and increased in later legislation. By 1970, however, the Congress had become convinced that minimum sentencing had had little or no effect on the problem of substance abuse and decided to repeal all minimum mandatory sentences. A report to the U.S. Senate Committee on the Judiciary, which was considering the CDAPCA, noted that:

> It had also become apparent that the severity of penalties including the length of sentences does not affect the extent of drug abuse and other drug-related violation. The basic consideration here was that the increasingly longer sentences that had been legislated in the past had not shown the expected overall reduction in drug law violations. The opposite had been true notably in the case of marihuana. Under Federal law and under many State laws marihuana violations carry the same strict penalties that are applicable to hard narcotics, yet marihuana violations have almost doubled in the last 2 years alone. (Controlled Dangerous Substances Act of 1969 1969, 2)

Federal Legislation since the Controlled Substances Act

For almost a century, state, local, and federal legislators have been concerned about a substance abuse problem in the United States that seems not to have been amenable to control by prevention and treatment, educational programs, or punitive legislation. Since the adoption of the Controlled Substances Act in 1970, the U.S. Congress has continued to pass law after law, attempting to deal with this issue. State and local legislative bodies have generally followed suit, often acting even more aggressively than the federal government.

On one front, the U.S. Congress has continued to pass laws increasing penalties for substance abuse and expanding the scope of such laws. In 1984, for example, the U.S. Congress changed its views on the effectiveness of harsh penalties for the control of substance abuse, reversing the stand its predecessors had taken in the CDAPCA of 1970. In the federal Sentencing Reform Act of 1984, it ordered the Federal Sentencing Reform Committee to establish new minimum mandatory sentences for convictions for various types of substance abuse. It also established new mandatory minimum sentences for drug offenses committed near schools, mandated prison sentences for serious drug felonies, and created probationary penalties for less serious offenses (Simplification Draft Paper 2016). Two years later, Congress followed up on its new, harder line against substance abuse convictions by establishing new sentences for cocaine possession. Continuing a historical trend that singles out minorities in legislation of this kind, the Anti-Drug Abuse Act of 1986 provided for a mandatory minimum sentence of 5 to 40 years for cocaine possession, a sentence that could not be suspended nor was it subject to parole. The inequity in the law was based on the fact that the mandatory minimum sentence was required for possession of 500 grams of powder cocaine (by far the drug of choice among middle- and upper-class whites), or 5 grams of crack cocaine (much more popular among blacks and lower-income men and women) (Vagins and McCurdy 2006). Two years later, Congress extended this policy in the Omnibus Drug Abuse Act of 1988 by imposing a five-year mandatory sentence for possession of 3 grams of crack cocaine for second-time offenders and for possession of 1 gram of crack cocaine for third-time offenders (Stolz 1992).

While Congress has apparently remained convinced of the effectiveness of strong penalties against substance abuse, it has also had to deal with a change in the nature of that problem, specifically with the expansion of the number of chemicals similar in chemical structure and psychoactive properties to cocaine, heroin, and other traditional drugs of abuse, now available to the general public. These chemicals are often called *designer drugs*.

The term *designer drugs* has at least two meanings. First, it is used to describe new kinds of medications being developed for the treatment of a variety of specific diseases. The field of study out of which such drugs develop is called *pharmacogenomics*, a combination of two terms referring to the study of drugs (pharmacy) and the study of genetics (genomics).

Second, the term *designer drugs* is used to refer to a number of synthetic chemicals that are derivatives of legal drugs developed for use in recreational settings. Chemists (usually amateur chemists) who synthesize designer drugs usually do so primarily for the purpose of avoiding legal restrictions on the production and sale of compounds that have been declared illegal by the U.S. government. Such compounds have generally been classified by the government as Schedule I or Schedule II drugs, that is, drugs that have high potential for abuse, that have some or no currently accepted medical use in treatment in the United States, and that lack any accepted safety for use under medical supervision. Table 2.3 outlines the major classes of designer drugs that have been developed over the past few decades.

Table 2.3 Major Classes of Designer Drugs and Their Analogs

Class of Drugs	Examples	Street Names
Fentanyl analogs	Alpha-methylfentanyl Benzylfentanyl Carfentanil Remifentanil Thenyfentanyl Thiofentanyl	Apache China girl China town China white Good fellas Great bear Tango and Cash
Phenylethylamine analogs	3,4-methylenedioxyamphet- amine (MDA) 3,4 methylenedioxymetham- phetamine (MDMA) 3,4- methylenedioxymetham- phetamine (MDEA) 4-bromo-2,5-dimethoxy- phenethylamine 4-methylthioamphetamine (4-MTA)	Ecstasy Adam Eve Eden Flatliner Death drug Chicken powder Bromo Shamrock
Meperidine analogs	1-methyl-4-phenyl-4-propion- oxypiperidine (MPPP) I -(2-phenethyl)-4-phe- nyl-4-acetoxypiperidine (PEPAP)	New heroin Synthetic heroin

(Continued)

Table 2.3   (Continued)

Class of Drugs	Examples	Street Names
Flunitrazepam (Rohypnol)	(single compound)	Rowies Roachies Roofies Ropies Circles Forget-me-pill Mexican valium (also known as "date rape" pill)
Gamma-hydroxybutyric acid (GHB)	(single compound)	G Liquid E Fantasy Georgia Home Boy Liquid Ecstasy Easy Lay Salty Water Cherry Meth Organic Quaalude
Methaqualone	Quaalude	Ludes Mandrex Quad Quay

The federal government first became interested in controlling the production and use of designer drugs used for recreational purposes in the early 1980s when it became apparent that existing legislation was ineffective against the many new psychoactive compounds being produced by amateur chemists. In order to deal with this issue, Congress included a provision in the Comprehensive Crime Control Act of 1984 that allowed the administrator of the Drug Enforcement Administration (DEA) to place analogs of banned substances on Schedule I or Schedule II for a period of up to one year, with a six-month extension if necessary. The law was somewhat unusual in that no evidence of a compound's properties or possible risks was needed for such an action; the administrator's concerns about a substance were sufficient for listing. Two years later, Congress moved to make its ban on analogs even broader and more comprehensive in the Controlled Substances Analogue Enforcement Act of 1986. It provided, first of all, that:

A controlled substance analogue shall, to the extent intended for human consumption, be treated, for the purposes of any Federal law as a controlled substance in schedule I. (Part B— Authority to Control; Standards and Schedules 2016)

It then defined a "controlled substance analog" as any substance as:

1. the chemical structure of which is substantially similar to the chemical structure of a controlled substance in schedule I or II;

2. which has a stimulant, depressant, or hallucinogenic effect on the central nervous system that is substantially similar to or greater than the stimulant, depressant, or hallucinogenic effect on the central nervous system of a controlled substance in schedule I or II; or

3. with respect to a particular person, which such person represents or intends to have a stimulant, depressant, or hallucinogenic effect on the central nervous system that is substantially similar to or greater than the stimulant, depressant, or hallucinogenic effect on the central nervous system of a controlled substance in schedule I or II. (Part B— Authority to Control; Standards and Schedules 2016)

As with other illegal substances, designer drugs have been the subject of a number of other pieces of legislation since the mid-1980s. Most of these acts deal with specific substances, such as methamphetamine (Comprehensive Methamphetamine Control Act of 1996, Children's Health Act of 2000, and Combat Methamphetamine Epidemic Act of 2005) and MDMA (ecstasy; Illicit Drug Anti-Proliferation Act of 2003).

Since the mid-1980s, the U.S. Congress has also begun to focus on other aspects of the nation's substance abuse problem. In many cases, it has given more serious attention to other approaches to solving this problem, such as the educational, prevention, and treatment approaches discussed previously. One of the most famous of these efforts was the Just Say No program espoused during the administration of President Ronald Reagan by his wife, Nancy Reagan. After her husband's election to the presidency in 1981, Nancy Reagan announced that her primary field of interest was going to be substance abuse. She began visiting schools around the nation with the goal of educating young people about the risks associated with using illegal drugs. At one of these visits, to the Longfellow Elementary School in Oakland, California, in 1982, she was asked by a student what she should do if she were offered drugs. Mrs. Reagan's reply was that she should "just say no." That brief comment soon became the theme of a nationwide campaign to encourage young people to refuse to become involved in substance abuse. In some ways reflecting the efforts of early temperance workers, Mrs. Reagan and her associates visited dozens of schools across the country, encouraging students to sign agreements not to become involved with drugs. She also appeared on many television appearances; enlisted the help of the Girl Scouts of America, the Kiwanis Club, and other service organizations; and sponsored an international conference of 30 first ladies from around the world to support her efforts (First Lady Biography: Nancy Reagan 2016). Although for many years the best-known educational program on substance abuse, this campaign was hardly the only or even necessarily the most successful of its kind (McGrath 2016).

The U.S. Congress and many state legislatures also recognized the potential value of educating young people about the dangers of substance abuse and began to commit tax dollars to such programs. In 1998, for example, the U.S. Congress passed and President Bill Clinton signed the National Youth Anti-Drug Media Campaign Act. The purpose of this act was to "conduct a national media campaign in accordance with this subtitle for the purpose of reducing and preventing drug abuse among young people in the United States" (Public Law 105-277 1998, Sec. 102[A]). The Office of National Drug Control Policy, responsible for implementation of the act, was enthusiastic about its potential for reducing substance abuse among young adults (The National Youth Anti-drug Media Campaign Communication Strategy Statement [1998]), and the federal government eventually invested more than $1 billion in the program by 2003 (Eddy 2003, CRS-5). A number of studies found, however, that the program had little or no effect on substance abuse among young Americans, and the program was gradually phased out (only to be replaced by a somewhat similar program called Above the Influence; see Hornik 2008; Ingraham 2016.)

Specialized Legislation

A relatively recent trend in federal drug legislation has been the focus on specific psychoactive substances or specific aspects of the campaign against drug abuse, dependence, and addiction. One of the earliest examples of this type of legislation was the Comprehensive Methamphetamine Control Act of 1996 (CMCA). That act was passed in response to what experts in substance abuse regarded as a "meth epidemic" of unparalleled magnitude in the United States at the time. One article in *The North Dakota Law Review* began with the somewhat sensationalistic claim that "an epidemic of methamphetamine abuse and addiction has swept across our nation and the world. Its wake has destroyed families, devastated communities, caused property crimes to surge, and caused severe neglect of children" (Bovett 2007). Although arguably a bit extreme in light of the evidence, this view was reflected in a number of similar claims by law enforcement officials, substance abuse experts, state and federal legislators, and members of the general public (Quotes about Methamphetamine 2016).

The CMCA attempted to deal with the meth epidemic from a number of angles: It made access to the raw materials used in producing methamphetamine more difficult and more expensive to obtain; it instituted rules for the preparation and transfer of such chemicals; and it increased penalties for all aspects of the illegal production of methamphetamine (Prah 2005). It also created a Methamphetamine Interagency Task Force to monitor progress of the new legislation and develop suggestions for further actions against meth abuse. One consequence of the task force's research was the introduction of another anti-meth bill in 2000, which became the Methamphetamine Anti-Proliferation Act of 2000, followed five years later by yet another piece of legislation, the Combat Methamphetamine Epidemic Act of 2005. The best available evidence suggests that meth use remained relatively constant between 2002 and 2014 among individuals between the ages of 12 and 17 and older than 26, at about 0.2 percent of the general population throughout that period, while usage rates among those between the ages of 18 and 25 dropped significantly, from 0.6 percent in 2002 to 0.2 percent in 2014 (Hedden et al. 2015, Figure 10 Table, page 9). The 106th Congress (1999–2001) also considered a number of other bills focusing on specific substances, such as the Ecstasy Anti-Proliferation Act and the Club Drug Anti-Proliferation Act, neither of which was passed in its original form, but which were absorbed into other related bills.

A particularly striking bill of special significance, the Family Smoking Prevention and Tobacco Control Act was passed in 2009. The act provided for the first time specific authority of the FDA to treat tobacco and cigarettes as a substance with health risks worthy of governmental regulation. The act imposed new label and warning standards for tobacco products, banned flavored cigarettes, placed limits on advertising of tobacco products to young people, and required tobacco companies to obtain specific approval for the introduction of new products to the marketplace (Tobacco Control Act 2016).

The most recent focus of congressional discussions has been the nation's prescription drug abuse epidemic and related opioid abuse issues. A number of bills were introduced into the 114th Congress (2015–2017) calling for additional federal funding for research on prescription drug abuse and opioid addiction, improved programs of education for young adults about the dangers of prescription drugs, action on specific psychoactive substances (such as DMX), control and disposal of prescribed drugs, and guarantees for patients who need opioids for the treatment of pain (for examples of such bills, see Prescription Drugs 2016). As is generally the case with federal legislation, only a small handful of these bills ever received consideration by Congress as a whole. However, in an action that surprised many observers Congress passed a wide-ranging bill, the Comprehensive Addiction and Recovery Act, which was signed by President Obama on July 22, 2016. The bill provided for increased prevention, treatment, recovery, law enforcement, criminal justice reform, and overdose reversal programs and was widely hailed as "the most comprehensive effort undertaken to address the opioid epidemic" (Comprehensive Addiction and Recovery Act 2016).

Should Illegal Substances Be Legalized?

The premise underlying most of this chapter has been that the consumption of certain substances is potentially harmful and dangerous for the individuals who use them. Certainly the federal government and both state and local governments appear to have taken this stance over most of the last century. And yet, a number of individuals and organizations have long taken the position that governments should not be involved in legislating the psychoactive substances individuals choose to consume for recreational purposes. Since the 1960s, there has been an ongoing debate as to whether these substances should be made legal or not. The debate has been a somewhat unusual one, with liberal Democrats and conservative Republicans—and individuals at every point between these extremes—agreeing with each other on either one or the other position.

One of the fundamental issues involved in this debate involves the decriminalization versus legalization of drugs. Although the two terms are sometimes used synonymously, they actually have very different meanings. *Decriminalization* refers to the removal of all jail and prison sentences for possession or use of an illegal drug. A person may still receive a fine for such an action, but it is unlikely to appear on any permanent legal record or result in confinement. In this regard, drug decriminalization is similar to traffic fines or other misdemeanors that are regarded as relatively minor legal violations (The Difference between Legalisation and Decriminalization 2014). By contrast, *legalization* refers to the removal of all prohibitions on possession or use of an illegal drug, within certain specific boundaries. For example, in a state where the use of illegal drugs has been decriminalized, a person might be fined $100 for having 10 grams of marijuana in his or her possession; in a state where drug use has been legalized, there would be no penalty of any kind for the possession and use of such a small amount of the drug (although larger quantities would still be subject to penalties, some quite severe).

As of late 2016, 19 states and the District of Columbia have decriminalized the possession and use of marijuana, the only drug for which such action has been taken in the United States. An example of the terms of decriminalization is the Mississippi law, in which possession of 30 grams of marijuana or less results in a fine of $250. A second conviction for the same offense results in another $250 and, for a third conviction, a fine of $500. By contrast, possession of 500 grams to 1 kilogram of marijuana results in a fine of $250,000 and a prison term of 4 to 16 years (Mississippi Laws & Penalties 2016).

Arguments in Favor of Legalizing Drugs

The debate over decriminalization and/or legalization of drugs is based almost entirely today on a single currently illegal substance, marijuana. But arguments in favor of decriminalizing or legalizing other substances have long been, and are still being, made. Some of those arguments are as follows:

The decision as to whether or not to use a particular psychoactive substance is a personal decision in which the state should have no role

One of the fundamental principles of a democratic state is that people should be allowed to do with their own bodies whatever they want, provided they do no harm to other individuals. Having a marijuana cigarette or a Quaalude pill on a Saturday night may provide pleasure to the person who uses these substances without harming anyone else. As one blogger puts this argument:

> The war on drugs is more of a war on personal choice, a war on your right to decide how you live your life. If someone wants to ingest something; put it into their own body, their own property, and they aren't harming any other human being, animal or property, then where is the harm in that? How is the state justified in telling me that I cannot consume a natural substance? As long as your personal choice doesn't infringe on the freedom of others, then people should be allowed to be live and act freely. (Caufield 2013)

The cost of the war on drugs is much too expensive, especially in terms of the benefits received

In 1971, the year that President Richard M. Nixon first declared a "war on drugs," the federal budget to carry on that war was about $350 million annually ($2.14 billion in 2016 dollars). Five years later, that budget had increased nearly tenfold, reaching $760 million (Goldberg 1980). Those costs continued to rise over the next four decades, reaching a total federal expenditure in 2016 of $30.6 billion (National Drug Control Budget 2016, 2). And these numbers reflect only federal spending. The cost of fighting drug abuse on state and local levels adds substantially to these totals. According to one study conducted in 2010, states and local municipalities had spent $25,684,407,000 in 2008 on drug enforcement programs, almost twice the total spent by the federal government ($13.7 billion) for that year (Miron and Waldock 2010, Table 3, page 35; National Drug Control Strategy 2008).

The vast efforts by state, local, and federal governments to reduce substance abuse in the United States have been largely unsuccessful

A number of studies conducted since 1982 suggest that many (but certainly not all) efforts to reduce substance abuse by legal means have been a failure. Some examples of those findings have been cited earlier in this chapter. In 1996, a committee of the New York Country Lawyers Association, the oldest bar association in New York City, issued a report on state and federal drug policy. It concluded that "[n]otwithstanding the vast public resources expended on the enforcement of penal statutes against users and distributors of controlled substances, contemporary drug policy appears to have failed, even on its own terms, in a number of notable respects." It went on to suggest that that drug policy may actually have had more damaging effects on society as a whole than have the harmful effects of psychoactive substances and their abusers (Fischler et al. 1996).

That situation appears to continue today. A recent policy statement investigating the efficacy of federal "drug war" programs noted that

> despite the incarceration of tens of millions of Americans and more than a trillion dollars of spending, illegal drugs remain cheap, potent, and widely available. The harms associated with them—addiction, overdose and the spread of HIV/AIDS and hepatitis B and C—continue to persist in every community. Meanwhile the war on drugs is creating problems of its own—broken families, increased

poverty, racial disparities, wasted tax dollars, prison overcrowding and eroded civil liberties. (An Exit Strategy for the Failed War on Drugs 2013)

The war on drugs has created its own set of social issues and problems

Legal prohibitions on drugs have spawned the growth of a huge crime network and provide a significant financial asset for terrorist groups. Since cocaine, heroin, marijuana, and other recreational drugs are illegal, they can be obtained only through black markets. These black markets have become an important element of organized crime in almost every country of the world. Drug organizations maintain control over their operations by means of well-organized and efficient crime groups that involve distributors and enforcers. In addition, substance abusers themselves often turn to crime to earn the dollars they need to maintain their illegal habit. If the government controlled the distribution of substances that are now illegal, the primary motivation for drug cartels would disappear, and drug-related crime rates would decrease dramatically.

In addition, profits made from the sale of illegal substances such as cocaine, heroin, and marijuana are a major source of income for terrorist groups, many of whom control the source of production for such drugs. One report on this issue concluded that "[r]efusing to address the role of prohibition [of drugs] in financing terrorism will enable terrorist groups to continue to build the resources they need to engage in even more extensive acts of terrorism than we have witnessed to date" (Oscapella 2003, 2).

Proponents of the decriminalization of illegal substances also raise a number of other points in defending their position, such as the fact that many legal substances, such as alcohol and tobacco, are far more destructive than most illegal drugs; that some illegal substances have important practical applications in research, medicine, religion, and other fields; that some substance abusers become involved with drugs simply because they are illegal and they are attracted by the adventure of becoming involved in an illegal activity; that U.S. policies on illegal substances have proved to be disastrous for domestic policies in nations where these drugs are produced (such as Afghanistan, Colombia, Bolivia, and Mexico); and that governments should treat psychoactive substances consistently, not granting approval to some (such as tobacco and alcohol) and heavily penalizing others (such as marijuana and cocaine). (For an excellent overall review of the pro-legalization argument, see Cussen and Block 2000.)

Arguments in Opposition to Legalizing Drugs

In spite of these arguments, the thought of decriminalizing or legalizing drugs is still anathema to many people. Some of the arguments for maintaining current prohibitions on illegal substances are the following:

Illegal substances have been so classified at least partly because they are harmful to human health

Hardly anyone who has studied the health effects of drugs like cocaine, heroin, LSD, and MDMA would argue with the contention that the use of such drugs can have devastating short- and long-term effects on a person's health. The argument is less clear for other drugs, marijuana perhaps being the best example. In any case, the proponents of retaining prohibitions on Schedule I and Schedule II drugs often point to mortality and morbidity statistics for these drugs. The most recent data available for mortality in the United States found that 46,471 people died in 2013 from drug-induced causes (both legal and illegal). This number represented a 5.8 percent increase over the previous year and 143 percent over the death rate for 1999 (Xu et al. 2016, 10–11 and Supplemental Tables, Table 1–3, page 6).

Numerous studies about the health effects of individual psychoactive substances have been conducted over the years.

A general overview of this situation is provided on an annual basis in SAMHSA's Substance Abuse Treatment Episode Data Set study. According to the most recent data available, the substance responsible for the greatest number of emergency department (ED) admissions for drug-related issues is alcohol, accounting for 368,007 instances out of a total of 1,739,523 total drug-related admissions in that year, or 21.2 percent of all such admissions. Admissions involving alcohol with another drug accounted for an additional 280,935 admissions (16.2%). The next most common drugs responsible for ED admissions were heroin (334,163 admissions; 19.2%), marijuana (289,379 admissions; 16.6%), other opiates (161,332 admissions; 9.3%), amphetamines (140,334 admissions; 8.1%), and cocaine (all forms; 105,474 admissions; 6.1%). (A good review of the many health and medical consequences related to substance abuse is available at Medical Consequences of Drug Abuse 2012.)

Substance abuse is closely linked to crime and violence, so laws against the illegal use of drugs are needed to reduce crime and violence

This argument is similar to the one presented earlier in support of decriminalization of drugs in that it recognizes the close relationship between substance abuse and many kinds of crimes. Instead of arguing that legalizing drugs will reduce this problem, however, proponents of drug prohibition say that strong penalties are needed to keep a rein on crime arising out of drug abuse. The DEA claims that legalizing drugs would not eliminate the crimes associated with substance abuse because individuals under some age, such as 18 or 21, would still not be allowed to purchase or use certain substances, and that portion of the population is currently and has long been a major consumer of illegal substances. Therefore, a black market for the drugs would still exist, retaining most of the violent crimes now associated with illegal drug use.

Drug prohibition programs have worked

Those in favor of retaining strict penalties for the use of marijuana, cocaine, heroin, and other drugs argue that illegal drug use has decreased substantially as a result of stiff drug laws. The DEA reports that illegal drug use has dropped by a third in the last 20 years, and the use of cocaine by 70 percent during that time. The agency claims that "[s]ignificant progress has been made in fighting drug use and drug trafficking in America." It argues that efforts to legalize drugs as being the only workable alternative to the war on drugs are wrong and that "the facts are contrary to such pessimism" (Speaking Out against Drug Legalization [2010], 13).

Legalization of drugs will not achieve the objectives that proponents claim for it

Individuals who have argued against the decriminalization of drugs frequently point to previous efforts in this direction, which, they say, have always failed. These commentators tend to use a common set of facts to support their view, such as the claim that decriminalization of marijuana in California in 1976 led to an increase in arrests for driving under the influence of drugs in the state by 46 percent for adults and 71 percent for juveniles. They also point to decriminalization of marijuana by the states of Alaska and Oregon in the 1970s that resulted in a doubling of the use of the substance (see, for example, Maginnis 2016).

Opponents of decriminalization resort to a number of other arguments to support their position. Perhaps the best single source for these arguments is a booklet published by the DEA in May 2003 and revised in 2010, Speaking Out against Drug Legalization. In addition to the points made previously, this booklet suggests that the war against drugs requires a balanced approach that includes both prevention and treatment, but also requires laws prohibiting their use; that the drug war, although expensive, is only a minor part of the overall federal budget, which represents an important element in dealing with an important national social issue; that alcohol abuse has already caused the nation severe social and health problems, and that the legalization of drugs will only make that situation worse; and that, in any case, most people convicted of substance abuse do not go to prison but, instead, are referred to treatment programs (Speaking Out against Drug Legalization [2010]).

A Special Case: Marijuana

Within the general realm of substance abuse issues, one topic is currently of special interest: the legal use of marijuana. A movement appears to be developing throughout the nation that calls for the legalization of the use of marijuana, either for medical purposes only or for medical and recreational uses.

Medical Marijuana

Arguments over the legalization or prohibition of marijuana use are generally similar to those for other drugs, outlined in the preceding section. But proponents of legalization also point out that marijuana is probably the least dangerous of all substances listed under Schedule I of the Controlled Substances Act. If used in moderation, it almost certainly has fewer health effects than alcohol and tobacco, both of which are legal in the United States. It is also the least likely of all major drugs (tobacco, alcohol, cocaine, and opiates) to lead to addiction. In its 1999 exhaustive study, *Marijuana and Medicine: The Scientific Base*, the last major study on the subject, the Institute of Medicine found that about 9 percent of all individuals who had tried marijuana eventually became dependent on the drug, compared to 32 percent who became addicted to tobacco, 23 percent to heroin, 17 percent to cocaine, 15 percent to alcohol, and 9 percent to hypnotics and sedatives (Joy, Watson, and Benson 1999, 95).

Opponents of the decriminalization of marijuana often point to the possible role of the substance as a "gateway" drug. A gateway drug is a substance that, when used, leads to an increased risk of the use of other illegal substances. That is, some individuals say that a person who uses marijuana is more likely then to move on to cocaine, heroin, or other more serious drugs. For many years, the DEA has been using some form of this argument in its literature opposing the decriminalization and/or legalization of marijuana. At one point, for example, it cited a study conducted at Columbia University that "children (12 to 17 years old) who use gateway drugs—tobacco, alcohol and marijuana—are up to 266 times—and adults who use such drugs are up to 323 times—more likely to use cocaine than those who don't use any gateway drugs" (National Study Shows "Gateway" Drugs Lead to Cocaine Use 1994; Publications 1994). Over time, the DEA cut back on the magnitude of this gateway effect (Tandy 2005), but has continued to mention it as a major reason to continue listing marijuana as a Schedule I drug (Brosious 2016).

Other authorities hold different views about the role of marijuana as a gateway drug. In its 1999 study cited previously, the Institute of Medicine concluded on this subject that "marijuana is not the most common, and is rarely the first, 'gateway' to illicit drug use. There is no conclusive evidence that the drug effects of marijuana are causally linked to the subsequent abuse of other illicit drugs" (Joy, Watson, and Benson 1999, 6; for further research on this question, see also Gateway Theory 2016).

One of the issues of greatest concern about marijuana at the present time is its use for medical purposes. Evidence suggests that marijuana has been used for medicinal purposes for over 2,000 years. Some of the earliest mentions of these substances for medical uses occur in Chinese herbal and medical works dating to the first century CE, if not earlier (Abel 1980). In recent years, a number of medical benefits have been claimed for these substances.

One common way of categorizing these benefits is by the confidence in which medical experts have for each effect. One such scheme classifies the medical claims for marijuana into four major categories: established effects, relatively well-confirmed effects, less confirmed effects, and basic research stage. The disorders included in each of these categories are as follows:

Established Effects: Control of nausea and vomiting; treatment of anorexia and weight loss.

Relatively Well-Confirmed Effects: Treatment for spasticity, pain, movement disorders, asthma, glaucoma.

Less-Confirmed Effects: Treatment for allergies, inflammation, infections, epilepsy, depression, bipolar disorder, anxiety disorders, dependency, and withdrawal symptoms.

Basic Research Stage: Treatment of autoimmune diseases, cancers, fevers, blood pressure disorders, and protection of the nervous system (Russo and Grotenhermen 2006, 140–143; for an expanded and more current discussion of this topic, see 65170: Medical Marijuana and Other Cannabinoids 2016).

These claims have been sufficiently convincing, at least to some state legislators and parts of the general public that, as of 2016, 25 states and the District of Columbia have passed laws permitting the growing and sale of marijuana for medicinal purposes. The first state to pass such a law was California in 1996, later followed by Alaska (1998), Oregon (1998), Washington (1998), Maine (1999), Colorado (2000), Hawaii (2000), Nevada (2000), Montana (2004), Vermont (2004), New Mexico (2007), Rhode Island (2006), Michigan (2008), Arizona (2010), New Jersey (2010), Delaware (2011), Connecticut (2012), Massachusetts (2012), Illinois (2013), New Hampshire (2013), Maryland (2014), Minnesota (2014), New York (2014), Guam (2014), Ohio (2016), and Pennsylvania (2016) (State Medical Marijuana Laws 2016; this site is a good source for changes in and the current status of state medical marijuana laws).

There remains strong opposition to the use of marijuana, even for medical purposes. Probably the most common objection is that the substance is still listed as a Schedule I drug by the U.S.

government under the provisions of the Controlled Substances Act of 1970. That means that a person in California or Maine or New Mexico (or any other state that has approved the use of medical marijuana) may be able to purchase and use the drug in his or her own state, but will still be breaking federal law in doing so. As recently as November 2015, President Barack Obama's choice as the new chief of the DEA said that calling smoked marijuana a medicine was "a joke." "What really bothers me," he said, "is the notion that marijuana is also medicinal—because it's not. We can have an intellectually honest debate about whether we should legalize something that is bad and dangerous, but don't call it medicine—that is a joke" (Reid and Condon 2015).

Federal law enforcement officials have, of course, carried out DEA policy on the use of medical marijuana. During the administration of George W. Bush, for example, law enforcement officials raided marijuana dispensaries licensed to sell marijuana to individuals with a prescription and arrested individuals who grow marijuana for such dispensaries (see, for example, DEA's War on California 2002). Bush's first "drug czar," John Walters, frequently made clear his views on medical marijuana. Not only was marijuana an invalid tool for treating any medical condition, according to Walters, but, in fact, the push for marijuana dispensaries was really a tool for obtaining complete legalization for the substance. During one television interview, for example, he said, "In California, where medical marijuana has been used as a kind of a wedge issue, or kind of phony effort to try to say, 'It's only going to go to people who are sick.' It's not going to people who are sick. In fact, in San Francisco it has been reported in the news there are now more marijuana dispensaries than there are Starbucks in downtown San Francisco" (Anderson Cooper 360 Degrees 2009).

The administration of President Barack Obama, who took office in January 2009, has had a somewhat different—and somewhat inconsistent—view of this controversy. In October 2009, Attorney General Eric H. Holder, Jr., announced that the federal government would initiate a more lenient view with regard to individuals who distribute or use marijuana for medical purposes. "It will not be a priority to use federal resources to prosecute patients with serious illnesses or their caregivers who are complying with state laws on medical marijuana," Holder said, in a policy statement that represented a 180-degree change from that of the administrations of Presidents Bill Clinton and George W. Bush (Stout and Moore 2009). In confirming this new direction, Deputy Attorney General David W. Ogden sent out a memorandum to federal prosecutors in states with medical marijuana laws. That memorandum emphasized that the administration still held to the position that marijuana is "a dangerous drug, and the illegal distribution and sale of marijuana is a serious crime," which it intended to prosecute. On the other hand, the memo went on, the Department of Justice had limited resources, and it had to prioritize the crimes it chose to pursue. In general, therefore, investigators were directed to concentrate on marijuana-related crimes that met certain criteria, namely, those that involved the following:

- unlawful possession or unlawful use of firearms;
- violence;
- sales to minors;
- financial and marketing activities inconsistent with the terms, conditions, or purposes of state law, including evidence of money laundering activity and/or financial gains or excessive amounts of cash inconsistent with purported compliance with state or local law;
- amounts of marijuana inconsistent with purported compliance with state or local law;
- illegal possession or sale of other controlled substances; or
- ties to other criminal enterprises (Memorandum for Selected United States Attorneys 2009).

Most observers viewed the Ogden memo as a signal that federal agents would largely keep hands off legitimate use of medical marijuana in states where such use had been approved. Two years later, however, the Obama administration felt it necessary to issue a second memorandum clarifying (or, some say, reversing) its position on the issue. That memo, the so-called *Cole Memorandum* of 2011 (or Cole 2011), pointed out that the Ogden memo was not meant to imply that the federal government was simply going to turn its back on marijuana prosecutions. It was, Cole 2011 went on, "never intended to shield such activities from federal enforcement action and prosecution, even where those activities purport to comply with state law" (Memorandum for United States Attorneys 2011). The gates appeared to be open to more aggressive attacks by federal agents on state medical marijuana facilities, which shortly appeared to be the case as the number of such raids soon began to increase (Riggs 2011).

Fast forward two more years, and the situation appeared to change one more time. In a second memorandum by Deputy Attorney General James M. Cole (Cole 2013), the administration repeats the apparent message of the Ogden memo, namely, that the Department of Justice has decided to focus its limited resources on only certain types of marijuana-related activities, roughly corresponding with the list provided earlier (Memorandum for All United States Attorneys 2013). This most recent memo, then, appears to indicate that the Obama administration has decided essentially to ignore activities related to the use of marijuana for medical purposes in states where such use has been approved. (For a detailed background on the history of this issue, see Grim and Reilly 2013.)

Recreational Marijuana

Progress toward the legalization of marijuana for recreational use has occurred more slowly than it has for medical marijuana. The earliest steps in that direction took place in the 1970s when a handful of states decriminalized the use of marijuana for recreational purposes. The first such action, the Oregon Decriminalization Bill of 1973, made possession of one ounce of marijuana a violation (not a crime) punishable by a fine of $500 to $1,000 (Blachly 1976). Over the next four years, ten more states—Alaska, California, Colorado, Maine, Minnesota, Mississippi, Nebraska, New York, North Carolina, and Ohio—followed Oregon's lead in decriminalizing the use of recreational marijuana (Scott 2010).

It took nearly 40 years, however, to take the next step: outright legalization of marijuana. Then, in the general elections of November 2012, two states, Colorado and Washington, adopted legislation legalizing the recreational use of up to one ounce of marijuana. On November 4, 2014, two more states (Alaska and Oregon) and the District of Columbia also voted to legalize the use of small amounts of marijuana for recreational purposes. The precise wording of laws in each of the four states and the District varies to some extent (State Laws 2016).

The legalization of recreational marijuana in four states has permitted the conduct of a "grand experiment" about certain long-standing and fundamental questions regarding marijuana consumption, such as the following:

- How does legalization affect the prevalence and incidence of marijuana use in the general population?
- What is the effect of legalization on marijuana use among children and adolescents?
- How does legalization affect patterns of physical, mental, and other forms of health in the general population?
- To what extent are accident rates (such as vehicle crashes) affected by legalization?
- Are financial benefits to states, such as taxes on marijuana sales, comparable to those predicted by supporters of legalization?

None of these questions is easy to answer, and, as of early 2017, it is still too early to know what those answers might be. Nonetheless, officials in all four states are aware of the importance of such questions and the need to collect data about them. In Colorado, for example, the state legislature adopted legislation in 2013 requiring the state Division of Criminal Justice and the Department of Public Safety to collect data and prepare a report on the effects of marijuana legalization in a variety of fields. The following data are summarized from a report released in March 2016 pursuant to that charge. Among the trends noted in the report are the following (all data from Reed 2016, 5–9):

- The total number of marijuana-related arrests dropped from 12,894 in 2012 (the last year before legalization) to 7,004 (the first year after legalization), a decrease of 46 percent. The number of arrests for possession was reduced by half (47%) and for sales by a quarter (24%) with essentially no change for production (–2%).

- The number of court filings for marijuana-related cases dropped by 81 percent between 2012 and 2015, from 10,340 to 1,954. The rate for juveniles 10 to 17 fell 69 percent, for young adults 18 to 20 by 78 percent, and for adults 21 and over, by 86 percent.

- The number of summons issues by the Colorado State Police for marijuana-related offenses decreased by 1 percent between 2014 and 2015.

- The number of marijuana-related hospitalizations increased from 803 per 100,000 in the period 2001–2009 to 2,413 per 100,000 in the period 2014–June 2015.

- The number of marijuana-related visits to emergency departments increased 29 percent, from 739 per 100,000 in the period 2010–2013 to 956 per 100,000 in the period 2014–June 2015.

- The Healthy Kids Colorado Survey found a "slight decline" in the number of "30-day use" respondents after legalization of the drug.

- The rate of juvenile arrests for marijuana-related crimes increased by 2 percent (from 598 to 611) between 2012 and 2014.

- Total state revenue from taxes, licenses, and fees increased 77 percent from calendar year 2014 to 2015, going from $76,152,468 to $135,100,465. Essentially all of this increase resulted from marijuana-related activities.

- Tax revenue from marijuana-related activities in 2015 was $35,060,590, an increase of 163 percent over 2014 revenues of $13,341,001. Of the 2015 total, $8,626,922 was distributed to local schools.

Other states have prepared reports similar to Colorado's (see Dilley 2016; Monitoring Impacts of Recreational Marijuana Legalization: 2015 Baseline Report 2015), with results roughly similar to those from Colorado. Stronger statements about the effects on society of legalization marijuana, however, await the passage of time and more detailed studies of the issue.

Resistance to Legalization

As can be expected in the progress of any important social issue, the adoption of new laws or decisions by courts do not necessarily mark the end of the dispute over such issues (see, for example, the debates over abortion and same-sex marriage in the United States). Such has also been the case with the legalization of marijuana in Colorado, Washington, Alaska, Oregon, and the District of Columbia. The adoption of legislation permitting the use of marijuana for recreational purposes in these entities has not meant that opponents of legalization have ended their battle against the practice. In one instance, for example, residents of Pueblo County filed a lawsuit against the state because an adjacent crop of marijuana plants allegedly blocked their view. In another suit, a Holiday Inn hotel in Frisco, Colorado, filed a RICO (Racketeer Influenced and

Corrupt Organizations Act) suit against the state because, it claimed, a marijuana dispensary scheduled to open next to the property would interfere with its normal business activities. In yet a third case, a group of sheriffs and other law enforcement officials from Colorado, Kansas, and Nebraska sued the state, claiming that the legalization of marijuana violated state law, the Colorado constitution, and the U.S. Constitution. Plaintiffs lost in all three of these cases (Warner 2016).

The case that perhaps drew the greatest attention nationally was *Nebraska and Oklahoma v. Colorado* (U.S. Supreme Court docket #220144), in which Nebraska and Oklahoma sued Colorado. The two states argued that the legalization of marijuana in Colorado was likely to result in an increase in drug-related crimes in their own states and that the new Colorado law was, therefore, unconstitutional. In March 2016, the Supreme Court declined to hear the case, essentially bringing to an end this type of complaint about the new Colorado marijuana law (*Nebraska and Oklahoma v. Colorado* 2016). While the legal history of challenges to marijuana law has universally failed thus far, it is still early days in the history of marijuana legalization, and additional challenges in other states on a variety of issues are to be expected. (See, for example, Mapes 2015.)

References

Abel, Ernest L. 1980. *Marihuana, the First Twelve Thousand Years*. New York: Plenum Press.

"Above the Influence." 2016. http://abovetheinfluence.com/about/. Accessed on June 26, 2016.

"An Exit Strategy for the Failed War on Drugs." 2013. Drug Policy Alliance. https://www.drugpolicy.org/sites/default/files/DPA_Exit%20Strategy_Federal%20Legislative%20Guide.pdf. Accessed on June 27, 2016.

Anderson, Jordan. 2012. "This House Supports Random Drug-Testing in Schools." idebate.org. http://idebate

.org/debatabase/debates/culture/children/house-supports-random-drug-testing-schools. Accessed on June 23, 2016.

"Anderson Cooper 360 Degrees." 2009. CNN. http://transcripts.cnn.com/TRANSCRIPTS/0905/06/acd.02.html. Accessed on June 29, 2016.

"Are Recovery High School Really Working?" 2016. Recovery.org. http://www.recovery.org/are-recovery-high-schools-working/. Accessed on June 30, 2016.

Bielawski, Michael. 2015. "Marijuana Legalization Could Rewrite Employee Drug-Testing Rules." VermontWatch dog.org. http://watchdog.org/256084/drug-testing-vermont-marijuana-legalization/. Accessed on June 22, 2016.

Blachly, Paul H. 1976. "Effects of Decriminalization of Marijuana in Oregon." *Annals of the New York Academy of Sciences*. 282(1): 405–415.

Board of Education of Independent School District No. 92 of Pottawatomie County v. Earls. 2002. U.S. Supreme Court. http://www.supremecourt.gov/opinions/boundvolumes/536bv.pdf. Accessed on June 23, 2016.

Bonnie, Richard J., and Charles H. Whitebread. 1974. *The Marihuana Conviction*. Charlottesville: University of Virginia Press.

Bovett, Rob. 2007. "Meth Epidemic Solutions." *North Dakota Law Review*. 82(4): 1195–1216.

Brecher, Edward M., and the editors of Consumer Reports Magazine. 1972. *The Consumers Union Report on Licit and Illicit Drugs*. Boston: Little, Brown and Company. http://www.druglibrary.org/Schaffer/LIBRARY/studies/cu/cumenu.htm. Accessed on June 24, 2016.

Brody, Jane E. 2013. "Effective Addiction Treatment." *The New York Times*. http://well.blogs.nytimes.com/2013/02/04/effective-addiction-treatment/?_r=0. Accessed on June 22, 2016.

Brosious, Emily Gray. 2016. "White House Drug Czar Rallies against Marijuana Legalization, Argues 'Gateway' Theory." Sun Times Network. http://extract.suntimes.com/news/10/153/17947/white-house-drug-czar-michael-botticelli-fights-against-marijuana-legalization-claims-gateway-theory. Accessed on June 28, 2016.

Buxton, Julia. 2006. *The Political Economy of Narcotics: Production, Consumption and Global Markets.* London: Zed Books.

Caufield, M. 2013. "The War on Personal Choice." Exposing the Truth. https://www.exposingtruth.com/war-personal-choice/. Accessed on June 27, 2016.

Center for Substance Abuse Prevention. 2016. U.S. Department of Health and Human Services. Substance Abuse and Mental Health Services Administration. http://prevention.samhsa.gov/. Accessed on June 21, 2016.

Coats v. Dish. 2015. 2015 CO 44. Colorado Supreme Court. http://extras.mnginteractive.com/live/media/site36/2015/0615/20150615_085459_coats-vs-dish.pdf. Accessed on June 22, 2016.

Comprehensive Addiction and Recovery Act. 2016. CADCA. http://www.cadca.org/comprehensive-addiction-and-recovery-act-cara. Accessed on December 23, 2016.

"Controlled Dangerous Substances Act of 1969." 1969. Report of the Committee on the Judiciary. United States Senate. Report No. 91–613. 91st Congress, 1st Session. https://bulk.resource.org/gao.gov/91-513/000050F5.pdf. Accessed on June 25, 2016.

"Controlled Substances." 2016. Drug Enforcement Administration. http://www.deadiversion.usdoj.gov/schedules/orangebook/e_cs_sched.pdf. Accessed on June 25, 2016.

"Controlled Substances Act." 2009. U.S. Food and Drug Administration. http://www.fda.gov/regulatoryinformation/legislation/ucm148726.htm. Accessed on June 25, 2016.

Courtwright, David T. 1995. "The Rise and Fall of Cocaine in the United States." In Jordan Goodman, Paul E. Lovejoy, and Andrew Sherratt, eds. *Consuming Habits: Drugs in History and Anthropology*. London: Routledge.

Cussen, Meaghan, and Walter Block. 2000. "Legalize Drugs Now! An Analysis of the Benefits of Legalized Drugs." *American Journal of Economics and Sociology*. 59(3): 525–536.

D.A.R.E. 2016. http://www.dare.org/. Accessed on June 21, 2016.

"DEA's War on California." 2002. Americans for Safe Access. http://www.safeaccessnow.org/asanews172. Accessed on June 29, 2016.

DePillis, Lydia. 2015. "Companies Drug Test a Lot Less Than They Used To—Because It Doesn't Really Work." *The Washington Post*. https://www.washingtonpost.com/news/wonk/wp/2015/03/10/companies-drug-test-a-lot-less-than-they-used-to-because-it-doesnt-really-work/. Accessed on June 22, 2016.

"The Difference between Legalisation and Decriminalization." 2014. *The Economist*. http://www.economist.com/blogs/economist-explains/2014/06/economist-explains-10. Accessed on June 27, 2016.

Dilley, Julia, et al. 2016. "Marijuana Report: Marijuana Use, Attitudes and Health Effects in Oregon." Oregon Public Health Division. https://public.health.oregon.gov/PreventionWellness/marijuana/Documents/oha-8509-marijuana-report.pdf. Accessed on June 29, 2016.

Donohoe, Martin. 2005. "Urine Trouble: Practical, Legal, and Ethical Issues Surrounding Mandated Drug Testing of Physicians." *Journal of Clinical Ethics*. 16(1): 69–81.

"Drug Courts." 2016. National Institute of Justice. http://www.nij.gov/topics/courts/drug-courts/pages/welcome.aspx. Accessed on June 30, 2016.

"DrugFacts: Treatment Approaches for Drug Addiction."
2016. National Institute on Drug Abuse. https://www
.drugabuse.gov/publications/drugfacts/treatment-
approaches-drug-addiction. Accessed on June 22, 2016.

DuPont, Robert L. 2015. "Workplace Drug Testing in the
Era of Legal Marijuana." Institute for Behavior and Health,
Inc. http://www.drugfreebusiness.org/Media/documents/
IBH_workplacetesting.pdf. Accessed on June 22, 2016.

"Early History." 2016. Women's Christian Temperance
Union. http://www.wctu.org/history.html. Accessed on
June 24, 2016.

Eddy, Mark. 2003. "War on Drugs: The National Youth Anti-
Drug Media Campaign." CRS Report for Congress. http://
www.drugpolicy.org/docUploads/RS21490.pdf. Accessed
on June 26, 2016.

Engber, Daniel. 2015. "Why Do Employers Still Routinely
Drug Test Workers?" *Slate*. http://www.slate.com/articles/
health_and_science/cover_story/2015/12/workplace_drug_
testing_is_widespread_but_ineffective.html. Accessed on
June 22, 2016.

"First Lady Biography: Nancy Reagan." 2016. National First
Ladies Library. http://www.firstladies.org/biographies/
firstladies.aspx?biography=41. Accessed on June 26,
2016.

Fischler, Alan B., et al. 1996. *Report and Recommendations of
the Drug Policy Task Force. New York: New York Lawyers'
Association*. http://www.drcnet.org/nycla.html. Accessed on
June 27, 2016.

Forbes, David W., ed. 1998–2003. *Hawaiian National Bibliography*, 1780–1900. Honolulu: University of Hawaii
Press.

"Gateway Theory." 2016. DrugWarFacts.org. http://www
.drugwarfacts.org/cms/Gateway_Theory#sthash.iIjjF7fZ
.dpbs. Accessed on June 29, 2016.

Gfroerer, Joseph C., Wu Li-Tzy, and Michael A. Penne. 2002. "Initiation of Marijuana Use: Trends, Patterns, and Implications." Office of Applied Statistics. Substance Abuse and Mental Health Services Administration. http://citeseerx .ist.psu.edu/viewdoc/download?doi=10.1.1.187.6614&rep= rep1&type=pdf. Accessed on June 24, 2016.

Gieringer, Dale. 2000. "125th Anniversary of the First U.S. Anti-Drug Law: San Francisco's Opium Den Ordinance (Nov. 15, 1875)." http://www.drugsense.org/dpfca/opium law.html. Accessed on June 25, 2016.

Goldberg, Peter. 1980. "The Facts about Drug Abuse." The Drug Abuse Council. http://www.druglibrary.org/schaffer/ library/studies/fada/fada1.htm. Accessed on June 27, 2016.

Grim, Ryan, and Ryan J. Reilly. 2013. "Obama's Drug War: After Medical Marijuana Mess, Feds Face Big Decision on Pot." *Huffpost Politics*. http://www.huffingtonpost.com/ 2013/01/26/obamas-drug-war-medical-marijuana_n_ 2546178.html. Accessed on May 21, 2016.

Hamilton, Alexander. 1904. *The Works of Alexander Hamilton (Federal Edition)*, 12 vols. Edited by Henry Cabot Lodge. New York; London: G. P. Putnam's. http://oll.libertyfund .org/titles/hamilton-the-works-of-alexander-hamilton-fed eral-edition-vol-11. Accessed on June 24, 2016.

Hanson, David J. 2009. "National Prohibition of Alcohol in the U.S." Alcohol Problems and Solutions. http://www .alcoholproblemsandsolutions.org/Controversies/10911 24904.html. Accessed on June 24, 2016.

Harrison Narcotics Tax Act, 1914. 1914. Schaffer Library of Drug Policy. http://www.druglibrary.org/schaffer/history/ e1910/harrisonact.htm. Accessed on June 24, 2016.

Hedden, Sarra L., et al. 2015. "Behavioral Health Trends in the United States: Results from the 2014 National Survey on Drug Use and Health." HHS Publication No. SMA 15-4927, NSDUH Series H-50. http://www.samhsa.gov/

data/sites/default/files/NSDUH-FRR1-2014/NS
DUH-FRR1-2014.pdf. Accessed on June 18, 2016.

"Hemp Facts." 1997. North American Industrial Hemp
Council, Inc. http://www.naihc.org/hemp_information/
hemp_facts.html. Accessed on June 24, 2016.

Holland, Ellen. 2015. "Operation Golden Flow: America's
Urine Is Liquid Gold for Drug War Profiteers." *Cannabis
Now.* http://cannabisnowmagazine.com/current-events/
legal/operation-golden-flow-americas-urine-is-liquid-
gold-for-drug-war-profiteers. Accessed on June 22, 2016.

Hornik, Robert, et al. 2008. "Effects of the National Youth
Anti-Drug Media Campaign on Youths." *American Journal
of Public Health.* 98(12): 2229–2236. http://www.ncbi
.nlm.nih.gov/pmc/articles/PMC2636541/. Accessed on
June 26, 2016.

Ingraham, Christopher. 2016. "A New Anti-drug Campaign
Has a Wild Idea to Stop Kids from Drinking and Doing
Drugs." *The Washington Post.* https://www.washingtonpost
.com/news/wonk/wp/2015/07/16/the-newest-anti-drug-
campaign-is-written-entirely-in-emoji/. Accessed on June 26,
2016.

"International Opium Convention Signed at The Hague
January 23, 1912." 1912. *Telebit.* http://www.telebit.gr/
press/rss/files/almanak/1872-1912/opium1912.pdf.
Accessed on June 24, 2016.

James-Burdumy, Susanne, et al. 2010. "The Effectiveness
of Mandatory-Random Student Drug Testing." National
Center for Education Evaluation and Regional Assistance.
https://ies.ed.gov/ncee/pubs/20104025/pdf/20104025.pdf.
Accessed on June 23, 2016.

Johnson, Robert A., and Dean R. Gerstein. 1998. "Initiation
of Use of Alcohol, Cigarettes, Marijuana, Cocaine, and
Other Substances in US Birth Cohorts since 1919."
American Journal of Public Health. 88(1): 27–33.

Joy, Janet E., Stanley J. Watson, Jr., and John A. Benson, Jr., eds. 1999. *Marijuana and Medicine: Assessing the Science Base*. Washington, DC: National Academies Press.

Judge, J. W. 2007. "Workplace Drug Testing's Mixed Success." *Behavioral Healthcare*. 27(4): 14, 16.

King, Rufus. 1972. *The Drug Hang-Up; America's Fifty-Year Folly*. New York: Norton. http://www.druglibrary.org/special/king/dhu/dhumenu.htm. Accessed on June 25, 2016.

Levy, Sharon, Miriam Schizer, and Committee on Substance Abuse. 2015. "Adolescent Drug Testing Policies in Schools." *Pediatrics*. 135(4): 782–783.

Maginnis, Robert L. 2016. "Legalization of Drugs: The Myths and the Facts." http://www.slideshare.net/sevans-idaho/legalization-of-drugs. Accessed on June 28, 2016.

Mapes, Jeff. 2015. "Oregon Marijuana Law Could Face Legal Challenge, City and County Associations Say." *Oregon Live*. http://www.oregonlive.com/mapes/index.ssf/2015/03/oregon_marijuana_law_could_fac.html. Accessed on June 29, 2016.

"Marihuana and Social Policy." 1971. Marihuana: A Signal of Misunderstanding. National Commission on Marihuana and Drug Abuse. http://www.druglibrary.org/Schaffer/Library/studies/nc/ncrec1_9.htm. Accessed on June 21, 2016.

"The Marihuana Tax Act of 1937." 2016a. Schaffer Library of Drug Policy. http://www.druglibrary.org/schaffer/hemp/taxact/t10a.htm. Accessed on June 24, 2016.

"The Marihuana Tax Act of 1937." 2016b. Schaffer Library of Drug Policy. http://www.druglibrary.org/schaffer/hemp/taxact/mjtaxact.htm. Accessed on June 24, 2016.

McGrath, Michael. 2016. "Nancy Reagan and the Negative Impact of the 'Just Say No' Anti-drug Campaign." *The Guardian*. https://www.theguardian.com/society/2016/

mar/08/nancy-reagan-drugs-just-say-no-dare-program-opioid-epidemic. Accessed on June 26, 2016.

"Medical Consequences of Drug Abuse." 2012. National Institute on Drug Abuse. https://www.drugabuse.gov/related-topics/medical-consequences-drug-abuse. Accessed on June 28, 2016.

"Memorandum for All United States Attorneys." 2013. U.S. Department of Justice. https://www.justice.gov/iso/opa/resources/3052013829132756857467.pdf. Accessed on December 23, 2016.

"Memorandum for Selected United States Attorneys." 2009. U.S. Department of Justice. https://www.justice.gov/sites/default/files/opa/legacy/2009/10/19/medical-marijuana.pdf. Accessed on June 29, 2016.

"Memorandum for United States Attorneys." 2011. U.S. Department of Justice. https://www.justice.gov/sites/default/files/oip/legacy/2014/07/23/dag-guidance-2011-for-medical-marijuana-use.pdf. Accessed on June 29, 2016.

Miron, Jeffrey A., and Katherine Waldock. 2010. "The Budgetary Impact of Ending Drug Prohibition." Washington, DC: Cato Institute. http://object.cato.org/sites/cato.org/files/pubs/pdf/DrugProhibitionWP.pdf. Accessed on June 27, 2016.

"Mississippi Laws & Penalties." 2016. NORML. http://norml.org/laws/item/mississippi-penalties-2?category_id=868. Accessed on June 27, 2016.

Moberg, D. Paul, and Andrew J. Finch. 2008. "Recovery High Schools: A Descriptive Study of School Programs and Students." *Journal of Groups in Addiction & Recovery*. 2(2–4): 128–161.

"Monitoring Impacts of Recreational Marijuana Legalization: 2015 Baseline Report." 2015. Forecasting and Research Division. Washington State Office of Financial Management. http://www.ofm.wa.gov/reports/marijuana_impacts_2015.pdf. Accessed on June 29, 2016.

Musto, David E. 1987. *The American Disease: Origins of Narcotic Control*, rev. ed. New York: Oxford University Press.

"National Drug Control Budget." 2016. Office of National Drug Control Policy. https://www.whitehouse.gov/sites/default/files/ondcp/press-releases/fy_2017_budget_high lights.pdf. Accessed on June 27, 2016.

"National Drug Control Strategy." 2008. Office of National Drug Control Policy. https://www.whitehouse.gov/sites/default/files/ondcp/Fact_Sheets/FY2009-Budget-Sum mary-February-2008.pdf. Accessed on June 27, 2016.

"National Study Shows 'Gateway' Drugs Lead to Cocaine Use." 1994. Columbia University Record. http://www.columbia.edu/cu/record/archives/vol20/vol20_iss10/record2010.24.html. Accessed on June 28, 2016.

Nebraska and Oklahoma v. Colorado. 2016. SCOTUSblog. http://www.scotusblog.com/case-files/cases/nebraska-and-oklahoma-v-colorado/. Accessed on June 29, 2016.

Nephew, Thomas M., et al. 2002. *Surveillance Report #55: Apparent per Capita Consumption: National, State, and Regional Trends, 1977–98*. Rockville, MD: National Institute on Alcohol Abuse and Alcoholism, Division of Biometry and Epidemiology: Alcohol Epidemiologic Data System. http://pubs.niaaa.nih.gov/publications/surveil lanceArchive/CONS98.pdf. Accessed on June 24, 2016.

"The New D.A.R.E. Program—This One Works." 2014. D.A.R.E. http://www.dare.org/the-new-dare-program-this-one-works/. Accessed on June 21, 2016.

Newton, David E. 1999. *Drug Testing: An Issue for School, Sports, and Work*. Springfield, NJ: Enslow Publishers.

Newton, David E. 2014. *Steroids and Doping in Sports: A Reference Handbook*. Santa Barbara, CA: ABC-CLIO.

Normand, Jacques, Richard O. Lempert, and Charles P. O'Brien, eds. 1994. *Under the Influence: Drugs and the American Workforce*. Washington, DC: National Academies Press.

Olson, Dave. 2004a. "Advantages and Disadvantages of Work-place Drug Testing." Privacy, Freedom, and Security Program. Evergreen State College. http://www.uncleweed.com/words/essays/drugtesting-matrix.pdf. Accessed on June 22, 2016.

Olson, Dave. 2004b. "Privacy Issues in Workplace Drug Testing." Privacy, Freedom, and Security Program. Evergreen State College. http://uncleweed.net/words/essays/Work place-Drug-Testing.pdf. Accessed on June 22, 2016.

Oscapella, Eugene. 2003. "How Drug Prohibition Finances and Otherwise Enables Terrorism." Speech given at the Lisbon International Symposium on Global Drug Policy. http://www.ukcia.org/research/ProhibitionFinances Terrorism.pdf. Accessed on June 28, 2016.

"Part B—Authority to Control; Standards and Schedules." 2016. U.S. Code. Title 21. Chapter 13. Subchapter 1. http://uscode.house.gov/view.xhtml?path=/prelim@title21/chapter13/subchapter1/partB&edition=prelim. Accessed on June 26, 2016.

Pearce, David. 2016. "Vintage Wine." BLTC Research. http://cocaine.org/cocawine.htm. Accessed on June 24, 2016.

Pidd, Ken, and Ann M. Roche. 2014. "How Effective Is Drug Testing as a Workplace Safety Strategy? A Systematic Review of the Evidence." *Accident Analysis & Prevention.* 71(1): 154–165.

Prah, Pamela M. 2005. "Methamphetamine." *CQ Researcher.* http://library.cqpress.com/cqresearcher/document. php?id=cqresrre2005071500. Accessed on June 26, 2016.

Pratt, Timothy. 2015. "Marijuana Legalization Clashes with Drug Testing in the Workplace." *The Guardian.* http://www.theguardian.com/sustainable-business/2015/apr/19/marijuana-workplace-drug-testing-employers-employees-medical-recreational. Accessed on June 22, 2016

"Prescription Drugs." 2016. Govtrack.us. https://www.govtrack .us/congress/bills/subjects/prescription_drugs/6184. Accessed on June 27, 2016.

"Professional Sports and Their Drug Policies." 2016. *USA Today*. http://usatoday30.usatoday.com/sports/graphics/sports_steroids/flash.htm. Accessed on June 23, 2016.

Public Law 105–277. 1998. http://frwebgate.access.gpo.gov/cgi-bin/getdoc.cgi?dbname=105_cong_public_laws&docid=f:publ277.pdf. Accessed on June 26, 2016.

"Publications." 1994. National Criminal Justice Reference Service. https://www.ncjrs.gov/App/publications/abstract.aspx?ID=161247. Accessed on June 28, 2016.

Quinn, Elizabeth. 2015. "Steroids, Anabolic and Androgenic Steroids in Sports. Very Well. https://www.verywell.com/steroids-in-sports-3120518. Accessed on June 23, 2016.

"Quotes about Methamphetamine." 2016. Quotesgram. http://quotesgram.com/quotes-about-methamphetamine/. Accessed on June 26, 2016.

Reed, Jack K. 2016. "Marijuana Legislation in Colorado: Early Findings." Colorado Department of Public Safety. http://cdpsdocs.state.co.us/ors/docs/reports/2016-SB13-283-Rpt.pdf. Accessed on June 29, 2016.

Reid Paula, and Stephanie Condon. 2015. "DEA Chief Says Smoking Marijuana as Medicine 'Is a Joke.'" CBS News. http://www.cbsnews.com/news/dea-chief-says-smoking-marijuana-as-medicine-is-a-joke/. Accessed on June 29, 2016.

"Report of Committee on Acquirement of the Drug Habit." 1902. *Proceedings of the American Pharmaceutical Society*. https://books.google.com/books?id=QHICAAAAYAAJ&pg=PA572&lpg=PA572&dq=%22if+the+chinaman+cannot+get+along+without+his+dope%22&source=bl&ots=_Mp0NsjY1i&sig=EI-khMNxBLGFY770MM8m9Q137Zo&hl=en&sa=X&ved=0ahUKEwjH95SflsHNAhUT6GMKHVypC6AQ6AEIIzAB#v=onepage&q=%22if%20the%20chinaman%20cannot%20get%20along%20without%20his%20dope%22&f=false. Accessed on June 24, 2016.

"Results from the 2014 National Survey on Drug Use and Health: Detailed Tables." 2015. Research Triangle Park, NC: RTI International. http://www.samhsa.gov/data/sites/default/files/NSDUH-DetTabs2014/NSDUH-DetTabs2014.pdf. Accessed on June 22, 2016.

Riggs, Mike. 2011. "Obama Administration Overrides 2009 Ogden Memo, Declares Open Season on Pot Shops in States Where Medical Marijuana Is Legal." Reason.com. http://reason.com/blog/2011/06/30/white-house-overrides-2009-mem. Accessed on December 23, 2016.

Ringwalt, Chris, et al. 2008. "Random Drug Testing in US Public School Districts." *American Journal of Public Health*. 98(5): 826–828.

Robertson, Elizabeth B., Susan L. David, and Suman A. Rao. 2003. *Preventing Drug Use among Children and Adolescents: A Research-Based Guide for Parents, Educators, and Community Leaders*. Bethesda, MD: U.S. Department of Health and Human Services, National Institutes of Health: National Institute on Drug Abuse.

Russo, Ethan, and Franjo Grotenhermen. 2006. *Handbook of Cannabis Therapeutics: from Bench to Bedside*. New York: Haworth Press.

Schaffer, Cliff. 2016. "Did Alcohol Prohibition Reduce Alcohol Consumption and Crime?" Schaffer Library of Drug Policy. http://www.druglibrary.org/prohibitionresults.htm. Accessed on June 24, 2016.

Scott, Emilee Mooney. 2010. OLR Research Report. https://www.cga.ct.gov/2010/rpt/2010-R-0204.htm. Accessed on June 29, 2016.

"Simplification Draft Paper." 2016. United States Sentencing Commission. http://www.ussc.gov/research/research-and-publications/simplification-draft-paper-2. Accessed on June 26, 2016.

"65170: Medical Marijuana and Other Cannabinoids." 2016. NetCE. http://www.netce.com/coursecontent.php?courseid=1256#chap.7. Accessed on June 29, 2016.

"Speaking Out against Drug Legalization." [2010]. U.S. Drug Enforcement Administration. https://www.dea.gov/pr/mul timedia-library/publications/speaking_out.pdf. Accessed on June 28, 2016.

"State Industrial Hemp Statutes." 2016. National Conference of State Legislatures. http://www.ncsl.org/research/agricul ture-and-rural-development/state-industrial-hemp-statutes .aspx. Accessed on June 24, 2016.

"State Laws." 2016. NORML. http://norml.org/laws/. Accessed on June 29, 2016.

"State Medical Marijuana Laws." 2016. National Conference of State Legislatures. http://www.ncsl.org/research/health/ state-medical-marijuana-laws.aspx. Accessed on June 29, 2016.

Stolz, Barbara Ann. 1992. "Congress and the War on Drugs: An Exercise in Symbolic Politics." *Journal of Crime and Justice*. 15(1): 119–136.

Stout, David, and Solomon Moore. 2009. "U.S. Won't Prosecute in States That Allow Medical Marijuana." *The New York Times*. http://www.nytimes.com/2009/10/20/ us/20cannabis.html. Accessed on June 29, 2016.

Stuart, Susan P. 2010. "When the Cure Is Worse Than the Disease: Student Random Drug Testing & Its Empirical Failure." *Valparaiso University Law Review*. 44(4): 1055–1082.

Sznitman, S. R., and D. Romer. 2014. "Student Drug Test- ing and Positive School Climates: Testing the Relation be- tween Two School Characteristics and Drug Use Behavior in a Longitudinal Study." *Journal of Studies on Alcohol and Drugs*. 75(1): 65–73.

Tandy, Karen P. 2005. "Marijuana: The Myths Are Killing Us." U.S. Drug Enforcement Administration. https:// www.dea.gov/pubs/pressrel/pr042605.html. Accessed on June 28, 2016.

"Tobacco Control Act." 2016. U.S. Food and Drug Adminis- tration. http://www.fda.gov/TobaccoProducts/Guidance

ComplianceRegulatoryInformation/ucm246129.htm.
Accessed on June 27, 2016.

"2016–2017 NCAA Banned Drugs." 2016. http://www
.ncaa.org/sites/default/files/2016_17_%20Banned_%20
Drugs_%20Educational_%20Document_20160531.pdf.
Accessed on June 23, 2016.

Uncle Mike [pseud.]. 2008. "U.S. District Court, Denver,
Colorado Imposes First Federal Marihuana Law Penalties."
http://www.unclemikesresearch.com/u-s-district-court-
denver-colorado-imposes-first-federal-marihuana-law-
penalties/. Accessed on June 24, 2016.

Vagins, Deborah J., and Jesselyn McCurdy. 2006. "Cracks in
the System: Twenty Years of the Unjust Federal Crack
Cocaine Law." American Civil Liberties Union. https://
www.aclu.org/sites/default/files/field_document/cracksin
system_20061025.pdf. Accessed on June 26, 2016.

Vernonia School Dist. 47J v. Acton 515 U.S. 646. 1995. U.S.
Supreme Court. http://www.supremecourt.gov/opinions/
boundvolumes/515bv.pdf. Accessed on June 23, 2016.

Vimont, Celia. 2011. "Recovery High Schools: Giving
Students a Second Chance." Partnership for Drug-Free
Kids. http://www.drugfree.org/join-together/recovery-
high-schools-giving-students-a-second-chance/. Accessed
on June 30, 2016.

Wallace, Alicia. 2015. "Colorado Supreme Court: Employers
Can Fire for Off-Duty Pot Use." *Denver Post.* http://www
.denverpost.com/2015/06/15/colorado-supreme-court-em
ployers-can-fire-for-off-duty-pot-use/. Accessed on June 22,
2016.

Warner, Joel. 2016. "Marijuana Legalization Movement
Just Won Multiple Courtroom Battles, But Will That Be
Enough to Quash Future Legal Threats?" *International
Business Times.* http://www.ibtimes.com/marijuana-
legalization-movement-just-won-multiple-courtroom-bat
tles-will-be-enough-2342055. Accessed on June 29, 2016.

Whitebread, Charles. 1995. "The History of the Non-Medical Use of Drugs in the United States: A Speech to the California Judges Association 1995 Annual Conference." Schaffer Library of Drug Policy. http://www.druglibrary.org/schaf fer/history/whiteb1.htm. Accessed on June 25, 2016.

Xu, Jianquan, et al. 2016. "Deaths: Final Data for 2013." National Vital Statistics Report. Volume 64, Number 2. http://www.cdc.gov/nchs/data/nvsr/nvsr64/nvsr64_02. pdf. Accessed on June 28, 2016. Supplemental tables are at http://www.cdc.gov/nchs/data/nvsr/nvsr64/nvsr64_02_ta bles.pdf. Accessed on June 28, 2016.

Yamaguchi, Ryoko, Lloyd D. Johnston, and Patrick M. O'Malley. 2003. *Drug Testing in Schools: Policies, Practices, and Association with Student Drug Use.* Occasional Paper No. 2. Ann Arbor: Institute for Social Research. University of Michigan. http://www.yesresearch.org/publications/oc-cpapers/YESOccPaper2.pdf. Accessed on June 23, 2016.

Youth Violence: A Report of the Surgeon General. 2001. Public Health Service. Office of the Surgeon General. Washington, DC: Government Printing Office. http://www.ncbi.nlm. nih.gov/books/NBK44294/. Accessed on June 21, 2016.

Zimmer, Lynn. 1999. *Drug Testing: A Bad Investment.* New York: American Civil Liberties Union.

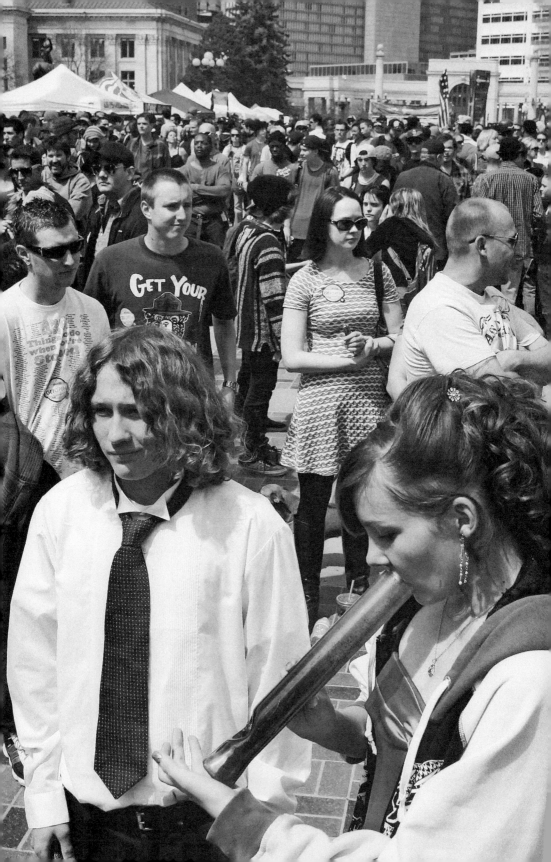

Introduction

A book about substance abuse can provide technical details, a historical review, a discussion of current issues in the field, a list of additional resources, and other aids in learning more about the topic. But this book also provides individuals with some special interest in the topic of substance abuse with an opportunity to express their personal views about some specific aspect of the problem. It also provides a human look on a topic that has never been and never can be a dry academic topic for discussion and debate.

Cannabis Use and Cannabis-Related Behaviors among Adolescents Following Legalization: Expelling the Myths
Candice Beathard

In 1996, California made global headlines by becoming the first state to legalize medical cannabis for qualifying patients. Within 20 years, 25 states legalized medical cannabis and 4 states legalized recreational cannabis, with more states expected to follow suit (ProCon 2016). Legalizing cannabis is a complex issue for many reasons, including conflicting federal and state laws, specifics related to growing and selling the substance,

Young adults attend a pro-marijuana rally held in Denver in April 2013. Marijuana is now legal in Colorado. (AP Photo/Brennan Linsley)

economic complexities, and the subsequent effects on "vulnerable" populations such as adolescents (National Conference of State Legislatures 2016).

Outspoken critics of legalizing cannabis raise concerns about adolescents and their cannabis-related behaviors with the implementation of such laws. Some critics speculate that legalizing cannabis increases the amount of cannabis in each state, leading to an increase in use of cannabis among youth. Opponents worry because cannabis remains the most commonly used substance among youth in the United States, and for the first time in its 40-year history, the 2015 Monitoring the Future Survey found that daily cannabis use exceeds daily tobacco use among 12- to 17-year-olds (National Institute on Drug Abuse 2015).

People were alarmed in 2015 when the media announced that high school students use more cannabis than cigarettes, but the media outlets did not present the full picture. Daily cannabis use is higher than daily cigarette use because tobacco use has continued to decline significantly among this age group (from 6.7 to 5.5% in one year, 2014–2015, for example). Daily cannabis use among 12- to 17-year-olds has remained stable since the early 2000s (Substance Abuse and Mental Health Services Administration 2015). Additionally, researchers discovered that medical cannabis laws do not increase—and in fact, sometimes decrease—adolescent usage of cannabis (see Beathard 2015 for a full literature review of the findings).

An increased supply of cannabis at the state level is another concern after passing medical cannabis legislation. Many people are worried that adolescents will have greater access to cannabis with an influx of cannabis in their state. Although limited research exists on this topic, some suggest that an increase in supply of medical cannabis actually decreases adolescents' approval of cannabis usage (Beathard 2015).

The second argument against legalizing cannabis with respect to adolescents is that it sends the wrong message to young people in the United States. They believe that adolescents' attitudes toward cannabis become more favorable following implementation. However, this argument is more complicated than a simple cause-and-effect relationship.

There is a clear inverse pattern between cannabis use and perceived risk among adolescents (University of Michigan 2016). In other words, as annual cannabis use increases, perceived risk of using cannabis decreases. This inverse pattern has persisted over decades, and is important because perceived risk is a significant determinant of cannabis use among high school students. In addition, data are showing a decline in perception of cannabis use as risky (National Institute on Drug Abuse 2015). However, passing medical cannabis laws does directly affect adolescent views on cannabis. Rather there is a national trend of youth taking a more permissive stance on medical cannabis (Schmidt and Spetz 2016, 1500–1502).

Each of the arguments presented above, although well intended, is not substantiated in the literature and research. It is clear that youth in the United States are using cannabis more than tobacco, and the more cannabis they use, the less risky they view the substance. However, medical cannabis laws do not increase cannabis use among adolescents. In fact, these laws sometimes decrease use of cannabis, decrease approval of cannabis, and do not directly affect adolescent views on cannabis.

Expelling these myths is important for policy makers and perhaps more critical for researchers studying the newly established recreational cannabis laws. Will these same results hold true for recreational cannabis policies? Cannabis policy is arguably the fastest evolving policy in the United States. Each year, the number of states passing medical cannabis policies increases, and within the next five years, additional states are expected to pass recreational cannabis laws. Evaluating the effects of these newly established policies on adolescent behavior is of paramount importance. No policy maker, no parent, no proponent, or critic of legalizing cannabis wants adolescents to use cannabis or have access to cannabis. With such a hotly debated, controversial topic, it is important to remember that everyone has this common goal.

References

Beathard, C. 2015. "Current Drug Policies in the United States: Using Research to Inform Policy." http://ir.library .oregonstate.edu/xmlui/handle/1957/56235. Accessed July 11, 2016.

National Conference of State Legislatures. 2016. "State Medical Marijuana Laws." http://www.ncsl.org/research/ health/state-medical-marijuana-laws.aspx. Accessed on July 21, 2016.

National Institute on Drug Abuse. 2015. "Drug Use Trends Remain Stable or Decline among Teens." https://www .drugabuse.gov/news-events/news-releases/2015/12/ drug-use-trends-remain-stable-or-decline-among-teens. Accessed on July 27, 2016.

ProCon. 2016. "25 Legal Medical Marijuana States and DC: Laws, Fees, and Possession Limits." http:// medicalmarijuana.procon.org/view.resource.php?resourceI D=000881&print=true. Accessed on July 7, 2016.

Schmidt, L. A., L. M. Jacobs, and J. Spetz. 2016. "Young People's More Permissive Views about Marijuana: Local Impact of State Laws or National Trends." *American Journal of Public Health*. 106(8): 1498–1503.

Substance Abuse and Mental Health Services Administration. Center for Behavioral Health Statistics and Quality. 2015. "Behavioral Health Trends in the United States: Results from the 2014 National Survey on Drug Use and Health" (HHS Publication No. SMA 15-4927, NSDUH Series H-50). http://www.samhsa.gov/ data/. Accessed July 7, 2016.

University of Michigan. 2016. "Monitoring the Future: A Continuing Study of American Youth." http://moni toringthefuture.org/data/12data/fig12_1.pdf. Accessed July 15, 2016.

Dr. Candice Beathard is a research analyst with an expertise in drug policy and substance use. She completed a postdoctoral research opportunity as the lead author of Senate Bill 844 Task Force Report: Researching the medical and public health properties of cannabis. Dr. Beathard received her PhD in Public Health Policy from Oregon State University, Corvallis, where she studied cannabis policy, adolescent attitudes regarding cannabis use, substance use and abuse among the homeless and welfare recipients, and driving while under the influence of cannabis policies.

The Religious and Spiritual Use of Cannabis in History
Jeffrey Brown

It is a fact that cannabis, also known as marijuana and hemp, has been used for thousands of years in many different religions and cultures. The weaving of hemp fiber began 10,000 years ago along with pottery making and prior to metal working. From very early in history the plant has been used for food, clothing, shelter, energy, medicine, insight and recreation.

In his book *The Dragons of Eden,* Carl Sagan has speculated that cannabis may have been the first crop planted by Stone Age man. He used the pygmies as an example of a group who were basically hunter-gatherers until they started planting cannabis, which they use for religious purposes. He stated that cannabis is their only cultivated crop and that "it would be wryly interesting if in human history this cultivation led generally to the invention of agriculture and thereby to civilization" (Sagan 1977, 201).

Richard E. Schultes, a prominent researcher in the field of psychoactive plants, has speculated in his article "Man and Marijuana" that early man in his search for seeds and oil certainly ate the sticky tops of the plant. This practice, he said, "may have introduced man to an 'other-worldly' plane from which emerged religious beliefs and perhaps even the concept of Diety." And, he continued, "the euphoric, ecstatic and hallucinatory aspects of the plant became accepted as a special 'gift of the gods', a sacred medium for communion with the spiritual world and as such it has remained in some cultures to the present" (Schultes 1973).

Another authority in the field, William A. Emboden, has noted in his book *The Ritual Use of Cannabis Sativa L.* that "[c]ertain older non-Western religious cults seem to employed cannabis as a euphoriant, which allowed the participant a joyous path to the 'ultimate,' hence appellations as 'heavenly guide'."

India appears to be the place where the most direct reference to cannabis use is recorded. Cannabis is mentioned as a medicinal and magical plant as well as sacred grass in the Atharva Veda (2000–1400 BCE), which also calls hemp one of the Five Kingdoms of Herbs that releases us from anxiety and is a source of happiness, joy-giver, and liberator. Other ancient names for the plant were Hero Leaved, Desired-in-the-Three-Worlds, God's Food, Fountain of Pleasures, and Shiva's Plant.

According to Hindu legends Shiva had a family squabble and went to the fields where upon sitting under a cannabis plant to be sheltered from the sun ate some of its leaves. He felt so refreshed that it became his favorite food and that is how he got his title, "The Lord of Bhang," bhang being a cannabis beverage.

According to shamanic tradition, Indra, king of the gods, discovered cannabis and sowed it in the Himalayas so that it would be available to the people. Tradition says Indra gave the herb to people to attain elevated states of consciousness. Early legends maintained that the angel of mankind lived in the leaves and it was so sacred that it was reputed to deter evil and cleanse its user of sin. Hemp was also thought to be a holy plant given to man for the welfare of mankind and was considered to be one of the Divine Nectars able to give mankind anything from good health, long life, to visions of the gods.

Cannabis is still being used in India for religious purposes. During the twentieth century, the Indian Hemp Drugs Commission was created to study the use of cannabis by the people of India. One of the commission's conclusions was that "cannabis alleviates fatigue, creates the capacity for hard work and the ability to concentrate and gives rise to pleasurable sensations, so that one is at peace with everyone." The commission also noted that one religious user claimed that "when we drank bhang and the Mystery I am He grew plain" (Young and Kaplan 1969). This is in reference to it being an entheogen, a substance used in the realization of the God or Goddess within.

There is also an early record of the religious use of cannabis in China. The Shen Nung Pharmacopeia, from the Han dynasty, classifies cannabis as among the "Superior Immortality Elixirs." "Eating Hemp flower tops," it says, "makes one become a Divine Transcendent" (as quoted in Conrad 1997, 15). As in India cannabis was a symbol of power over evil. A Chinese Taoist priest in the fifth century BCE wrote that cannabis was used in combination with ginseng to set forward time to reveal future events. It is also recorded that in the first century AD the Taoist recommended adding cannabis to their incense burners as a means of achieving immortality. In early Taoist ritual, fumes and odors of incense burners were said to have produced a mystic exaltation and contribution to well-being.

In ancient Japan cannabis was used in ceremonial purification rites and for driving away evil spirits. Clothes made of hemp were worn especially during formal and religious ceremonies due to its traditional association with purity. By the first century Taoists used cannabis in incense burners. A fifth-century booklet stated that "Hemp and Mulberry have long been used in worshiping the Gods" (Ancient Asia 2016).

There is tradition of cannabis use in Africa in religious ceremony. Cannabis is held to be sacred and is connected with many religious and social customs. Cannabis is regarded by some sects as a magic plant possessing universal protection against all injuries to life and is symbolic of peace and friendship. Certain tribes consider its use a duty.

The mystical Sufi Muslims believed spiritual enlightenment was attainable through a state of ecstasy or altered consciousness and used hashish for that purpose. Hashish was sacramental, a portal through which to commune directly with Allah. Early Arabic texts referred to cannabis as "The Bush of Understanding," "Shrub of Emotion," "Blissful Branches," and "Morsel of Thought."

The modern-day Jamaican Rasta religion is where I, the author of this piece, became aware of the use of cannabis in religion. I joined and accepted the Rasta religion on faith and later researched and became aware of the history of its religious use by many others. Cannabis, called ganja by Jamaicans, is not a drug but a "Holy Herb." Among Rastas it is known as "Wisdom Weed" and the "Spiritual Meat" of the movement. Symbolically, ganja grew out of the grave of King Solomon and has the power to "Heal the Nations." It is the "Holy Eucharist" and "Spiritual Intensifier" with biblical justification for its use on the first page of the Bible, where Genesis 1:29 approves usage of "every herb bearing seed." Rastas, through the use of ganja, feel themselves to be divinely inspired, experiencing the same magnificence of spirit and oneness with nature, which Moses must have experienced "high" on the mountain top in the form of the "burning bush," as did Jesus "high" on top of Mount Sinai.

References

"Ancient Asia." 2016. U.S. Hemp Museum. http:// ushempcomuseum.com/ancient-asia/. Accessed on June 11, 2015.

Campbell, J. M. 1894. On the Religion of Hemp. Indian Hemp Drugs Commission Report. London: Government Central Printing Office.

Conrad, Chris. 1997. *Hemp for Health: The Medicinal and Nutritional Uses of Cannabis Sativa*. Rochester, VT: Healing Arts Press.

Emboden, William A., Jr. 1972. "Ritual Use of Cannabis Sativa L.: A Historical-Ethnographic Survey." In Peter T. Furst, ed. *Flesh of the Gods*. Prospect Heights, IL: Waveland Press, Chapter 8.

Sagan, Carl. 1977. *The Dragons of Eden: Speculation on the Evolution of Human Intelligence*. New York: Random House.

Schultes, Richard E. 1973. "Man and Marijuana." *Natural History*. 82(7): 59–65, 80–82.

Young, W. Mackworth, and John Kaplan. 1969. *Marijuana. Report of the Indian Hemp Drugs Commission, 1893–1894*. Silver Spring, MD: Thos. Jefferson Publishing Company.

Jeffrey Brown grew up in Miami, Florida, and joined a Jamaican Rasta church when he was about 20 years old. The church uses cannabis or ganja as its sacrament. Jeff went on to write a book, Marijuana and the Bible, *which goes into the sacramental use of cannabis by many different religions with a special emphasis on the Rasta church he joined.*

Marijuana Use and Intelligence
Nicholas J. Jackson

Our social and legal perspectives on marijuana are changing. Some places in the United States have legalized the recreational use of marijuana, and many others are considering legalization. Proponents and opponents of legalization both point to research to support their beliefs, despite its scarcity and the lack of scientific consensus on the subject. What is clear to researchers is that the younger a person is when he or she begins using marijuana, the more likely he or she is to have worse physical and mental health as well as to obtain less education as an adult (Hall 2015). It is unclear, however, whether these poorer outcomes occur as a direct result of marijuana use or if substance use in early adolescence is a symptom of dysfunction in the child's environment, which can also lead to these same negative outcomes in adulthood. Researchers are currently debating the impact that marijuana use in adolescence has on long-term changes in intelligence.

Adolescence may be a particularly vulnerable time for marijuana's effects on the brain. Our cells have receptors for cannabinoids, which naturally circulate in our bodies and aid in various cognitive abilities such as memory and planning (Pacher, Bátkai, and Kunos 2006). Adolescence can be a period of increased sensitivity to external cannabinoids found in marijuana because we undergo major developmental changes to our endocannabinoid system during puberty. As a result, marijuana's impact on cognition may be greatest during this time period, as studies on rats have demonstrated (Renard et al. 2013). However, unlike rats, humans choose to use marijuana. This choice may result from any number of environmental factors that could impair cognitive ability independently of marijuana use.

Cross-sectional studies, in which marijuana use and intelligence are assessed at the same time, have demonstrated a negative effect of marijuana on intelligence. However, these deficits are often limited to knowledge acquired through education and experience, such as vocabulary. This type of intelligence, called crystallized intelligence, may be affected by environmental conditions that existed prior to marijuana involvement (Solowij et al. 2011; Pope et al. 2003). Longitudinal studies, which measure an individual's intelligence before ever using marijuana, can be used to compare the changes in intelligence over time for those who used marijuana and those who abstained. The most influential of these studies, by Meier et. al. (2012), showed a dramatic drop in intelligence from ages 13 to 38 for those who used marijuana in early adolescence. While these authors attributed this drop to a neurotoxic effect of marijuana, the majority of longitudinal research on the topic supports a more nuanced view. Researchers Fried, Watkinson, and Gray (2005) found significant declines in intelligence for current heavy users of marijuana but no decline in those who had quit using marijuana, suggesting that the effects on intelligence are related to recent use only. Recent research by Jackson et al. (2016) suggests that marijuana users have lower crystallized intelligence prior to marijuana use. Later declines in intelligence were found to be similarly limited to acquired knowledge. Most importantly, the authors found that identical twins (who share the same genes) did not differ in their intelligence when one twin was a marijuana user and the other was not. This suggests that it is not the marijuana use per se that results in intelligence declines, but rather environmental factors that predispose an individual both to perform worse on tests of acquired knowledge and to use marijuana. Other recent longitudinal studies by Mokrysz et al. (2016) and Auer et al. (2016) provide support for this notion by demonstrating either no effect of marijuana or, again, effects limited to acquired knowledge.

Although recent human subject research suggests that the marijuana–intelligence association is likely the result of underlying environmental factors, the truth is more nuanced. Animal research clearly indicates a neurotoxic effect of marijuana. The question is how large this effect is in humans and, most importantly, if this effect is greater than environmental risk factors that are also associated with long-term intelligence decline. While more research needs to be done on the topic, when considering the effects of marijuana on intelligence, we should also consider the reasons that have led to an adolescent choosing to use marijuana and the role these factors play in the development of their intelligence.

References

Auer, R., et al. 2016. "Association between Lifetime Marijuana Use and Cognitive Function in Middle Age: The Coronary Artery Risk Development in Young Adults (CARDIA) Study." *JAMA Internal Medicine*. 176(3): 352–361.

Fried, P.A., B. Watkinson, and R. Gray. 2005. "Neurocognitive Consequences of Marihuana—A Comparison with Pre-Drug Performance." *Neurotoxicology and Teratology*. 27(2): 231–239.

Hall, W. 2015. "What Has Research Over the Past Two Decades Revealed about the Adverse Health Effects of Recreational Cannabis Use?" *Addiction.* 110(1): 19–35.

Jackson, N. J., et al. 2016. "Impact of Adolescent Marijuana Use on Intelligence: Results from Two Longitudinal Twin Studies. *Proceedings of the National Academy of Sciences.* 113(5): E500–E508.

Meier, M. H., et al. 2012. "Persistent Cannabis Users Show Neuropsychological Decline from Childhood to Midlife." *Proceedings of the National Academy of Sciences.* 109(40): E2657–E2664.

Mokrysz, C., et al. 2016. "Are IQ and Educational Outcomes in Teenagers Related to Their Cannabis Use? A Prospective Cohort Study." *Journal of Psychopharmacology.* 30(2): 159–168.

Pacher, P., S. Bátkai, and G. Kunos. 2006. "The Endocannabinoid System as an Emerging Target of Pharmacotherapy." *Pharmacological Reviews.* 58(3): 389–462.

Pope, H. G., et al. 2003. "Early-Onset Cannabis Use and Cognitive Deficits: What Is the Nature of the Association?" *Drug and Alcohol Dependence.* 69(3): 303–310.

Renard, J., et al. 2013. "Long-Term Cognitive Impairments Induced by Chronic Cannabinoid Exposure during Adolescence in Rats: A Strain Comparison." *Psychopharmacology.* 225(4): 781–790.

Solowij, N., et al. 2011. "Verbal Learning and Memory in Adolescent Cannabis Users, Alcohol Users and Non-Users." *Psychopharmacology.* 216(1): 131–144.

Nicholas Jackson is a statistician in the Department of Medicine at the University of California–Los Angeles and a doctoral student in quantitative psychology at the University of Southern California. He holds a master of public health in biostatistics and a master of arts in quantitative psychology.

A Young Man's Story
Jackie Lien

This is the story, in his own words, of a 17-year-old male who is currently in the adolescent substance abuse treatment program at Phoenix Counseling Center in Phoenix, Oregon.

It all started with the death of my pops when I was 9. I didn't know what to do after he was gone. I was too young with no guidance. My mom started drinking when pops died, and I felt like I lost both parents at the same time. I first tried marijuana when I was 10. After that I brought it to school. I started hanging out with "hooligans," because I had the weed. I did illegal stuff, popped Xanax, and joined a gang. I tried meth when I was 12 with my gang. Those homies ended up doing me dirty, so I changed my friend group. I started smoking weed all the time. In middle school I got into fights and bailed on sports practices just to smoke weed.

Once I got into high school, I started experimenting. I messed with meth and Percocets, I drank a lot, and smoked weed every day. I started jumping people for drugs and traded everything I had for meth. I had a good girlfriend, but, to me, meth was more important. I robbed cars, stole from my family, and I hurt those I loved just to get drugs and get my fix. At this point I was 16. I didn't care what happened to me. I just wanted to be high. I traded expensive stuff I had even though I liked it, and I screwed my little brother over even though I loved him.

Then I got put on probation. I started doing acid and drinking, because I knew they wouldn't show up in a urinalysis. The acid really messed my mind up. I started hallucinating when I wasn't even high. Meth was my drug of choice, but I couldn't risk getting away with using it, so I tried other things. I was a legit addict.

I wanted to change my mind state, because I was so hurt on the inside. My mom had been drinking since my pops passed away, and no one was there for me except the drugs. I was with a number of different girlfriends during all this; I cheated on some of them; some of them left me because of my drug use. I ended up getting locked up for a bad alcohol relapse.

After that I met a girl on Facebook who was into meth. I felt like she really liked me, and I was going to keep her forever. We ended up getting high for a week straight even though I was on probation and she was in drug treatment. We fell in a weird sort of love that happened too fast. I went on the run with her and had plans to get married in Las Vegas. We were using weed and all sorts of different pills. My mom found out where I was and called the police. After two weeks I turned myself in and went to detention. I was put into rehab but soon got fed up with the rehab process. I ran with my girlfriend-straight to my friend's house where I knew I could get some meth. We used for the first time in a month and a half. Two days later the police caught up with us. We were chased by six cops. I ran on foot hoping not to get caught, but I eventually gave up, because I was done running. They took me to juvenile detention where I cried and cried until I knew my girlfriend was safe. She ended up going back to rehab. I stayed in a cell until I got transferred into a program for kids who could not manage being in society without breaking the law.

Instead of hating where I was at, I learned to have a positive perspective on my situation in life. I was able to catch up on a ton of school credits, and I made some friendships that will be irreplaceable. I got back together with an old girlfriend who didn't use drugs. I learned to trust people again, and I learned to love myself. I learned what a real Narcotics Anonymous participant was. Anybody who needed help could go. I had a completely different understanding of life with seven months clean.

I've drank a little since then, but my life is so different now that I know what living clean is like. It's a new experience that I would say is worth trying if your life seems like it isn't going anywhere. That's where my life was going before I got significant clean time and before I started counseling to try to figure out why I was the way I am. I have found out that everything gets better eventually as long as I stay away from drugs.

This young man was adopted at birth after being removed from his home by Child Welfare due to the fact that both of his parents were addicted to meth. When he refers to his "pops" and mom, he is talking about his adoptive parents. He has had no contact with his biological parents. After being in and out of a number of different treatment programs, he has been consistently attending our program for the past four months, doing both individual and group counseling. While in counseling, he has realized that when his "pops" died, he felt abandoned that caused him to act out in negative ways, including using drugs, to try to get attention from his mom. His drug use also blotted out his feelings of abandonment, grief, and loss. Counseling has helped him make sense of why he has behaved the way he has and why he feels what he feels. He is a rapper and uses rap to express himself. Now with some good clean time behind him, he has completed high school and has plans to attend the local community college.

Jackie Lien, MA, is a licensed professional counselor who has a passion for working with individuals who are struggling with addiction. She is currently executive director and clinical director at Phoenix Counseling Center, Inc., a nonprofit agency providing heart-centered counseling for addiction and trauma in Phoenix, Oregon.

A Recovery High School
Michelle Lipinski

A little over a decade ago I was asked to start the first recovery high school in Massachusetts. I had no idea what a recovery school was, let alone how to operate one. I was given a building. There were no staff, no students, no curriculum, no furniture, no technology, and no set of rules. The recovery high school concept had been operating in a few states under the leadership of some of the most compassionate and mission-driven leaders I have ever met. Many of these leaders are still fighting the fight today. They are desperately trying to keep their schools open amid threats of budget cuts at the local, state, and national levels. They show up every day to find innovative ways to keep students moving toward their matriculation requirements, keeping students focused on their recovery goals and trying their damnedest to keep these children on this earth and not underneath it. So my journey into the complex world of adolescent addiction began.

If someone had told me a quarter of a century ago when I first became a high school biology teacher that I would be working with some of the most brilliant minds in the fields of substance use and education to help understand the create solutions to this opioid crisis, I would have thought them a bit insane. If someone had told me I would have days when I cry tears of joy for my students who managed to stay sober for just 24 hours for the first time in two years, I would have never thought it possible. If someone had told me I could be a leader in creating a place where students actually heal from the scars caused by their real or perceived trauma, by their diagnosed mental illness, by their intergenerational substance use, by being both the victim and the bully, by numbing their pain for so long they can no longer live in their own skin without a hit, high, or sip of their poison . . . and then I get to watch them walk across my stage in their caps and gowns beaming with pride because THIS diploma means more than passing the MCAS. Everyone in the audience at graduation, all of the family members, the friends, the sponsors, the treatment providers, the probation officers, the school officials, the law enforcement and community partners, they all know what it means to receive a Northshore Recovery High School diploma and they cheer, they applaud, and mostly they cry that these beautiful young people get to participate in a rite of passage that most never thought possible. In fact, most of the people in the audience thought these children would end up in jail, institutions, or be no longer on this earth.

We cherish our students. My staff and I know how precious their lives are because we are burying our students and graduates at an alarming rate. We have planned funerals, eulogized the children, sang songs of bereavement for those sweet children who sat in our desks and laughed at our futile attempts to make them smile amid their battle. We memorialize them by advocating and literally begging our elected officials to understand what is happening to this generation and how it feels to be on the front lines of this epidemic. We celebrate our victories when our senators come and serve us Thanksgiving dinner, when our students receive a standing ovation at the statehouse on Recovery Day, or when the governor signs the largest opioid bill in the country and we are standing right behind him when he openly weeps on national television because the words of our students have made an impact on him. One of my first hires as the principal of Northshore was my English teacher, Michaela Gile. When we moved sites last year out of our decade-long "home" I remembered the words she had posted on social media. Her words more than resonated with me. I try and explain to people I meet why I stay in this field despite all of setbacks and perceived hopelessness. Michaela expressed this perfectly:

As I am emptying out my desk (fine, I am weeping a little), to get ready for our big move, I found a reflection I wrote in back in 2007. Here it goes:

Since I started working at Recovery High School in August of 2006, I have undergone profound changes.

I used to think that all children could be saved by education, that it was my duty to help them reach a tangible outcome to measure success—something spectacular and creative, preferably—and that I had to hoist them up to levels of learning they had not previously reached. But I have learned—and I still struggle with it—that it is the little things that measure progress. . . that relating on a personal level exceeds academic achievement. . . that sometimes, just reading something or having an insightful conversation in a safe environment means more than a vocabulary test. I have learned that I should not take this work home, but I do anyway. I have learned that I have the means to control my frustration and that every moment, every kind word counts. I have learned that when I struggle with loving a kid, I have to work harder at it because they're just overgrown toddlers who need to be cherished. I have learned that sometimes, I just have to wait until it gets better. . . that there are things I cannot control, but I have yet to learn how to deal with that. My dreams are filled with suffering children, and although I know (I hope, I pray) that most of them will be fine eventually, I also fear that some of them won't, and that's what keeps me up at night. I hope that we can build a foundation, a sanctuary, a safe place to which they can retreat, because dear God, to be so young and create such change. . . I hope that the power of community that our students experience will stay with them and give them room to breathe when life gets hard. . . and I hope life will be gentle for them. (Michaela Gile, English Teacher, Northshore Recovery High School)

If only everyone could see that our students, our children, need more compassion. Some have called me an enabler. Some have called me soft. Some have called me much stronger names because I demand that we don't give up. When they challenge us with every trick in the book (and trust me I know them all), we love them harder. When they are hurling obscenities at the highest decibels, we see their pain and we do everything in our power to get small and hold them both literally and figuratively and we don't give up. We don't suspend them for showing us they are sicker than we knew, we have them amend and restore themselves. We built a place where there are 365 fresh starts for every student. We need to build more places where these broken children can heal and find hope. We need to put all of the resources we can find toward helping our sick children before they disappear. We DO have the chance to save this generation. We just need to listen to them, treat them, teach them, and love them unconditionally.

Michelle Lipinski is the principal of the North Shore Recovery High School in Beverly, Massachusetts.

Pins and Needles: Treating Cravings with Acupuncture
Cassandra Newell

I didn't know the real meaning of "cravings" until I got sober. In the days, weeks, and months that followed, I craved alcohol viscerally, with every cell in my body. I craved everything about it, from its taste to the funny numb feeling my face would get after eight or ten drinks. Then the obsession would set in, and I'd spend hours reliving my drinking days, weighing the relative merits of beer versus wine, constructing a mental map of the nearest liquor stores.

When my therapist suggested acupuncture as a supplemental (adjunct) treatment option, I was more than desperate enough to give it a try. I'd already tried treating my anxiety with guided meditation, breathing exercises, and aromatherapy, among other things, but never noticed much of an effect. But within minutes of the needle insertion, I experienced a strange physical sensation, like my skull was expanding at my temples, relieving the pressure caused by my racing, repetitive thoughts. The tension that seemed to completely permeate my body dissipated. When I left, I was finally calm. As I continued to receive acupuncture treatment over the coming weeks, my interest in the science behind this approach grew.

Although the practice of acupuncture is thousands of years old, its application to addiction recovery is relatively recent. In 1972, a surgeon in Hong Kong was using acupuncture to treat postoperative pain in a patient who also happened to be an opium addict (NADA Brochure 2016). He found that the treatment relieved not only the patient's pain but also his withdrawal symptoms. A few years later, several doctors at Lincoln Hospital in the South Bronx, New York, began developing an acupuncture protocol designed specifically for addiction recovery, now called the National Acupuncture Detoxification Association (NADA) protocol (Bemis 2013b). Today, this protocol is used as a supplement to conventional treatment approaches in over 40 countries, including at 1,000 treatment centers in the United States and Canada alone (NADA Brochure).

Nevertheless, acupuncture remains controversial, both in general and in the context of addiction treatment. Many, many people, myself included, have reported a relief of cravings, anxiety, and withdrawal symptoms when treated with the NADA protocol, in which five needles are placed in each outer ear for 30–45 minutes. However, scientists don't yet understand how acupuncture works: how do these needles change the chemistry of the brain to relieve these symptoms? Moreover, there isn't actually a consensus on whether acupuncture itself has an effect, or whether patients' positive experiences are just a placebo effect induced by the expectation of a positive experience.

Scientists designing experiments to investigate the efficacy of acupuncture for addiction treatment face numerous challenges. Sample sizes are often small due to funding and logistical issues, which make it difficult to obtain statistically significant results. Furthermore, it is difficult to create double-blind conditions, in which neither the subjects nor the researchers know which subjects are in the experimental group and which are in the control group. Double-blind conditions are critical for obtaining meaningful results, as they protect against the placebo effect (because the subjects are unaware of whether they're receiving the true treatment) and researcher bias. Many studies create single-blinding by treating the control group with "sham" acupuncture, in which needles are placed in the skin, but not at accepted acupuncture points. However, it is difficult to blind the experimenter (placing the needles), as anyone trained in acupuncture or familiar with the research topic will recognize which needle locations are "true" acupuncture points.

Conclusive evidence regarding the effectiveness of acupuncture for addiction treatment, though elusive, would greatly benefit clinicians and patients alike. If its effectiveness is disproved, the resources currently being used to provide acupuncture services could be directed to other addiction treatments. However, if acupuncture is effective, efforts should be made to further promote it, as it offers unique benefits when used as an adjunct to other treatments. For example, acupuncture is relatively low cost, as needles are inexpensive and many U.S. states and Canadian provinces allow the NADA protocol to be performed by non-acupuncturists (such as social workers, correctional officers, and disaster responders) (NADA Brochure). The NADA protocol is also nonverbal and can thus be used with nonverbal patients or across language barriers (Bemis 2013a).

Tens of millions of Americans will suffer from addiction at some point in their lives, and addiction is responsible for tens of thousands of deaths each year (Sederer 2015). Acupuncture is poised to be a powerful ally in this fight, but further clinical studies and fundamental research are needed to determine what its role should be.

References

Bemis, Ryan. 2013a. "Ear Acupuncture and Humanitarian Aid: History, Application, and Improvement of the NADA Model." Laramie, WY: National Acupuncture Detoxification

Association (NADA) Literature Clearinghouse. http://www
.acudetox.com/about-nada/resources-and-research/category/
36-resources-research-outreach?download=176:ear-acupun
cture-and-humanitarian-aid. Accessed on July 31, 2016.

Bemis, Ryan. 2013b. "Evidence for the NADA Ear
Acupuncture Protocol: Summary of Research." National
Acupuncture Detoxification Association. http://www
.acudetox.com/phocadownload/Research_Summary_
2013%20(2).pdf. Accessed on July 31, 2016.

"NADA Brochure." 2016. National Acupuncture
Detoxification Association. http://www.acudetox.com/
phocadownload/NADAbrochure_Final2016Revised.pdf.
Accessed on July 31, 2016.

Sederer, Lloyd. 2015. "A Blind Eye to Addiction." US News
and World Report. http://www.usnews.com/opinion/
blogs/policy-dose/2015/06/01/america-is-neglecting-its-
addiction-problem. Accessed on July 31, 2016.

*Cassandra Newell is a scientist-turned-writer, a former MIT
chemistry PhD student, and a graduate of Colby College. Happily
sober, Cassandra lives in Somerville, Massachusetts, with her two
catbeasts.*

Creating Recovery-Supportive Campuses
John Ruyak

Heading to college is an exciting opportunity for many students, but those in recovery from a substance use disorder
(SUD) may have a different experience. For students in recovery the decision to go to college may be a difficult choice, one
that may put their recovery at risk. These students often have to
choose between sobriety and attending college. Many make the
choice to postpone college in order to maintain their health.
Still, there are some who choose to pursue a college degree.

At a college with 30,000 undergraduate students, it is esti-mated that there can be as many as 450 students seeking help for a substance abuse issue (Harris and Thompson 2005, 7). Imagine you are one of these students. You came to college straight out of inpatient treatment for an alcohol-related SUD. You spent 90 days working an intensive program, building resiliency and prioritizing health rather than your next drink. As you move into your residence hall you hear hall mates plan-ning what they will drink at tonight's party; you know others drink, but already the drinking culture surrounds you. Mid-week as class is wrapping up, your professor normalizes alcohol use by imploring everyone to study at least a little before going out. What you haven't heard is anyone talking about not drink-ing. Later that week there is a football game and open contain-ers of alcohol are allowed on campus during games. Thousands of people are on campus, many drinking from open bottles of beer while moving between pop-up bars in the back of pickup trucks.

The truth is that the college environment is one that is absti-nent hostile (Cleveland et al. 2003, 13). For people in recovery, this is what they must brave if they wish to obtain a degree at a traditional college. College campuses are steeped in traditions that perpetuate the widespread use of alcohol; in fact, accord-ing to the National College Health Assessment 2015 survey, 57.2 percent of undergraduate student's report drinking alco-hol in a 30-day period (American College Health Association 2016, 7). Whether this use is being perpetuated by the media, at certain on-campus events, or by student organizations, stu-dents in recovery face this everyday as they attempt to maintain their recovery and do well in school.

When students in recovery advocate for themselves they are often met with stigma from their friends as well as the univer-sity. They hear things like "It isn't addiction if you are in col-lege." They feel ostracized as teachers say, "watch out for this one" after they disclose their condition. They feel let down as administrators refuse to provide support because the university avoids acknowledging that students on their campus may have SUDs and that this may be connected to the campus's culture of alcohol use. So students remain isolated as they weather environments entrenched with alcohol and other substance use.

Fortunately, colleges can support students in recovery. Across the nation many colleges support students in recovery by formally integrating CRPs (collegiate recovery programs) into their operations. This can include dedicated spaces where students can gather and find support from like-minded peers. In some cases, campuses are able to provide dedicated faculty, scholarships, and recovery-specific housing and academic courses to create comprehensive CRPs. These schools are saying, "Students in recovery are welcome on this campus, they have unique needs and we will support them." Unfortunately, among the thousands of colleges there is a paltry number of officially recognized CRPs. There are 4,726 institutions of higher education with about 170 collegiate recovery support efforts, including formalized CRPs and fledgling efforts, currently in the United States (U.S. Department of Education 2016; Collegiate Recovery Asset Map 2016).

The evidence to support the effectiveness of CRPs is growing. Programs report that their CRPs have low returns to use, and higher GPAs and higher graduation rates than the general student population (Laudet et al. 2014, 6). The promise of these programs should compel administrators to develop recovery support programs. However, students and their allies still struggle to obtain the resources necessary to start sustainable CRPs.

To bring comprehensive recovery support to every campus, institutions must start accepting the disease model of SUDs. Medically speaking, SUDs are diagnosable and treatable diseases. Every student, regardless of his or her health status, has the right to attend college. However, without recovery support college systems continue to endanger the health and well-being, as well as the success of someone with a disease. This would be a social justice issue in any other context. This framework should be applied to those suffering or recovering from SUDs because it is unjust to threaten the right to education because of a diagnosable disease.

Many colleges provide comprehensive recovery support for their students, and the number is growing. If administrators and professionals at colleges start to view recovery support as an essential resource on their campuses, much like resources for veterans and LGBTQ communities, a culture of caring, understanding, and acceptance for those affected by SUDs will start to take shape. Students would no longer have to choose between maintaining their recovery and obtaining a degree. This should be the aim of our schools, to create systems where no person is hindered from successfully obtaining a degree because of a disease that they did not choose to have.

References

American College Health Association. 2016. American College Health Association—National College Health Assessment II: Undergraduate Reference Group Executive Summary Fall 2015. Hanover, MD: American College Health Association. http://www.acha-ncha.org/docs/NCHA-II_FALL_2015_UNDERGRADUATE_REFERENCE_GROUP_EXECUTIVE_SUMMARY.pdf. Accessed on July 31, 2016.

Cleveland, H., et al. 2003. "Characteristics of a Collegiate Recovery Community: Maintaining Recovery in an Abstinence-Hostile Environment." *Journal of Substance Abuse Treatment*. 33(1): 13–23.

"Collegiate Recovery Asset Map." 2016. Transforming Youth Recovery. https://collegiaterecovery.capacitype.com/map. Accessed on July 31, 2016.

Harris, K., A. Baker and A. Thompson. 2005. "Developing a Collegiate Recovery Community: Project 1." Center for Collegiate Recovery Communities. http://www.depts.ttu.edu/hs/csa/docs/1.pdf. Accessed on July 31, 2016.

Laudet, A., et al. 2014. "Collegiate Recovery Communities Programs: What Do We Know and What Do We Need to Know?" *Journal of Social Work Practice in the Addictions.* 14(1): 84–100.

U.S. Department of Education, National Center for Education Statistics. 2016. Digest of Education Statistics, 2014 (NCES 2016-006), Table 105.50.

John Ruyak, MPH, is the alcohol, drug and recovery specialist at Oregon State University's Student Health Services Department. He leads the campus's CRP, as well as helps run the school's alcohol and drug harm reduction programs. He is an ally of students in recovery and a proponent of sound policy and programming aimed at reducing the prevalence of high-risk drinking on college campuses.

Five Days
Ed and Marnie Semeyn

Our daughter Stephanie's substance abuse spanned over half of her 41 years. Her drug use began experimentally, but over the years progressed to increasingly more addictive substances. Ultimately, her "drug of choice" was heroin. Her years of substance abuse were a roller-coaster ride, the bottom marked by a lifestyle of addiction, and the upswing marked by the climb to recovery, only to be followed by another downward cycle into the wasteland of addiction. Over her years of substance abuse Stephanie had been through at least four different drug rehab programs.

Although she had not been living with us for the last ten years, we maintained sporadic contact by phone since she lived in the same town. Whenever we were convinced she had again fallen into vise of addiction, we severed all contact, having learned all too well the pitfalls of enabling. On the other hand, whenever Stephanie entered a drug recovery program, we provided as much support and loving care as possible. We participated in numerous counseling and group therapy sessions.

Stephanie well knew we were her strongest supporters in her climb to recovery, but she also knew that we would completely divorce ourselves from any involvement with her when she fell back into the oblivion of addiction.

TUESDAY: A phone message was left by one of our local hospitals, informing us that a woman had been admitted earlier that day. No further information was provided. Upon our arrival at the hospital, we were given directions to what we soon learned was the CCU (Critical Care Unit). The doctors immediately briefed us on what they knew about the circumstances leading up to Stephanie's arrival at the hospital. Apparently, Stephanie had passed out in somebody's house, and whoever was with her couldn't get her to respond. An ambulance was called, and Stephanie was rushed to the hospital, sweating profusely and barely uttering a few unintelligible words.

After providing the doctors with as much history as we could about our daughter's years of substance abuse, we were then updated on her present condition. Stephanie had been stabilized for the present, but her life signs were extremely weak. Her heart rate and blood pressure were dangerously low, requiring the implementation of a respirator along with a number of IV lines.

After our consultation with the medical staff, we entered the softly lit room and saw our daughter for the first time in weeks. Her head was turned slightly to the side, and apart from the mechanical sound of the respirator, the room was oppressively quiet. One of the IVs, we were told, administered potent antibiotics to combat a virulent blood infection (MRSA). As one of the doctors explained, a "vegetable matter" of infection had formed on Stephanie's heart valves, the result being that the doctors could not make progress against the infection because as the blood recirculated through the valves of her heart, the effect of the antibiotics was being compromised by the MRSA that had attached to her heart valves and was reinfecting her blood. We suspect that Stephanie contracted MRSA from contaminated drugs or possibly dirty needles.

We were also told that Stephanie was being administered what the doctors said was a "suppressor," which had the effect of narrowing her blood vessels. This was being done to help maintain her blood pressure, and reduce the strain on her already weakened heart.

We remained with our daughter for a few hours, trying to process what we had learned. We knew her condition was serious, but how serious? What was the prognosis? Should we look ahead to an eventual recovery, or was there a darker future in store? The doctors were noncommittal, because, no doubt, they likewise were unsure about what the future held. We left the hospital that day with nothing to cling to except our hopes and our prayers.

WEDNESDAY: As we entered the CCU, the doctors asked us to meet with them in a nearby conference room. Once seated, we were told that two further developments in Stephanie's condition had occurred since the previous day. First, Stephanie was experiencing some swelling of her brain and we were asked if we would sign a medical release permitting the insertion of a shunt into the back of her skull to drain off some fluid, thereby lowering the pressure on her brain. We immediately complied. Next we were told that the downside of using a "suppressor" was that circulation was frequently cut off to the small blood vessels in the extremities (fingers and toes), the result being a gradual blackening of Stephanie's fingers and toes, and the possibility that some of them might have to be removed.

We were shocked as well as stunned by both disclosures. It was as if each new day brought an additional setback, and the hope for our daughter's recovery increasingly remote. We left the hospital that day hollow and emotionally drained.

THURSDAY. Two days had passed since Stephanie was hospitalized. She remained completely unresponsive, and now her condition was further complicated by brain swelling and the very real possibility of losing some of her appendages, all while her life remained dependent on a respirator, and MRSA continued to rage through her bloodstream (despite the antibiotics).

We arrived at the hospital to learn that Stephanie's brain swelling had gone down. We grabbed on to this news as it seemed to offer the first glimmer of hope. The first sign of something positive to cling to. Was this, perhaps, the beginning of a gradual turnaround, eventually leading to some measure of recovery? Unfortunately, no other promising news was forthcoming.

At home that evening, my wife had finally reached the breaking point. She told me she wanted to meet with the entire medical staff involved in caring for Stephanie. She wanted answers to questions concerning the possibility of Steph's recovery.

Throughout this ordeal our two younger daughters were kept fully informed about each day's developments. Anne is three years younger than Stephanie, while Courtney is six years younger. Both sisters were just as distraught as we were about their sister's condition.

FRIDAY. We arrived at the hospital, accompanied by our pastor, and immediately requested to meet with the medical staff (three doctors and two critical care nurses). We wanted to know what the prospects were for our daughter's recovery. They could speculate, but not speak to the possibility of recovery with any certainty. One of the nurses said that Stephanie could very possibly be on a respirator for the rest of her life. We talked, we cried, we prayed. At this lowest point, our pastor provided immeasurable comfort and support. Her presence was truly a blessing.

As the meeting drew to a close, we wanted to know what would happen were Stephanie to be removed from the respirator. The response was predictably clinical, our response: despair. Before we left the hospital we expressed to the medical staff what we, as a family, had finally decided.

Late that evening I was sitting on our back porch trying to distract myself by attempting to read. Unable to focus my attention

I paused, and as I gazed out at the enveloping darkness, I heard a barely audible voice. "It's OK Dad, you can let me go."

SATURDAY. Our daughter, Anne, drove in from the other side of the state. Courtney, the youngest sister, lived in Montana, unable to arrive before our request was carried out.

As explained by the doctors on Friday, when the respirator was turned off Stephanie's heart rate would likely continue normally for 5–10 minutes. Shortly thereafter there would be a gradual weakening as well as lengthening of seconds between heart beats. As this occurred, my wife and I, along with our daughter Anne, sat quietly watching the heart monitor.

Courtney had called Stephanie's room on Anne's cell phone, tearfully demanding to talk to her sister. As Stephanie's heart rate weakened, Anne held her cell phone to Stephanie's ear, while Courtney cried out her love for her sister.

Fifteen to 20 minutes after the respirator was turned off, the shock of what had just happened overwhelmed us. Our beloved daughter/sister was gone. A mother, father, and daughter stood at the foot of Stephanie's bed, our arms wrapped tightly around each other as our grief poured out in heart-wrenching sobs. Four lives forever diminished.

Ed Semeyn: For most of my boyhood years I spent my summers playing softball and baseball at a local park where David Newton, the author of this book, was both my coach and mentor. Professionally, I spent 33 years teaching social studies at our local high school, after which I worked part-time in a public library. Now I am fully retired.

Marnie Semeyn: Over the years my wife has enjoyed a rich and varied career: aerobics and racquetball instructor, owner and operator of a tanning salon business ("Oasis Tanning"). For the past several years she has pursued her passion—gardening and runs a small gardening enterprise of 20 clients. She is also actively involved in church work, and volunteers at a local hospital guild.

Psychiatric Disorders and Substance Abuse: Comorbidity, Correlation, and Causation
Teagan Wall

Over 20 million Americans have been diagnosed with some form of substance abuse disorder, classified as the use of one or more substances causing a disruption of one's life and/or mental and physical distress. On top of that, almost 8 million of those people were diagnosed with another form of mental disease or disorder (Mental and Substance Use Disorder 2016). The co-occurrence of mental disorders and substance abuse disorder has been studied from the onset of both or each disorder to the progression and treatment of the diseases. Understanding how mental health and substance abuse interact with one another can help prevention organizations better educate the public and help doctors design better treatment plans.

Addiction is defined as compulsively engaging in destructive or detrimental rewarding stimuli, despite the negative consequences of those actions. Under this definition, anything as common as sugar or video games can be thought of as addictive, depending on the level of compulsion and the negative effect of the behaviors on the individual's life. Substance abuse disorder, on the other hand, requires the ingestion or use of a mind-altering or psychoactive substance. The difference between these two issues is thus not behavioral, but physiological. Substance abuse disorder often stems from a combination of addictive behaviors and physiological changes or impulses resulting from previous substance use.

Contrary to popular belief, not all substance use and addiction is illegal, or even necessarily socially unacceptable. The most common example is nicotine addiction. Over 15 percent of Americans smoke cigarettes (Centers for Disease Control and Prevention, 2015). Despite the fact that almost 70 percent of smokers want to quit smoking, and the fact that the health risks of smoking are well documented and studied, thousands of teenagers under the age of 18 smoke their first cigarette every day (U.S. Department of Health and Human Services 2014).

For these teens, smoking is strongly associated with other mental health disorders later in life, including major depression and anxiety disorders. The relationship between substance abuse, even for substances like nicotine, and mental health is a prevalent and important one.

One question scientists often ask is whether individuals with underlying mental health conditions are more likely to use psychoactive drugs and develop substance abuse disorder, or whether the mental conditions are caused, or at least greatly exacerbated, by drug use. The answer may vary depending on both the type of mental illness, and the type of drug used. Psychologists and academics use a measure called the Sensation Seeking Scale (SSS) to look at a person's level of sensation seeking impulses and desires. This scale has four subscales: thrill seeking, disinhibition, experience seeking, and boredom susceptibility. The results of this test can be used to support or confirm certain psychiatric diagnoses, including impulse control disorder, attention deficit hyperactivity disorder (ADHD), depression, and anxiety. Additionally, several studies have shown high levels of correlation between overall SSS levels and drug use, as well as between subscale levels and the use of specific subtypes of psychoactive drugs.

For a more specific example, one study (Andrucci et al. 1989) found that use of amphetamine (a powerful stimulant) among teenagers is highly correlated with overall SSS levels and all subscale levels except boredom seeking, with which it has only a much weaker correlation. This result is especially interesting because boredom-seeking measures are often used to support ADHD diagnoses, and amphetamine is commonly prescribed to treat ADHD. One possibility is that amphetamine is less pleasurable in the ADHD brain compared to people without ADHD, and thus is less commonly used by people with that disorder. This possibly indicates that the presence of psychiatric disorders or predispositions is not only a predictor of substance abuse, but is also potentially indicative of which drugs an individual is likely to abuse.

This particular example and set of tests suggests that psychiatric disorders may precipitate drug use and substance abuse disorders. Other examples, including the relationship between schizophrenia and smoking (schizophrenics smoke more, and absorb more nicotine when smoking, compared to non-schizophrenic smokers, apparently as a form of self-medication), support this claim (Schizophrenia and Smoking 1995). However, it may not be the whole story. Drug use may trigger the onset or worsening of certain psychiatric disorders as well. One study (Lahti et al. 1995) showed that even very low doses of ketamine, an anesthetic and sedative, could trigger severe psychotic symptoms. A previously undiagnosed and apparently healthy individual, who is highly predisposed to schizophrenia, could therefore potentially trigger a psychotic episode, or accelerate the onset of the disease, by using these drugs. Additionally, chronic drug use or substance abuse disorder can permanently alter brain chemistry, potentially resulting in psychiatric disorders such as depression and anxiety later in life.

Exactly why individuals, especially adolescents, begin using psychoactive substances recreationally, knowing the risks to their physical and mental health, their neurodevelopment, and potentially their criminal record, is still not well understood. Lack of temporal reasoning, an inability to properly weight small but extremely costly risks, and a reduced capability to comprehend the complete set of pros and cons likely play an important role, as well as the mental health status of those individuals prior to drug use. Improving our understanding of the relationship between typical decision-making abilities at various stages of the brain's development versus disordered sensation-seeking behavior can help create and target improved drug prevention and intervention programs for both teens and adults.

References

Andrucci, Gay L., et al. 1989. "The Relationship of MMPI and Sensation Seeking Scales to Adolescent Drug Use." *Journal of Personality Assessment*. 53(2): 253–266. doi: 10.1207/s15327752jpa5302_4.

Centers for Disease Control and Prevention. 2015. "Current Cigarette Smoking among Adults—United States, 2005–2014." *Morbidity and Mortality Weekly Report.* 64(44): 1233–1240. http://www.cdc.gov/mmwr/preview/mmwrhtml/mm6444a2.htm?s_cid=mm6444a2_w. Accessed on July 31, 2016.

Lahti, A. C., et al. 1995. "Subanesthetic Doses of Ketamine Stimulate Psychosis in Schizophrenia." *Neuropsychopharmacology.* 13(1): 9–19.

"Mental and Substance Use Disorders." 2016. Substance Abuse and Mental Health Services Administration. http://www.samhsa.gov/disorders. Accessed on July 31, 2016.

"Schizophrenia and Smoking: An Epidemiological Survey in a State Hospital." 1995. *American Journal of Psychiatry.* 152(3): 453–55.

U.S. Department of Health and Human Services. 2014. "The Health Consequences of Smoking—50 Years of Progress: A Report of the Surgeon General." Atlanta: U.S. Department of Health and Human Services, Centers for Disease Control and Prevention, National Center for Chronic Disease Prevention and Health Promotion, Office on Smoking and Health. http://www.surgeongeneral.gov/library/reports/50-years-of-progress/full-report.pdf. Accessed on July 31, 2016.

Dr. Teagan Wall received her PhD in computation and neural systems from Caltech, where she studied the behavioral neuropharmacology of nicotinic compounds in the Lester Lab. She is passionate about educating the public on the mechanisms and inherent biases in decision making and has addressed this topic on various podcasts, YouTube channels, blogs, and television programs.

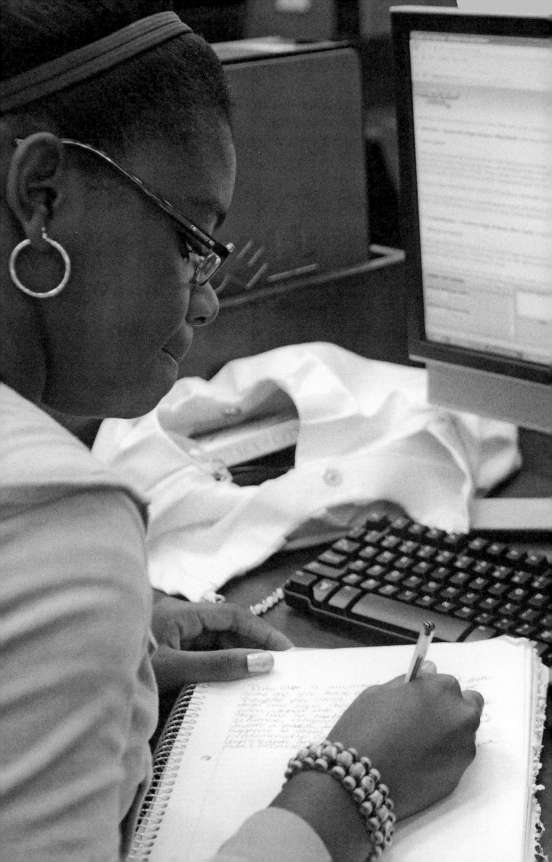

Introduction

Any history of drugs, substance abuse, alcoholism, smoking, and the political, legal, and social issues surrounding these topics must include a long list of women and men who have had a significant impact on that history. Some individuals have conducted research on these substances; others have advocated for or against their use; still others have devoted their lives to developing prevention programs or methods of treatment; and many have been involved in the development of local, state, national, or international policy with respect to substance use and abuse. This chapter provides biographies of a number of individuals, with a review of their contribution to the history of substance abuse, as well as a brief biographical sketch of each person.

Much the same can be said for a host of organizations that have been created to deal with substance-related issues. Groups such as the Partnership for Drug-Free Kids, the National Institute on Drug Abuse, the Substance Abuse and Mental Health Services Administration, and Alcoholics Anonymous have saved countless numbers of lives, as well as helping to shape local, state, and national policies on substance abuse issues. Brief sketches of some of these organizations are also included in this chapter.

Michelle Ngwafla, 16, takes notes on the answer she was given by government scientists at the National Institute on Drug Abuse to her online questions during class at Rockville High School in Rockville, Maryland, on October 7, 2008. (AP Photo/Kevin Wolf)

Al-Anon/Alateen

Al-Anon was founded in 1951 by Lois W., wife of Bill W., founder of Alcoholics Anonymous, and Anne B. The organization grew rapidly and was incorporated in 1954 under the name of Al-Anon Family Group Headquarters, Inc. The purpose of the organization was to assist family members in dealing with the problems they faced as loved ones of alcoholics. A year later, the group published its first book, *The Al-Anon Family Groups, A Guide for the Families of Problem Drinkers*. In 1957, a similar support group was formed for and by the children of men and women with alcohol problems, a group that was given the name Alateen. A year later, the board of directors of Al-Anon decided to establish an Alateen Committee and in 1964, a special staff person was hired to work with Alateen groups. Today, Al-Anon sees itself as an organization not designed to give advice or to work toward changing people's alcohol issues, but as an opportunity for those whose lives are affected by alcoholism to share their personal experiences with each other. It has outreach programs not only to spouses and children, but also to parents, grandparents, and siblings of alcoholics.

Al-Anon's regular magazine is *The Forum*. Since its founding, the organization has produced more than 100 books and pamphlets on topics such as *Discovering Choices* (book); *Dilemma of the Alcoholic Marriage* (book); *Hope for Today* (book); *One Day at a Time* (book); *Blueprint for Progress* (book); *Al-Anon/Alateen Service Manual* (booklet); *When I Got Busy, I Got Better* (booklet); *The Best of Public Outreach* (booklet); "Al-Anon is for Men" (pamphlet); "Alcoholism: The Family Disease" (pamphlet); "So You Love an Alcoholic" (pamphlet); "The Twelve Steps and Tradition" (pamphlet); "Alateen Newcomer Packet" (kit); and "Courage to Change" (CD-ROM).

Alcoholics Anonymous

Alcoholics Anonymous was founded by two men attempting to deal with their alcoholism, William Griffith ("Bill") Wilson and Robert Holbrook ("Bob") Smith. The traditional date for the founding of the organization is set at June 10, 1935, the date on which Smith had his last drink. Although the organization keeps no formal records, it has estimated that, as of January 1, 2016, it had 1,262,542 members in 60,698 groups in the United States, and 50,555 groups overseas, with 705,850 members. The total number of groups worldwide was estimated at 117,748. The organization is very simple in concept, with no membership dues or requirements, other than the desire to quit drinking. It is perhaps best known for its twelve-step program for dealing with problems of alcoholism.

Among its more than 150 books, pamphlets, guides, and other materials are *Alcoholics Anonymous* (book); *Experience, Strength, and Hope* (book); *Twelve Steps and Twelve Traditions* (book); *As Bill Sees It* (book); *Living Sober* (book); *Young People and A.A.* (book); "44 Questions" (pamphlet); "Do You Think You're Different?" (pamphlet); "A.A. and the Armed Services" (pamphlet); "A Newcomer Asks" (pamphlet); "A.A. and the Gay/Lesbian Alcoholic" (pamphlet); and *Box 459* (newsletter).

Richard Alpert (Ram Dass; 1931–)

During the 1960s, Alpert was involved in research on psychoactive substances at Harvard University, along with his good friend and colleague Timothy Leary. He later spent time studying spiritualism in India and devoted the greatest part of his life to studying and teaching about this subject in the United States.

Richard Alpert was born on April 6, 1931, in Newton, Massachusetts. His father was a prominent attorney; president of the New York, New Haven, and Hartford railroad; and a founder of Brandeis University and the Albert Einstein College of Medicine in New York City. Alpert received his BA from Tufts University, his MA in motivation psychology from Wesleyan University, and his PhD in human development from Stanford University. He then accepted a teaching and research post in the Department of Social Relations and the Graduate

School of Education at Harvard University. While at Harvard, he met Timothy Leary, from whom he learned about the psychoactive effects of a number of substances. Between 1960 and 1961, Alpert and Leary began a series of experiments on psilocybin, using graduate students at their subjects. The direction of these experiments was sufficiently troubling to Harvard administrators that both men were dismissed from their academic positions. That move was of little concern to Alpert, who later said that he had already become disillusioned with academics as a "meaningless pursuit."

In 1967, Alpert traveled to India, where he met his spiritual teacher, Neem Karoli Baba, and received his new name, Ram Dass, or "servant of God." He has spent the rest of his life studying a variety of spiritualistic philosophies, including Hinduism, karma, yoga, and Sufism. He is probably best known today not for his early studies of psychoactive substances, but for his 1971 book, *Be Here Now*. His other publications include *The Psychedelic Experience: A Manual Based on the Tibetan Book of the Dead* (with Leary and Ralph Metzner); *Doing Your Own Being* (1973); *The Only Dance There Is* (1974); *Journey of Awakening: A Mediator's Guidebook* (1978); *Compassion in Action: Setting Out on the Path of Service* (with Mirabai Bush; 1991); *Still Here: Embracing Aging, Changing and Dying* (2000); *Paths to God: Living The Bhagavad Gita* (2004); *Be Love Now* (with Rameshwar Das; 2010); and *Polishing the Mirror: How to Live from Your Spiritual Heart* (with Rameshwar Das; 2013). In 1997, Alpert suffered a stroke that paralyzed the right side of his body and left him with Broca's aphasia, a brain condition that makes speech difficult. Nonetheless, he continues to write, teach, and lecture, as his condition permits.

American Society of Addiction Medicine

The American Society of Addiction Medicine (ASAM) had its origins in the early 1950s, largely through the efforts of Dr. Ruth Fox, who initiated a series of meeting with fellow physicians interested in the research and clinical aspects of alcoholism and its treatment. In 1954, this group formalized its existence by creating the New York Medical Society on Alcoholism (NYMSA). The organization's work was funded primarily by the U.S. Alcohol, Drug Abuse, and Mental Health Administration, predecessor of today's Substance Abuse and Mental Health Services Administration (SAMHSA). In 1967, NYMSA decided to extend its work nationwide and changed its name to the American Medical Society on Alcoholism (AMSA).

As interest in medical aspects of drug abuse and addiction grew in the 1970s, a second organization began operation in California, the California Society for the Treatment of Alcoholism and Other Drug Dependencies (CSTAODD), expanding traditional alcohol treatment programs to include those dependent on or addicted to drugs. Over time, the two groups at opposite ends of the country, AMSA and CSTAODD, began to collaborate with each other, eventually leading to their union in 1983 under AMSA's name. In 1988, AMSA was accepted by the American Medical Association (AMA) as a national medical specialty society and adopted its present name of the American Society of Addiction Medicine (ASAM). Today, the organization consists of more than 3,200 physicians and related health providers interested primarily in issues of substance abuse. It has state chapters in 36 states and the District of Columbia, along with regional chapters in northern New England and the Northwest that include states that do not have their own separate chapters.

The work carried out by ASAM can be divided into four major categories: education, advocacy, research and treatment, and practice support. The organization's education component is designed to provide physicians and other health care workers with the most up-to-date information on basic issues in addiction treatment. In 2015, for example, ASAM offered a review course in addiction medicine and courses on buprenorphine treatment, state-of-the-art in addiction medicine, and opioid risk evaluation and mitigation strategies. The advocacy element in ASAM's program is aimed at influencing state and federal policies involving substance abuse to reflect the organization's goals and objectives. Some examples of the types of action it has taken include pushing for insurance coverage of mental health and addiction disorders, working for the repeal of alcoholism exclusions in insurance policies, expanding treatment for substance abuse among veterans, and regulating the sale of tobacco and alcohol to minors.

The research and treatment feature of ASAM's work aims to provide health care providers with a wide range of informational materials on all aspects of addiction and substance abuse. Some of the materials it provides are a Common Threads Conference on Pain and Addiction; clinical updates from the International Association for the Study of Pain; a joint statement on pain and addiction from the American Pain Society, the American Academy of Pain Medicine, and the American Society of Addiction Medicine; and a variety of publications on prescription drug abuse from federal agencies. The area of practice support is designed to provide materials that will help addiction physicians and other providers with the best available information about best practices in the field of addiction medicine. These materials include guidelines and consensus documents, such as the National Practice Guideline for Medications for the Treatment of Opioid Use Disorder; "how to's" and practice resources, such as the Drug Enforcement Administration document, "How to Prepare for a DEA Office Inspection"; standards and performance measures, such as the ASAM Standards of Care for the Addiction Specialist Physician Document; and "ASAM Criteria," a comprehensive set of guidelines for placement, continued stay, and transfer/discharge of patients with addiction and co-occurring conditions.

ASAM produces and provides a wide variety of print and electronic publications for the addiction physician and health care worker, such as the books *Principle of Addiction Medicine* and *The ASAM Essentials of Addiction Medicine; Journal of Addiction Medicine,* the association's official peer-reviewed journal; *ASAMagazine,* a publication containing news and commentary; and "ASAM Weekly," an online publication intended for both members and nonmembers who are interested in issues of addiction medicine.

Americans for Nonsmokers' Rights

Americans for Nonsmokers' Rights (ANR) was founded in 1976 for the purpose of protecting nonsmokers from the hazards posed by secondhand cigarette smoke, to prevent young people from becoming addicted to tobacco products, and to act as a counterforce to the tobacco industry in efforts to reduce the use of tobacco products in the United States. The organization is primarily member-supported and works to support all types of regulation of secondhand smoke, including voluntary, legislative, and regulatory policies. It also works to support legislative and regulatory efforts to limit the influence of the tobacco industry in the development of national policies on smoking and tobacco use. ANR's sister organization, the American Nonsmokers' Rights Foundation, was founded in 1982 to develop programs for school-age youth on the importance of smoke-free spaces in American society. The organization publishes a quarterly newsletter, *UPDATE!,* and has available on its website numerous fact sheets on topics such as secondhand smoke; economic impact of secondhand smoke; ventilation; preemption by the tobacco industry; going smoke-free at home, work, and in the community; smoke-free travel; legal issues; and target populations.

Americans for Safe Access

Americans for Safe Access (ASA) calls itself the "largest national member-based organization of patients, medical professionals, scientists and concerned citizens promoting safe and legal access to cannabis for therapeutic use and research." The organization has more than 30,000 members and chapters in 40 states. Founded in 2002, ASA lists a number of important accomplishments in its brief history, including organizing legal support for more than 30 individuals being accused of illegal marijuana use, conducting training tours on individual rights in the field of medical marijuana, organizing protest rallies against state and local actions against the medical uses of marijuana, filing suit against laws prohibiting the cultivation of marijuana for medical purposes, and working on the sponsorship of legislation to protect the rights of individuals who use marijuana for medical purposes.

On its web page, ASA has separate sections with specialized information about medical marijuana for medical patients, legal professionals, medical professionals, policy makers, and producers and providers. The website also provides news stories on recent events in the field of medical marijuana.

Harry J. Anslinger (1892–1975)

Anslinger was appointed the first commissioner of the Federal Bureau of Narcotics when it was established in 1930. He held that office for 32 years, one of the longest tenures of any federal official in modern history. He was consistently a strong advocate for severe penalties against the manufacture, distribution, sale, and use of certain drugs, especially marijuana.

Harry Jacob Anslinger was born in Altoona, Pennsylvania, on May 20, 1892, to Robert J. and Rosa Christiana Fladt Anslinger, immigrants from Switzerland and Germany, respectively. Upon completing high school, Anslinger attended the Altoona Business College before taking a job with the Pennsylvania Railroad. He received a leave of absence from the railway that allowed him to matriculate at Pennsylvania State College (now Pennsylvania State University), where he received his two-year associate degree in engineering and business management. From 1917 to 1928, Anslinger worked for a number of private and governmental agencies on problems of illegal drug use, a job that took him to a number of countries around the world. He has been credited with helping to shape drug policies both in the United States and in the foreign countries where he worked or consulted.

In 1929, Anslinger was appointed assistant commissioner in the United States Bureau of Prohibition, a position he held only briefly before being selected as the first commissioner of the newly created Federal Bureau of Narcotics in 1930. He assumed that post at a time when state and federal officials were debating the need (or lack of need) for regulations of hemp and marijuana. Both hemp and marijuana are obtained from plants in the genus *Cannabis*, the former with many important industrial applications, and the latter used as a recreational and medicinal drug. Historians have discussed the motivations that may have driven Anslinger's attitudes about the subject, but his actions eventually demonstrated a very strong opposition to the growing, processing, distribution, and use of all products of the cannabis plant. He was instrumental in formulating federal policies and laws against such use that developed during the 1930s.

Anslinger remained in his post until 1970, staying on even after his 70th birthday until a replacement was found. He then served two more years as U.S. representative to the United Nations Narcotic Convention. By the end of his tenure with the convention, he was blind and suffered from both angina and an enlarged prostate. He died in Hollidaysburg, Pennsylvania, on November 14, 1975, of heart failure.

Association for Medical Education and Research in Substance Abuse

The Association for Medical Education and Research in Substance Abuse (AMERSA) has more than 300 physician members from a number of specialty areas, along with nurses, social workers, psychologists, pharmacologists, dentists, and other professionals. The organization was founded in 1976 by members of the Career Teachers Program, which was then funded by the National Institute on Alcohol Abuse and Alcoholism and the National Institute on Drug Abuse for the purpose of developing faculty members with special training in the area of substance abuse. Members of AMERSA have developed, implemented, and evaluated curricula, educational programs, and faculty development programs and clinical and research measures for substance abuse services and professional education, and have conducted research related to substance abuse education, clinical service, and prevention. AMERSA sponsors an annual conference on substance abuse education, provides a speakers' bureau on the topic, and currently has a task force on physician education in the field of substance abuse. The organization publishes a quarterly peer-reviewed journal, *Substance Abuse*, and a regular newsletter, *About AMERSA*.

Bill W. (1895–1971)

Bill W. was cofounder with Dr. Bob of Alcoholics Anonymous (AA), an organization devoted to helping alcoholics attain sobriety. He had his last alcoholic drink on December 11, 1934, shortly after cofounding AA, and maintained his sobriety ever after that time.

Bill W. is the name preferred by William Griffith Wilson because it reflects and emphasizes the anonymity that AA asks of and offers to its members as they fight their battle against alcohol addiction. He was born on November 26, 1895, in East Dorset, Vermont, to Gilman Barrows Wilson, a womanizer and heavy drinker, and Emily Griffith Wilson, a strong-willed and abusive mother. His father abandoned the family in 1905, and his mother decided to do the same, choosing to study for a career in osteopathic medicine. Bill W. then became the ward of his maternal grandparents, with whom he spent the rest of his childhood.

After graduating from high school, Bill entered Norwich University, but remained there for only a short time, partly because of his shyness and lack of social skills, and partly because of his own misconduct and that of other classmates. It was during these years that he had his first drink, before rapidly becoming an alcoholic with many "lost weekends" in his life. He eventually was readmitted to Norwich, from which he graduated with a degree in electric engineering in 1917. He then served as a second lieutenant in the U.S. Army, a time during which his drinking became even more of a problem. When he returned at the end of the war, he took a job in the insurance department of the New York Central Railroad, while attending the Brooklyn Law School at night. He earned his law degree in 1920, but is said to have been too drunk to pick up his diploma.

Over the next decade, Bill worked as a field investigator for a number of financial firms, traveling over most of the United States to complete his assignments. Eventually, his drinking problem became so severe that he was unable to hold a job and he was admitted to the Charles B. Towns Hospital for Drug and Alcohol Addictions in New York City. Bill experienced his first, short-lived recovery in 1934 when he met an old drinking friend, Ebby Thacher, and learned that he (Thacher) had become sober largely through the efforts of an evangelical Christian organization known as the Oxford Group. Bill's own efforts to achieve a similar result failed, however, and he was returned to the Towns Hospital a second time. Finally, in May 1935, on a business trip to Akron, Ohio, Bill met another alcoholic who was going through struggles similar to his own, Robert Holbrook Smith ("Dr. Bob"), with whom he developed plans for a new group to help themselves and other alcoholics like themselves. That organization eventually grew to become the largest and most successful group for the treatment of alcoholism in the world. Bill spent the rest of his life serving in one role or another in AA. In 2009, *Time* magazine named Bill one of the 100 most important people of the twentieth century.

Bill was a heavy smoker throughout his life and developed emphysema in the 1960s, a condition from which he eventually died on January 24, 1971, while en route for treatment in Miami, Florida.

Hale Boggs (1914–1972/1973)

Boggs was a Democratic member of the U.S. House of Representative from Louisiana's Second Congressional District from 1947 to 1973. He was majority whip of the House from 1962 to 1971 and House Majority Leader from 1971 to 1973. In the years following the end of World War II, Boggs was one of the leading spokespersons for a more rigorous approach to sentencing for drug-related crimes. His position on the topic reflected that of many legislators, law enforcement officers, and members of the general public who believed that the use of illegal drugs had begun to skyrocket after the end of the war, and that some judges were treating the "drug epidemic" much too casually with overly generous fines and prison sentences. In 1951, Boggs submitted a bill to the Congress that dramatically increased the penalties for drug use and drug trafficking and, for the first time in U.S. history, applied those penalties equally to both narcotic drugs and marijuana. It also imposed mandatory sentencing for individuals convicted of drug-related crimes more than once. In 1956, Boggs also sponsored the Narcotic Control Act, which increased penalties even further.

Thomas Hale Boggs, Sr., was born on February 15, 1914, in Long Beach, Mississippi. He attended public and parochial schools in Jefferson Parish, Louisiana, before matriculating at Tulane University, in New Orleans, from which he received his bachelor's degree in journalism in 1934 and his law degree in 1937. He established his own law practice in New Orleans, but soon became interested in politics. He ran for the U.S. House of Representatives from the Second District of Louisiana in 1941 and was elected, but failed to receive his party's nomination for the same post a year later. He then returned to his law practice in New Orleans before enlisting in the U.S. Naval

Reserve in November 1943, after which he was assigned to the Potomac River Naval Command. He was discharged from the service in January 1946, ran for Congress again, and was once more elected to the U.S. House of Representatives. He served in that body until October 16, 1972, when he was lost on a flight from Anchorage to Juneau, Alaska, working for the campaign of Rep. Nick Begich. Neither the wreckage of the plane itself nor any of its passengers were ever found, and Boggs was declared legally dead on January 3, 1973, to allow the election of his successor, who, it turned out, was his wife, Lindy Boggs. Mrs. Boggs was then reelected eight more times, serving in the House until 1991.

Center for Lawful Access and Abuse Deterrence

The Center for Lawful Access and Abuse Deterrence (CLAAD) was founded in 2009 "to prevent prescription drug fraud, diversion, misuse, and abuse while advancing consumer access to high-quality health care." Funding for the organization is provided by a coalition of about a dozen commercial members (pharmaceutical companies) such as Allergan, Mallinckrodt Pharmaceuticals, Millennium Laboratories, Purdue Pharmaceuticals, and Zogenix. In addition to its commercial members, the organization includes a number of governmental and nonprofit organizations, including the Alliance for Safe Online Pharmacies, Allies in Recovery, American Pharmacists Association, American Society for Pain Management Nursing, American Society of Addiction Medicine, American Society of Anesthesiologists, Community Anti-Drug Coalitions of America, Drug Free America Foundation, Healthcare Distribution Management Association, International Nurses Society on Addictions, Johns Hopkins Bloomberg School of Public Health, National Alliance for Model State Drug Laws, National Association of Attorneys General, National District Attorneys Association, National Family Partnership, National

Governors Association, National Sheriffs' Association, Northeastern University, and the 15th Judicial Circuit of Florida.

CLAAD activities fall into three major categories: policy leadership, information and analysis, and coalition building. Policy leadership involves the development of laws, regulations, and other provisions that ensure that efforts to prevent the abuse and misuse of prescription drugs are effective without impeding the access of individuals to the medication they need for dealing with their own real medical problems. Some examples of actions taken within this context include the preparation of a document titled "Abuse-Deterrent Formulations: Transitioning the Pharmaceutical Market To Improve Patient and Public Health and Safety," which discusses the pros and cons of various ways of developing alternative drug formulations to achieve both drug safety and efficacy; federal legislative recommendations, a form of draft legislation that, "if enacted, would effectively reduce prescription drug abuse," and that was presented to majority and minority staffs of the U.S. Senate Health, Labor, Education, and Pensions Committee in 2014; proposed draft legislation offered to the state of Florida as an aid for dealing with its prescription drug abuse problems; and letters to various federal and state legislators and agencies on specific bills under consideration at both levels for ways of preventing prescription drug abuse. CLAAD has also made presentations or attended dozens of meetings at which prescription drug abuse was being considered, such as the 25th annual meeting of the National Association of Drug Diversion Investigators, the U.S. Food and Drug Administration Public Meeting on the Development and Regulation of Abuse-Deterrent Opioid Medications, the Partnership for Safe Medicines Interchange, the Generation Rx University Conference, the National Rx Drug Abuse Summit, and the National Sheriffs' Association 2014 Winter Conference. All policy decisions and positions made by CLAAD are required to be approved by at least 80 percent of nonprofit members of the organization.

Community Anti-Drug Coalitions of America

Community Anti-Drug Coalitions of America (CADCA) was founded in 1992 on the suggestion of Jim Burke, then chair of the President's Drug Advisory Council, as a possible mechanism for dealing with the growing problem of substance abuse throughout the United States. Today, CADCA claims to be "the premier membership organization representing those working to make their communities safe, healthy and drug-free." It works with more than 5,000 local communities to prevent tobacco use among youth, underage drinking of alcohol, and the use of illicit drugs. The coalition carries out its work in cooperation with about 30 partners from government, nonprofit organizations, the business world, and international associations and organizations. Some of those partners are the Centers for Disease Control and Prevention; Drug Enforcement Administration; and Departments of Education, Health and Human Services, Homeland Security, Justice, Labor, and State; National Institute on Drug Abuse; international drug prevention groups, such as FEBRAE (Brazil), MENTOR and SURGIR (Colombia), FUNDASALVA (El Salvador), SEC-CATID (Guatemala), ANCOD (Honduras), CEDRO and CRESER (Peru), and SANCA AND TASC (South Africa); the American College of Pediatrics; National Association of Counties; National Sheriffs Association; Students against Destructive Decisions; Consumer Healthcare Products Association; DIRECTV; Krispy Kreme; M&T Bank; the Robert Wood Johnson Foundation; and Xerox.

CADCA offers seven types of core services to communities: public policy and advocacy, training and technical assistance, research dissemination and evaluation, special events and conferences, communications, international programs, and youth programs. In the area of policy and advocacy, the group works with its partners to promote legislation and rulemaking that promotes drug prevention efforts that it supports. Recently, it has encouraged members and the general public to write letters to members of the U.S. Congress in support of four pieces of legislation, the Comprehensive Addiction and Recovery Act; Drug-Free Communities Program; Preventing Abuse of Cough Treatments Act; and Sober Truth on Preventing Underage Drinking Act. The CADCA training program has resulted in the training of more than 13,000 individuals from over 900 coalition members and over 150 coalition graduates from the organization's year-long National Coalition Academy. The coalition has also conducted more than 1,200 technical assistance sessions for its member coalitions. In addition to the National Coalition Academy, CADCA holds three other major training sessions, the Mid-Year Training Institute, National Leadership Forum, and National Youth Leadership Initiative.

Some of the organization's priority efforts are organized into ongoing events, programs, and campaigns on very specific topics. Some of the recent topics have been 17th Annual Drug-Free Kids Campaign Awards Dinner, Annual Survey of Coalitions, Drug-Free Kids Campaign, GOT OUTCOMES!, National Medicine Abuse Awareness Month, Tobacco Initiatives, and VetCorps. In connection with its efforts related to prescription drug abuse, CADCA has produced the "Prevent Rx Abuse" toolkit. The toolkit consists of four elements, the most basic of which is Prevention Strategies, seven methods of prevention that make use of access to information, enhancement of skills, provision of support, changes in access and barriers, changes in consequences, changes in physical design, and modification and change in policies. (Additional detailed information about the toolkit is available online at http://www.preventrxabuse.org/.)

The CADCA website is a rich source of reference materials on virtually every aspect of alcohol and drug prevention. These materials can be accessed by way of an interactive index at http://www.cadca.org/resources.

The primary element of the CADCA research function is the organization's Annual Survey of Coalitions, which attempts to identify coalitions around the country and learn more about what they are doing to address substance abuse problems in their communities. One result of the survey is the selection of a handful of local coalitions that have been most successful in achieving position outcomes in their communities. These results are published in a publication called GOT OUTCOMES!

In 2005, CADCA began to expand its work to others parts of the world and has since that date helped to establish 130 community anti-drug coalitions in 22 countries, including most of Central and South America, the Cape Verde Islands, Italy, Senegal, South Africa, Ghana, Kenya, Tanzania, Kyrgyzstan, Tajikistan, Iraq, and the Philippines. The organization offers essentially the same training, research, resource, and other services provided to domestic coalitions.

A useful overview of the structure and work of the coalition is available in its "Handbook for Community Anti-Drug Coalitions," which can be accessed online at http://www.cadca .org/sites/default/files/files/coalitionhandbook102013.pdf.

Thomas De Quincey (1785–1859)

De Quincey was an English author best known for his autobiographical work, *Confessions of an Opium Eater*. He also wrote a number of other works, including novels, essays, critical reviews, and additional autobiographical sketches.

Thomas De Quincey was born on August 15, 1785, in Manchester, England. After his father died in 1796, De Quincey's mother moved the family to Bath, where he was enrolled in King Edward's School. He was an outstanding scholar, able to read Greek and compose poems in the language as a teenager. His home life was difficult, however, and he ran away to Wales at the age of 17, with the blessings and minimal financial support of his mother and uncle. Eventually he found his way to London, where he nearly died of starvation and survived only because of the kindness of a 15-year-old prostitute whom we now know of only as "Anne of Oxford Street."

In 1804, he was found by friends in London and returned to his family, who arranged for him to enroll at Worcester College,

Oxford. It was at Oxford that he first took opium, in the form of laudanum, for a painful and persistent toothache. He soon became addicted to the drug, an addiction that persisted to a greater or lesser degree for the rest of his life. He describes his years of addiction in *Confessions*, as well as its effects on his life and writing and his efforts to overcome his addiction. From time to time, he was able to withdraw from use of the drug but, a point noted by some of his biographers, the quantity and quality of his literary work suffered significantly during these periods of abstinence.

In 1816, De Quincey married Margaret Simpson, who was eventually to bear him eight children. She has been described as the "anchor" in his life, and, after her death in 1837, De Quincey's use of opium increased significantly. De Quincey survived for most of his life after about 1820, partially through the financial support of his family and partially through his own literary efforts. In the early 1820s, he moved to London, where he worked as a novelist, essayist, translator, reporter, and critic. Publication of *Confessions* in 1821 essentially made his career as a writer, although he never again produced a work with such wide popularity. In addition to his opium addiction, De Quincey spent most of his life battling financial problems, and he was convicted and imprisoned on five occasions for nonpayment of his debts.

Biographers have noted De Quincey's substantial influence on later writers and artists, including Edgar Allan Poe, Charles Baudelaire, Nikolai Gogol, Aldous Huxley, William Burroughs, and Hector Berlioz, whose *Symphonie Fantastique* is reputedly loosely based on *Confessions*. The most recent collection of De Quincey's works was published in 21 volumes between 2000 and 2003. De Quincey died in Glasgow on December 8, 1859.

Drug Policy Alliance

The Drug Policy Alliance (DPA) was created in July 2000 as a result of the merger of the Lindesmith Center and the Drug

Policy Foundation. The Lindesmith Center, in turn, had been formed in 1994 as a think tank for the consideration of alternatives to existing policies and practices for dealing with drug issues, while the Drug Policy Foundation had been established in 1987, an organization established to work for drug reform, largely through the provision of grants to advance further studies on drug policies. The DPA now claims to be "the world's leading drug policy reform organization of people who believe the war on drugs is doing more harm than good." The organization currently claims to have nearly 30,000 members, with an additional 70,000 individuals receiving its online e-newsletter and action alerts.

DPA organizes its work under the rubric of about a half dozen major issues: Reforming Marijuana Laws, Fighting Injustice, Reducing Drug Harm, Protecting Youth, Defending Personal Liberty, and Making Economic Sense. Each of these general topics is further divided into more specific issues. The Reforming Marijuana Laws topic, for example, covers issues such as developing a legal regulatory market for marijuana, helping individuals who have been arrested for marijuana possession, and providing information about the potential health and social effects of marijuana use. The topic of Protecting Youth is further divided into efforts to deal with drug testing in schools and zero-tolerance policy in some school districts, as well as providing information and materials on "reality-based" drug education. The Making Economic Sense topic deals in more detail with subjects such as problems of supply and demand for marijuana, the problem of drug prohibition and violence, and the economic benefits of legalizing and taxing the sale of marijuana.

An important part of the DPA efforts on behalf of marijuana issue is a series of Action Alerts, through which members and friends of the association are encouraged to contact legislators, administrative officials, and other stakeholders about specific issues of concern to the organization. During 2012, for example, the DPA sponsored Action Alerts on protection of medical marijuana patients directed to members of the U.S. Senate, a campaign to influence President Barack Obama to work harder to protection of medical marijuana patients, efforts to lobby members of the U.S. Congress to end criminalization of marijuana use and possession, and a campaign to encourage Congress to reduce federal sending on the enforcement of existing marijuana laws.

The DPA publishes a number of reports, fact sheets, and other print and electronic materials on the topic of marijuana legalization. Members receive the tri-annual newsletter *The Ally*, which provides information on the organization's current activities and successes. Other publications include *Safety First: A Reality-Based Approach to Teens and Drugs*, a tool designed to help parents evaluate and discuss strategies for protecting teenagers from drug abuse; *Crime and Punishment in New Jersey: The Criminal Code and Public Opinion on Sentencing*, a report on the legal status of marijuana in that state; *Drug Courts Are Not the Answer: Toward a Health-Centered Approach to Drug Use*, an analysis of existing laws on marijuana possession; *Overdose: A National Crisis Taking Root in Texas*, a report on the growing number of overdose deaths in that state and the United States; *Arresting Latinos for Marijuana in California: Possession Arrests in 33 Cities, 2006–08*, a report on the special risk faced by Latinos in California for marijuana offenses; and *Healing a Broken System: Veterans Battling Addiction and Incarceration*, dealing with the special problems of marijuana use faced by veterans returning from service in Iraq and Afghanistan.

The DPA also provides an excellent resource dealing with drug facts on its website. Some of the topics covered on this page include fundamental facts about marijuana and other drugs, some new solutions for dealing with the nation's drug problems, the relevance of federal and state drug laws for individuals, a summary of individual rights in connection with existing drug laws, statistical information about the nation's war on drugs, and drug laws around the world.

European Monitoring Centre for Drugs and Drug Addiction

The concept of an all-European agency to deal with the growing problem of substance abuse on the continent was first proposed by French president Georges Pompidou in the late 1960s. That idea languished for about two decades before it was raised once more in 1989 by French president François Mitterrand. Mitterrand suggested a seven-step program that would involve establishing a common method for analyzing drug addiction in the European states; harmonizing national policies for substance abuse; strengthening controls and improving cooperation among states; finding ways of implementing the 1988 UN Convention against Illicit Traffic in Narcotic Drugs and Psychotropic Substances; coordinating policies and practices between producing and consuming countries; developing a common policy dealing with drug-related money laundering; and designating a single individual in each country responsible for anti-drug actions within that country.

Mitterrand's suggestion led to a series of actions within the European Community that eventually resulted in 1993 in the creation of the European Monitoring Centre for Drugs and Drug Addiction (EMCDDA) under Council Regulation (EEC) no. 302/93. The general administrative structure was established the following year, consisting of an Executive Director, a Management Board, and a Scientific Committee. The Management Board is the primary decision-making body for EMCDDA. It meets at least once a year and is composed of one representative from each member state of the European Union, two representatives from the European Commission, and two representatives from the European Parliament. The board adopts an annual work program and a three-year work program that guides the organization's day-to-day operations. The three-year program is developed with input from a wide variety of sources, including the general public (through the organization's website). The 2013–2015 program focused on topics such as data collection, analysis and quality assurance; monitoring and understanding drug use and problems: key indicators and epidemiology; monitoring demand reduction responses to drug-related problems; monitoring drug supply and supply reduction interventions; monitoring new trends and developments and assessing the risks of new substances; improving Europe's capacity to monitor and evaluate policies; and communicating the EMCDDA's findings to external audiences.

The Scientific Committee consists of 15 members appointed by the Management Board for the purpose of advising the board on scientific issues related to substance abuse. The first meeting of the Management Board was held in April 1994 at its Lisbon headquarters, where its administrative offices remain until today. Much of the work of EMCDDA takes place within eight units of the Scientific Committee. The eight units focus on prevalence, consequences and data management; supply reduction and new trends; interventions, best practice and scientific partners; policy, evaluation, and content coordination; Reitox and international cooperation; and communication; information and communication technology; and administration. Reitox is the name given to a network of human and computer links among the 27 nations that make up the EMCDDA operation.

The EMCDDA website is one of the richest resources available on nearly every aspect of substance abuse issues in the world. It contains information on a wide variety of topics, such as health consequences (deaths and mortality, infectious diseases, treatment demand, and viral hepatitis); prevalence and epidemiology (general population surveys, drug trends in youth, problem drug use, key indicators, and wastewater analysis); best practice (prevention, treatment, harm reduction, standards and guidelines), Exchange on Drug Demand Reduction Action, and Evaluation Instruments Bank; drug profiles (amphetamine, barbiturates, benzodiazepines, BZP and other piperazines, cannabis, cocaine and crack, fentanyl, hallucinogenic mushrooms, heroin, khat, LSD, MDMA, methamphetamine, *Salvia divinorum*, synthetic cannabinoids and 'Spice,' synthetic cathinones, synthetic cocaine derivatives, and volatile substances); health and social interventions (harm reduction, prevention of drug use, social reintegration, and treatment of drug use); policy and law (EU policy and law, laws, and public expenditure); new drugs and trends (action on new drugs); supply and supply reduction (interventions against drug supply, interventions against diversion of chemical precursors, interventions against money laundering activities, supply reduction, markets, and crime and supply reduction indicators); resources by drug (cannabis thematic page, cocaine and crack thematic page, and opioids and heroin thematic page); drugs and society (crime, driving, social exclusion, women and gender issues, and young people); and science and research (addiction medicine, neuroscience, and research in Europe).

Over the decades, the EMCDDA has produced a plethora of publications on virtually every imaginable aspect of substance abuse, including http://www.emcdda.europa.eu/attachements. cfm/att_136906_EN_TDAB11001ENN_FINAL_Web.pdf; "European Drug Report (2016)"; European Drug Markets Report (2016)"; "Drug Use, Impaired Driving, and Traffic Accidents"; "Hepatitis C among Drug Users in Europe"; "New Psychoactive Substances in 2015"; "Drug Related Infectious Diseases in Europe"; "Health Responses to New Psychoactive Substances"; "A Cannabis Reader"; and "Harm Reduction: Evidence, Impacts, and Challenges."

Harm Reduction Coalition

Harm Reduction Coalition (HRC) was founded in 1993 by a group of drug users, advocates, and needle exchange providers. The organization's goal is to challenge the persistent stigma on users of illegal substances and to work for reform of national, state, and local drug laws. HRC accepts as a reality that substance abuse is and always will be a part of human society, and that rather than working to completely eliminate this problem, governments should work to reduce the harm produced by substance abuse. The organization conducts most of its work through about a dozen specific programs, including the California Syringe Access Project, which promotes efforts to expand syringe exchange programs in the state; opiate overdose prevention projects, which provides educational programs in shelters, jails, treatment programs, and other facilities designed to serve substance abusers; Harm Reduction Training Institute, which offers training programs in Oakland and New York City for professionals and volunteers who work with substance abusers; and the Brick Rebuilding Project, which focuses on educating at-risk youth about the risks and dangers of substance abuse. HRC publishes a quarterly journal, *Harm Reduction Communication*, as well as a variety of brochures, booklets, pamphlets, videos, and posters in English and Spanish, such as "H Is for Heroin," "Hepatitis ABC," "Overdose: Prevention and Survival," "HRC Hepatitis C Reader," "9 Tips for Treating Hepatitis C in Current and Former Substance Users," and "To Do No Harm."

Francis B. Harrison (1873–1957)

Harrison is probably best known today as author of the Harrison Narcotics Tax Act of 1914, an act that was passed, somewhat ironically, only after Harrison himself had left office. The act did not specifically prohibit any illegal substance, but it provided for the registration and taxation of "all persons who produce, import, manufacture, compound, deal in, dispense, sell, distribute, or give away opium or coca leaves, their salts, derivatives, or preparations, and for other purposes." Law enforcement officers and the courts immediately began to interpret the law as restricting physicians from writing prescriptions for the nonmedical use of opiates, and they began arresting, prosecuting, and convicting individuals for such activities. To a significant extent, then, the Harrison Act marked the beginning of a national campaign against the use of certain substances for other than medical uses.

Francis Burton Harrison was born in New York City on December 18, 1873, to Burton Harrison, an attorney and private secretary to Jefferson Davis, president of the Confederate States, and Constance Cary Harrison, a novelist and social activist. He attended the Cutler School in New York City, and Yale University, from which he received his BA in 1895. He then earned his LLB at New York Law School in 1897. Harrison was elected to the U.S. Congress from New York's 13th District, but resigned after one term to run (unsuccessfully) for lieutenant governor of New York.

After a brief hiatus in the private practice of law, he ran for Congress again in 1907, this time from New York's 20th district, and was elected. He served for three terms in Congress before accepting an appointment as governor general of the Philippine Islands, where he remained until 1921. Following his service in the Philippines, Harrison essentially retired from public life, spending extended periods of time in Scotland and Spain. He returned to the Philippines on a number of occasions, however, as consultant and advisor, especially when the islands were granted their independence in 1934. Harrison was married six times, with five of those marriages ending in divorce. He died in Flemington, New Jersey, on November 21, 1957.

Albert Hofmann (1906–2008)

Hofmann discovered the psychedelic compound lysergic acid diethylamide (LSD) and experienced its hallucinogenic effects in 1943. He later studied chemicals present in so-called magic mushrooms also responsible for hallucinogenic effects and synthesized the most important of these, psilocybin.

Albert Hofmann was born in Baden, Switzerland, on January 11, 1906, to Adolf Hofmann, a toolmaker, and Elisabeth

Schenk Hofmann. He attended Zürich University, from which he received his bachelor's degree in chemistry in 1929 and his doctorate in the same subject in 1930. He then accepted an appointment as research chemist at Sandoz Pharmaceuticals, a company with which he remained for the rest of his professional career.

The event in Hofmann's life for which he is best known and that has now been recounted endlessly occurred on April 16, 1943. At the time, Hofmann was involved in a long-term study of some naturally occurring psychedelic plants, including the fungus ergot and the herb squill. He was working in particular with a chemical found in a number of these plants, known in German as Lysergsäure-diethylamid, and in English as lysergic acid diethylamide (LSD). In particular, he was studying LSD-25, that is, the 25th preparation of the substance. During his research, Hofmann spilled a small amount of LSD-25 on his hands and, before long, began to feel mentally disoriented. After a period of time, he found he could no longer continue working and jumped on his bicycle to ride home. That bicycle ride, as Hofmann has recounted the event on a number of occasions, was such a bizarre experience that he thought for some time that he had perhaps lost his mind. After about six hours of "extremely stimulated imagination . . . a dreamlike state . . . and an uninterrupted stream of fantastic pictures, extraordinary shapes with intense, kaleidoscopic play of colors" (as he later described the experience), Hofmann returned to normal, but with a desire to learn more about the compound he had discovered.

Much of Hofmann's career was devoted to further studies of LSD and other psychedelic compounds, research that was supported and encouraged by Sandoz because of its potential for application in the treatment of psychological disorders. In 1962, for example, Hofmann and his wife traveled to Mexico to collect the psychoactive herb Ska Maria Pastora (*Salvia divinorum*) for study and analysis. He also identified the most important active agent in another psychedelic plant, the Mexican morning glory (*Rivea corymbosa*), a close relative of LSD, lysergic acid amide.

Hofmann retired from Sandoz in 1971 but continued a career of writing, public speaking, and participation in a variety of professional organizations. Perhaps his most popular book is his own account of his research on LSD and its psychedelic effects, *LSD: My Problem Child* (1980). Hofmann died on April 29, 2008, in the village of Burg im Leimental, near Basel, Switzerland, at the age of 102.

Hon Lik (1951–)

Hon Lik (also Han Li) is a pharmacist and inventor, known internationally as the inventor of the modern electronic cigarette. He pursued the concept of a tobacco-free cigarette in the early twenty-first century partly over concerns of his own high levels of smoking (two packs a day) and partly because of his own father's fate, death from lung cancer arising out of his addiction to cigarette smoking also. Hon decided that there had to be a technical means for enjoying the pleasures of tobacco smoking without actually burning tobacco and producing the host of harmful components it contains. By 2004 he had developed such a device and applied for a patent for an "electronic atomization cigarette." The device works by vaporizing a solution that contains nicotine and other components in a small cartridge. The user then inhales the vapor produced (a process that has come to be called *vaping*) to enjoy the stimulus provided by nicotine along with artificial flavors and aromas that have been added to the cartridge solution. Hon eventually received Chinese, European, and U.S. patents for this device.

Hon and others founded the Ruyan company in China to market his invention, which, at first, was a huge success (it being the only company in China to manufacture such a device). Before long, however, Ruyan's business began to decline, a trend that Hon later attributed to resistance by Chinese tobacco and cigarette firms that worried about competition from the e-cigarette. Eventually Ruyan's sales fell from a near-monopoly of the Chinese market to about 5percent. Throughout all his travails, Hon has remained optimistic. "From the day my invention worked," Hon told a reporter from the French newspaper *Libération* in 2013, "where I could satisfy my nicotine without ruining my health, I realized that I opened a great debate. For my invention is a turning point for the hundreds of millions of smokers and for the future of the global tobacco industry" (in translation). Rights to the electronic cigarette are now owned by the British firm of Imperial Tobacco, although Hon has yet to see any royalties from sales of the product.

Hon Lik was born on September 26, 1951, in Shenyang, Liaoning, China. He attended the Liaoning College of Traditional Chinese Medicine, where he majored in pharmacy. After graduation, he joined the Liaoning Academy of Traditional Chinese Medicine, where he focused on the study of the ginseng plant, a popular aphrodisiac. As a result of this line of research, Hon was able to found his own company, Chenlong Baoling Longevity Ginseng products, to patent and sell his discoveries. In 1990, he was also appointed vice-superintendent for technology development at the Liaoning Academy. In order to commercialize his invention of the e-cigarette, Hon founded the Golden Dragon company in 2005, where he served as chief executive officer until 2013. He then was appointed head of the Chinese Research and Development team of Fontem Ventures, a division of Imperial Tobacco focusing on the development and sales of electronic cigarettes.

John W. Huffman (1932–)

Huffman is best known for having developed a group of synthetic compounds that produce physiological effects similar to those caused by Δ^9-tetrahydrocannabinol (THC), the principal psychoactive component of marijuana. These synthetic cannabinoids are chemical analogs of THC; that is, they have the same basic structure as THC, but differ in groups that have been substituted on the basic molecule. The compounds are known by abbreviations such as JWH-007, JWH-081, and JWH-398, where the "JWH" part of the name are Huffman's own initials. Huffman spent a significant portion of his academic career working on the development of these compounds, which are used primarily for two research purposes. First, they can be used to obtain additional information about cannabinoid receptors in the endocannabinoid system. (The endocannabinoid system is a collection of fatty acid derivatives that occur in animal bodies and the receptor sites to which they bond. The endocannabinoid system is implicated in a number of fundamental physiological responses, such as appetite, pain-sensation, mood, and memory.) Scientists now know that cannabinoids produce their psychoactive effects by attaching to receptor sites in the brain and peripheral nervous system, setting off a chain of chemical reactions. What they know relatively little about is the chemical structure of those receptors. The chemical structure of Huffman's synthetic cannabinoids can be used to solve that problem by finding out which compounds (and therefore which structures) activate receptor sites, thereby elucidating the three-dimensional structure of the receptor sites. The second purpose of the research, arising out of these discoveries, is the development of new pharmaceuticals that can produce cannabis-like physical effects, such as increasing one's appetite, reducing nausea, and treating glaucoma.

Huffman's research has been enormously useful in providing researchers with a better understanding of the way the endocannabinoid system works. But that research has also gained a level of notoriety among the general public because of its use in developing new types of psychoactive drugs used for recreational purposes. These drugs are incorrectly known as synthetic cannabis when, in fact, they often consist of a mixture of traditional herbs with mild mood-altering properties (such as *Canavalia maritima*, *Nymphaea caerulea*, and *Scutellaria nana*) coated with one or more of Huffman's synthetic cannabinoids. The resulting product may have psychoactive effects more than a hundred times greater than that of THC. They are sold under a variety of names, including Spice, K2, Chronic Spice, Spice Gold, Spice Silver, Stinger, Yucatan Fire, Skunk, Pulse, and Black Mamba. When they first became available to the general public, they were legal because they contained no THC or other banned substance. Over time, however, a number of states in the United States and countries around the world have banned products of this kind.

Huffman himself has spoken out strongly about the risks involved in using synthetic cannabinoids as recreational drugs. The compounds were prepared, he points out, for research purpose, and little is known about their general effects on the body. Indeed, public health officials have reported emergency room visits as a result of using Spice, K2, and its analogs, a fact responsible for most of the bans now being adopted. The problem is that most of the now-illegal compounds are still generally available on the Internet.

John William Huffman was born in Evanston, Illinois, on July 21, 1932. He attended Northwestern University, which granted his BS in chemistry in 1954. He then continued his studies at Harvard University, where he earned his AM and his PhD in chemistry in 1956 and 1957, respectively. At Harvard, he studied under probably the century's greatest synthetic organic chemist, Robert B. Woodward. Huffman's first job was as assistant professor of chemistry at the Georgia Institute of Technology. He left Georgia Tech in 1960 to take a position at Clemson University as assistant professor of chemistry. Over time, he rose to the position of associate professor and then, in 1967, full professor at Clemson. He remained at Clemson until his retirement in 2005. He then continued to work at the university as research professor until he took full retirement in 2011. He also spent one a year as visiting professor of chemistry at Colorado State University in 1982. During his career, Huffman published more than 100 papers in peer-reviewed journals.

Among the honors and awards granted to Huffman have been a National Institutes of Health (NIH) Career Development Award for 1965–1970, a Senior Scientist Award from the National Institute on Drug Abuse, Clemson University Alumni Association Award for Outstanding Research Accomplishments, and Raphael Mechoulam Annual Award in Cannabinoid Research.

In June 2011, Huffman talked with ABC News about the dangers of synthetic cannabinoids as recreational drugs. It would make more sense, he said, to legalize the use of marijuana, which has been thoroughly studied and whose effects are now well known. "The scientific evidence is," he explained, "that it's not a particularly dangerous drug," and, in any case, it is much less dangerous than the poorly understood and potentially highly risky synthetic cannabinoids.

Aldous Huxley (1894–1963)

Huxley is probably best known as the author of the novel *Brave New World*, which describes a world in which the state takes control of every aspect of a person's individual life. He is perhaps somewhat less well known among the general public as an enthusiastic advocate of the use of psychedelic drugs, arguing that all of the world's great beliefs arise out of hallucinogenic experiences of their founders and early disciples.

Aldous Leonard Huxley was born in Godalming, Surrey, England, on July 26, 1894. The Huxley family was then one of the most famous in Great Britain. Huxley's brother, Julian, was an eminent biologist; his father was a successful author; and his grandfather, T. H. Huxley, had been a great defender of Charles Darwin's theory of evolution, earning himself the accolade of "Darwin's Bulldog." After an early period of home schooling, Huxley attended the Hillside School before enrolling at Eton College. In 1911, he developed a case of keratitis punctata, an eye condition that left him essentially blind for more than two years and which, incidentally, disqualified him for service in World War I. When he recovered, Huxley enrolled at Balliol College, Oxford, from which he graduated in 1916.

After leaving Oxford, Huxley taught briefly at Eton and worked for a short time at a chemical plant in Billingham, but he was not very successful or happy in either job. It gradually became clear that his real career was in the arts, specifically, as a writer. He produced his first book of poems in 1916 (*Burning Wheels*), his first book of short stories in 1920 (*Limbo*), and his first novel in 1921 (*Chrome Yellow*). He was eventually to produce many more novels, books of poetry, travel writings, essays, short story collections, magazine articles, biographies, and plays.

Huxley may have been introduced to psychedelic drugs as early as 1930, although his first real experimentation dates to the 1950s. He is said to have taken his first dose of mescaline in 1950 and his first dose of LSD in 1953, after which he became a firm advocate of psychedelics as a key to out-of-body experiences that could be of enormous value to a person. He described and discussed these experiences in his collection of essays, *Doors of Perception* (1954), which was named after a book by William Blake and which served as an inspiration for the name of a rock band of the time, The Doors. He is said to have been a favorite writer of many hippies of the 1960s and a spiritual guide for other researchers in psychedelic substances, including Timothy Leary and Richard Alpert. Huxley is said to have requested an intramuscular injection of LSD on his deathbed, a believer in the psychedelic experience to the very end. He died in Los Angeles on November 22, 1963, which was also the date on which John F. Kennedy was assassinated and C. S. Lewis died.

International Council on Alcohol and Addictions

The International Council on Alcohol and Addictions is one of the oldest—if not the oldest—international nongovernmental organizations devoted to issues of alcoholism and substance abuse. It was organized in 1907 during the 11th International Conference against Alcoholism in Stockholm, Sweden. It was originally called the International Bureau against Alcoholism, and was formed because attendees at the conference realized that there was a need for a formal, ongoing, international resource of reliable information about the dangers of alcoholism. In 1964, the organization changed its name to the International Council on Alcohol and Alcoholism (ICAA), and four years later, it changed its name again, this time to recognize its interest in issues of substance abuse and addiction, to the International Council on Alcohol and Addictions. The ICAA's main activity is its annual international conference, at which a wide variety of papers and sessions on alcohol and substance abuse are offered. It also offers training sessions for specialists working in the field. The council is also joint sponsor with the German Archive for Temperance and Abstinence Literature of the Archer Tongue Collection for cultural studies on alcohol, currently located at the University of Applied Sciences Magdeburg–Stendal, at Magdeburg, Germany.

C. Everett Koop (1916–2013)

Koop served as U.S. surgeon general under President Ronald Reagan from 1982 to 1989. During his tenure, he was a vigorous advocate for a number of public health programs, perhaps the best known of which was his campaign against smoking.

Charles Everett Koop was born in Brooklyn, New York, on October 14, 1916. He earned his BA from Dartmouth College in 1937 and his MD from Cornell Medical College in 1941. He then took a position at the University of Pennsylvania, where he held a number of posts over the next 35 years, including surgeon-in-chief at the university's Children's Hospital (1948–1981) and professor of pediatric surgery (1959–1989). In 1981, President Reagan asked Koop to become deputy assistant secretary for health in the U.S. Public Health Service, with the understanding that he would be eventually be promoted to surgeon general, a promise that was kept in January 1982. Koop remained in that position until almost the end of Reagan's second term of office, leaving his post in October 1989.

Koop's term of service as surgeon general was marked by aggressive campaigns on a number of public health fronts, smoking perhaps being the most notable. His first public action as surgeon general, in fact, was to issue a report, *Report on Smoking and Health*, that summarized the association between smoking and cancer of the lung, oral cavity, larynx, esophagus, stomach, bladder, pancreas, and kidneys. He used that report as the basis for a national program that he called the Campaign for a Smoke-Free America by the Year 2000. As an integral part of the campaign, Koop called for legislation requiring very specific notices about the health effects of smoking on all cigarette packages, legislation that was adopted by the U.S. Congress in 1984. In spite of pressure from tobacco-state legislators, Koop continued his antismoking crusade throughout his term of office. In 1986, he issued an important report on the effects of secondhand smoke, *The Health Consequences of Involuntary Smoking*, which demonstrated that secondhand smoke was not simply an inconvenience, but a quantifiable health risk.

After leaving federal service, Koop became president of the National Safe Kids Campaign, a post he held until 2003. He also accepted an offer to return to Dartmouth College, where he served as Elizabeth DeCamp McInerny Professor of Surgery at Dartmouth Medical School and senior scholar at the C. Everett Koop Institute at Dartmouth College. He continued to write and speak on a variety of medical and health topics, and was the author of more than 200 books and articles of such topics. Koop died on February 25, 2013, in Hanover, New Hampshire.

Timothy Leary (1920–1996)

In his *New York Times* obituary, Leary was remembered as the man who "effectively introduced many Americans to the psychedelic 1960s." He is perhaps best remembered for having coined the phrase "turn on, tune in, drop out."

Timothy Francis Leary was born in Springfield, Massachusetts, on October 22, 1920. After graduating from Springfield Classical High School, he entered the College of the Holy Cross in Worcester, Massachusetts, where he spent two years. He then transferred to the University of Alabama, where he also remained only briefly. He is reputed to have had disciplinary problems at both institutions, and did not receive his bachelor's degree (in psychology) from Alabama until 1943. During World War II he served in the Medical Corps. After completing his studies at Alabama, he studied for his master's degree at Washington State University, which he received in 1946, and then continued with his doctoral studies at the University of California at Berkeley, which awarded him his PhD in psychology in 1950. Over the next decade, Leary followed a somewhat traditional academic pathway, serving as assistant professor at Berkeley from 1950 to 1955, director of psychiatric research at the Kaiser Family Foundation, in Menlo Park, California, from 1955 to 1958, and lecturer in psychology at Harvard University from 1958 to 1963.

The turning point in Leary's life came in August 1960, when he first consumed psilocybin mushrooms on a visit to Cuernavaca, Mexico. He later said that, as a result of this experience, he "learned more about . . . (his) brain and its possibilities . . . (and) more about psychology in the five hours after taking these mushrooms than . . . (he) had in the preceding fifteen years of studying doing research in psychology." For the rest of his life, Leary devoted his energies to learning more about psychedelic substances and spreading the word about his discoveries to the world.

After his return from Mexico in 1960, Leary decided to incorporate his new passion into his research and teaching at Harvard. Along with his colleague, Richard Alpert, Leary enlisted prison inmates and graduate students in a series of experiments using psychedelic substances to determine how they might be used in the treatment of psychological and psychiatric disorders. The university was somewhat less than enthusiastic about Leary's research and out-of-classroom activities, and it eventually terminated his contract on May 6, 1963, for failing to show up for his scheduled classes. Harvard also terminated Alpert at about the same time for providing psychedelic substances to an undergraduate in an off-campus setting.

After leaving Harvard, Leary and Alpert moved to an estate furnished to them by a wealthy admirer at Millbrook, New York. Although planned as a research institute, the facility soon became better known as a "hippie hangout" where all types of drugs were used. Over the next two decades, Leary fell afoul of the law a number of times, sometimes spending time in prison, and, on occasion, having to flee the country to escape prosecution and further imprisonment. During the last two decades of his life, Leary spent his time writing and lecturing. He was the author of nearly three dozen books, including *Interpersonal Diagnosis of Personality*; *Jail Notes*; *Design for Dying*; *Flashbacks: An Autobiography*; *The Politics of Ecstasy*; *High Priest*; *Confessions of a Hope Fiend*; and *Turn On, Tune In, Drop Out*. Leary died in Los Angeles at the age of 75 on May 31, 1996.

Otto Loewi (1873–1961)

Loewi was a German physician and pharmacologist who discovered that nerve messages are transmitted between neurons by means of specific chemicals, now known as neurotransmitters. Loewi gave to the first of the chemicals of this type that he discovered the name *Vagusstoff* ("vagus material"). The substance was later shown to be acetylcholine, one of the most important of all neurotransmitters. An understanding of the function of neurotransmitters is absolutely fundamental to an interpretation of the way drugs work in the human body. For his work on neurotransmitters, Loewi was awarded a share of the 1936 Nobel Prize in Physiology or Medicine.

Otto Loewi was born at Frankfurt-am-Main on June 3, 1873. He attended the University of Strasbourg, from which he received his medical degree in 1896. He then worked for a period of time at University College in London, the University of Vienna, and the University of Graz (Austria), where he remained for nearly three decades. It was at Graz that Loewi conducted the work on neurotransmitters for which he is best known.

Like many prominent Jewish scientists of the time, Loewi was increasingly at professional and personal risk as the Nazi party came to power in Germany and, later, Austria. In fact, he was the only Jewish professor hired at Graz between 1903 and the end of World War II. On the evening of March 11, 1938, Loewi and two sons were arrested by Nazi authorities and were allowed to leave the country only under the condition that they give up all of their personal property and possessions. Loewi moved to Belgium, where he served as professor of pharmacology for one year at the University of Brussels. He then moved on to the University of Leeds in England, before accepting an appointment in 1940 as professor of pharmacology at New York University (NYU). He served at NYU until 1955, when he retired. Loewi died in New York City on December 25, 1961.

Mothers Against Drunk Driving

Mothers Against Drunk Driving (MADD) was founded in 1980 by Irving, Texas, resident Candace ("Candy") Lightner after her 13-year-old daughter was killed in a hit-and-run accident by a man who already had previously been convicted of drunk driving. The organization went through a period of internal debate in the mid-1980s over the question as to whether drunk driving or the consumption of alcohol itself was the core issue with which it was concerned. At that point, in 1984, the organization changed its name from Mothers Against Drunk Drivers to Mothers Against Drunk Driving to reflect its broader concerns. (In disagreement with this revised view, Lightner resigned from the organization she had founded.) Over the years, MADD has sponsored a number of campaigns to reduce drunk driving, including an effort to change the drinking age to 21 in all states, a recommendation for widespread use of random roadblocks to catch drinking drivers, and the creation of a victim/survivor help line. Its current emphasis is on a Campaign to Eliminate Drunk Driving that consists of four basic elements: high-visibility law enforcement, ignition interlocks for convicted drunk drivers, advanced automotive technologies to prevent drunk driving, and expanded grassroots support for the organization and its programs.

National Coalition Against Prescription Drug Abuse

The National Coalition against Prescription Drug Abuse (NCAPDA) was founded in June 2010 following the death of Joseph John (Joey) Rovero, III, the son of April and Joseph Rovero. Rovero was a student at Arizona State University when he died from a lethal combination of alcohol and prescription medications, provided by prescription from Dr. Hsiu-Ying "Lisa" Teng, of Rowland Heights, California. Teng was later charged with second-degree murder in the deaths of Rovero and two other students, Vu Nguyen and Steven Ogle. Today, April Rovero serves as CEO of NCAPDA and Joseph Rovero is the organization's treasurer.

NCAPDA is a 501(c)3 nonprofit volunteer organization whose purpose it is to create nationwide awareness about the dangers of prescription drug misuse and abuse. It has developed partnership with a number of other institutions and organizations, including schools, colleges, community organizations, medical associations, law enforcement agencies, and other groups interested in the prescription drug abuse problem. Among NCAPDA's current partners are the Discovery Counseling Center of San Ramon Valley, SRV Community Against Substance Abuse, Teen Esteem, the Troy and Alana Pack Foundation, and the Sacramento Youth Drug and Alcohol Coalition. One of the organization's primary goals is to work for policy changes and new state and federal laws designed to combat the current prescription drug abuse epidemic.

The primary activities of NCAPDA are speaking engagements, panel discussions, and roundtable discussions conducted at a variety of venues to increase awareness of the prescription drug abuse problem and its prevention. Some examples of the programs offered include the showing of two documentary films, "Out of Reach" and "Behind the Orange Curtain" about prescription drug abuse; presentation of the original play, "Pharming," on the topic; lectures on "Overdosed America," "Adolescent Subcultures and Current Drug Trends"; prescription drug take-back days at local police stations; candlelight vigils held in memory of those lost to prescription drug problems; and Addiction by Prescription panel discussions. These presentations are made at a wide variety of venues, including local middle and high schools, service clubs, governmental offices, social clubs, restaurants and bars, and police stations.

The NCAPDA website has a number of useful resources for those interested in the prescription drug abuse problem, some designed specifically for parents, and others specifically for young adults. In addition to background information on potentially dangerous drugs and the nature of drug addiction, the Resources section of the website provides a number of valuable links to other sources of information and a collection of downloadable files on the topic of prescription drug abuse. The Stories section of the website also offers essays relating to the personal experiences of individuals who have lost relatives and friends to prescription drug causes and an option for adding one's own story to the collection.

National Council on Alcoholism and Drug Dependence, Inc.

The National Council on Alcoholism and Drug Dependence, Inc. (NCADD) was founded in 1944 by Marty Mann, the first woman who is said to have achieved sustained sobriety through the Alcoholics Anonymous program. Inspired by the work of reformer Dorothea Dix, who had developed a breakthrough program in mental health care, Mann wondered if she could create a similar program for alcoholics, like herself. She was able to obtain a modest grant from the Yale University Center of Alcohol Studies to establish such an organization, which she called the National Committee for Education on Alcoholism (NCEA). Over the years, the organization evolved into a variety of formats, eventually becoming the National Council on Alcoholism and, in 1990, adding "and Drug Dependence" to its name, to reflect an emphasis that had been added to the organization's mission three years earlier.

Mann created the NCEA on three simple principles, which continue to guide the organization's work today:

- Alcoholism is a disease and the alcoholic is a sick person.
- The alcoholic can be helped and is worth helping.
- This is a public health problem and therefore a public responsibility.

In its literature today, NCADD points out that it was formed at a time when the public perception of alcoholism and drug dependence was very different, one in which the attitude was one of "let[ting] the existing population of alcoholics and addicts die off and prevent the creation of future alcoholics and addicts by legally prohibiting the sale of alcohol and legally controlling the distribution of opium, morphine and cocaine." Mann's approach, of course, was entirely different from that view, and it is one that continues to inspire the organization today.

The mission of the NCADD focuses on a half-dozen major themes, the most important of which is the message to alcoholics and drug addicts to "get help," an offer that is fleshed out by the organization with a number of specific suggestions for dealing with one's addiction. Additional themes focus on becoming educated about the nature of alcohol and drugs, with special recommendations for parents, youth, friends and family, and those in recovery. The organization's website contains a very useful section on prescription drug abuse, which talks about the types of drugs most commonly abused and their character-istic features and effects, the nature of the problem for various age groups, methods of prevention and treatment, and useful resources on the topic.

National Inhalant Prevention Coalition

The National Inhalant Prevention Coalition (NIPC) was founded in 1992 by Synergies, a nonprofit corporation based in Austin, Texas. The organization began two years earlier as a statewide program called Texas Prevention Partnership, as an effort to educate school children in Texas about the dangers of inhalant abuse. Today, NIPC is operated by a branch of Syn-ergies in Chattanooga, Tennessee. Currently, the organization sponsors the National Inhalants & Poisons Awareness Week during the third week in March to better educate students and the general public about the dangers of using inhalants for the purpose of recreation. The NIPC also provides on its website an array of information about the medical, social, economic, and other risks of using inhalants.

National Institute on Drug Abuse

The origins of the National Institute on Drug Abuse (NIDA) date to 1935 when the U.S. Public Health Service established a research facility on drug abuse in Lexington, Kentucky. In 1948, that facility was officially renamed the Addiction Research Center. Research on drug abuse was facilitated in the site of the original facility, called "Narco," which was adjacent to a prison that held drug offenders and was run cooperatively with the Federal Bureau of Prisons. The federal government's interest in drug abuse was expanded in 1971 when President Richard M. Nixon established the Special Action Office of Drug Abuse Prevention within the White Office. A year later, the Special Action Office initiated two programs, the Drug Abuse Warn-ing Network (DAWN) and the National Household Survey on

Drug Abuse (NHSDA), both of which continue today. DAWN is a public health surveillance system that monitors emergency department drug-related admissions. It is now a part of the Substance Abuse and Mental Health Services Administration (SAMHSA). NHSDA is now known as the National Survey on Drug Use and Health and is also located in SAMHSA. Its function is to provide national- and state-level data on the use of illegal drugs, tobacco, alcohol, and mental health to researchers and the general public.

The NIDA itself was created by the act of Congress in 1974 for the purpose of promoting research, treatment, prevention, training, services, and data collection on the nature and extent of drug abuse. In general, the activities of the NIDA can be classified into one of two major categories: the conduct and support of research on a variety of issues related to drug abuse and dissemination of this information both for the purposes of future research and to improve programs of prevention and treatment of drug abuse, as well as to inform decisions by state, local, and the federal government on drug abuse policies and practices. The agency's organizational charts reflect the way in which these activities are organized. Three of the main NIDA offices deal with extramural affairs (funding of outside research), science policy and communications, and management. The agency also consists of a number of divisions that deal with intramural research (research within the agency); basic neuroscience and behavioral research; clinical research and behavioral research; epidemiology, services, and prevention research; and pharmacotherapies and medical consequences of drug abuse. Special programs, working groups, consortia, and interest groups focus on more specific topics, such as HIV/AIDS; childhood and adolescence issues; community epidemiology; women and sex/gender differences; nicotine and tobacco; neurosciences; and genetic issues.

The direction of NIDA activities over the period 2016–2020 has been laid out in the agency's *Strategic Plan*, published in December 2015. That report describes in detail the elements of the agency's four-pronged program over the coming five years: identifying the biological, environmental, behavioral, and social causes and consequences of drug use and addiction across the lifespan; developing new and improved strategies to prevent drug use and its consequences; developing new and improved treatments to help people with substance use disorders achieve and maintain a meaningful and sustained recovery; and increasing the public health impact of NIDA research and programs. This publication is available online athttps://www.drugabuse .gov/sites/default/files/nida_2016strategicplan_032316.pdf.

The NIDA budget has remained relatively constant over the first decade of the twenty-first century. It rose slightly from 2011 ($1,048,776) to 2012 ($1,052,114) to 2013 ($1,054,001), with also a relatively constant number of full-time employee equivalents (386, 386, and 382, respectively). About 90 percent of that budget goes for extramural research ($902,696 in 2013), with the largest fraction of that designated for basic and clinical neuroscience and behavior research ($478,902).

As indicated previously, dissemination of information is a major focus of the work carried out by the NIDA. Its publications include educational curricula, facts sheets, guidelines and manuals, journals, administrative and legal documents, posters, presentations, promotional materials, and reports. These publications can be reviewed on the agency's website at http://www.drugabuse.gov/publications by audience (students, teachers, parents, researchers, and health and medical professionals), by drug of abuse (e.g., alcohol, amphetamines, club drugs, LSD, marijuana, and steroids), by drug topic (such as addiction science, comorbidity, criminal justice, drugged driving, medical consequences, and relapse and recovery), by series (among which are Addiction Science and Clinical Practice, Brain Power, DrugFacts, Mind over Matter, and Research Reports), and by type.

The NIDA website also provides links to a number of resources for additional information about the subject of drug abuse and about the agency itself, including sections on NIDA in the News, NIDA Notes, meetings and events related to drug abuse topics, news releases, podcasts of NIDA-related programs, and electronic newsletters. The website is also available in Spanish.

Albert Niemann (1834–1861)

During his short life, Niemann made two important discoveries. The first was the active ingredient in coca leaves responsible for their psychoactive properties, a compound that he named *cocaine*. The second was a powerful gas produced by reacting ethylene (C_2H_4) with sulfur dichloride (SCl_2). The product became known as *mustard gas*, a chemical agent used widely during World War I.

During the late 1850s, Niemann was studying for his doctoral degree in chemistry at the University of Göttingen under the great chemist Friedrich Wöhler. For some years, Wöhler had been interested in the chemical composition of coca leaves brought back to Germany from South America, but had been unable to find the active ingredient for the plant's extraordinary psychoactive properties. When he received a shipment of fresh leaves in 1859, he assigned to Niemann the task of analyzing the natural product. Niemann responded successfully to this assignment, extracting from the leaves a white powder that he described as having a bitter taste (like other alkaloids, of which this compound was an example), promoting the flow of saliva, and having a numbing effect on the tongue. Niemann gave the name *cocaine* to the new substance, a combination of the plant name from which it came ("coca") and the traditional suffix used by chemists for all alkaloids ("-ine").

Niemann's research on cocaine earned him his PhD from Göttingen in 1860. In the same year, Niemann described his research on mustard gas (chemically, 1,1'-thiobis[2-chloroethane]; also known as sulfur mustard). He said that the gas caused terrible burns that festered for a long period of time and were very painful. Following his research on mustard gas,

Niemann's health deteriorated rapidly, and he returned to his home in Goslar, Germany, where he died on January 19, 1861, at the age of 26. Although some uncertainty surrounds the circumstances of his death, some historians believe that his exposure to mustard gas may have been a contributing factor. Two years after his death, a colleague at Göttingen, Wilhelm Lossen, determined the chemical formula for cocaine.

NORML (National Organization for the Reform of Marijuana Laws)

NORML is one of the relatively few organizations much better known by its acronym than by its full and official name, the National Organization for the Reform of Marijuana Laws. The group was formed in 1970 with an original grant of $5,000 from the Playboy Foundation. Founder of the organization was Keith Stroup, an attorney and a strong advocate of the legalization of marijuana, the cause for which NORML has worked for more than 45 years. Stroup served as executive director of the organization until 1979, a period during which 11 states decriminalized the use of marijuana and other states significantly reduced penalties for its use. NORML currently claims to have 135 chapters throughout the country and a legal staff of more than 500 attorneys to assist with the writing of legislation and legal action on behalf of its primary mission, the decriminalization of marijuana use nationwide. In addition to providing information about marijuana and its legalization to the general public, the organization lobbies state and federal legislators, sponsors an annual national conference, and has spawned a nonprofit foundation, the NORML Foundation, which is committed to educating the general public about marijuana and its legalization. NORML's website is an excellent source of information on a wide range of topics, including background information on cannabis itself, state laws, and general legal information, along with an extensive collection of books, pamphlets, articles, and other resources on marijuana.

Office of National Drug Control Policy

The Office of National Drug Control Policy (ONDCP) was established in 1988 as one provision of the Anti-Drug Abuse Act of 1988. It is the primary agency in the executive department for developing and executing policy on the use and abuse of illegal drugs in the United States. It is responsible for developing the National Drug Control Strategy, which outlines national policy on drug control, establishes a budget for this effort, and coordinates the work of federal, state, and local authorities in the fight against substance abuse. The office uses a three-pronged attack on drug abuse that focuses on prevention, treatment, and interdiction of drug sources.

The ONDCP has issued more than 1,000 pamphlets, brochures, reports, and other publications dealing with virtually every aspect of the substance abuse problem in the United States and other parts of the world, such as "2007 National Money Laundering Strategy"; "ADAM [Arrestee Drug Abuse Monitoring] II Report Fact Sheet 2008"; "Afghanistan Opium Winter Rapid Assessment Survey 2008"; "The DASIS [Drug and Alcohol Services Information System] Report: Adolescent Admissions Reporting Inhalants, 2006"; "The NSDUH [National Survey on Drug Use and Health] Report: Risk & Protective Factors for Substance Use among American Indian or Alaska Native Youths"; and "The War on Meth in Indian Country."

Quanah Parker (ca. 1845–1911)

Parker was the last chief of the Quahadi Comanche Indian tribe and a leading proponent of the melding of Christian and Native American Church movements, in which peyote is incorporated into traditional forms of worship. His most famous commentary is probably his comment that "The White Man goes into his church and talks about Jesus. The Indian goes into his Tipi and talks with Jesus."

The details of Quanah Parker's birth, as well as some other aspects of his life, are somewhat unclear. He is thought to have been born in the mid-1840s somewhere in the present state of Oklahoma. He himself claimed to have been born on Elk Creek, south of the Wichita Mountains, although other places have also been mentioned as a probable birthplace. His parents were Comanche warrior Noconie, (also known by the Indian name of Tah-con-ne-ah-pe-ah and called Peta Nocona by the whites) and Cynthia Ann Parker (later given the Indian name of Nadua, or "the found"), who had been captured by the Comanche during a raid on Fort Parker in Texas.

Parker apparently grew up in a traditional Native American community, replete with tribal customs. After his father was killed in 1860, Parker took shelter with a subgroup of the Comanches, the Quahadi tribe. Over time, he grew in respect and responsibility within the tribe and became its leader. From the mid-1860s to the mid-1870s, Parker fought against surrender to or assimilation by whites who were committed to taking over Native American lands and property. He eventually lost that fight at the battle of Adobe Walls, and was resigned to retiring to the reservation to which his tribe had been assigned.

Parker's connection with peyote is reputed to stem from 1884, when he fell very ill from an infection. Although he had, by then, become thoroughly absorbed by white culture, the medicines available to him from white practitioners were of no use. Only when he was provided with a concoction of peyote did he recover. The experience proved to be life-changing for him, convincing him of the value of native traditions (and native drugs) even in the modern world of the reservation. He spent much of the rest of his life in developing and promoting the National American Indian church movement, which incorporates elements of both white Christianity and traditional Native American beliefs and practices. Largely through his efforts, the modern Native American church still includes the use of peyote in its rituals.

Partnership for Drug-Free Kids

The Partnership for Drug-Free Kids was formed in 1986 with a grant provided by the American Association of Advertising Agencies. The organization was originally known as the Partnership for a Drug-Free America and changed its name to its current title in 2010. The original plan for the organization was to conduct a three-year effort to deal with the growing problem of substance abuse and addiction in the United States by way of an aggressive and sophisticated advertising campaign. At the end of that three-year period, however, a decision was made to continue the program. Perhaps the most famous element of the Partnership advertising program was its now-famous "fried egg" ad, which showed an egg before and during frying with the message "This is your brain; This is your brain on drugs." The centerpiece of the Partnership's current efforts is a website, drugfree.org, which attempts to translate the latest and most reliable information produced by research into tips and suggestions for teenagers about the risks posed by substance abuse. The organization also operates a number of specific educational campaigns, such as the Parent Campaign; Check Yourself, for teenagers; Get Help for Drug Problems; RX/OTC Abuse; Meth; Inhalants; Cough Medicine Abuse; and Steroids. Detailed information about all of these programs is available on the organization's website. Much of the organization's work is carried out through four major theme programs: the Parent Support Network, which offers assistance to parents who are interested in or concerned about teenage substance abuse; Medicine Abuse Project, which focuses specifically on problems association with prescription drug abuse; Youth Programming, which concentrates on efforts to prevent teenagers from starting on substance abuse activities; and Public Education Campaigns, which direct efforts to broader programs for educating the general public about substance abuse issues in the United States.

Friedrich Sertürner (1783–1841)

While still a young pharmacist's apprentice, Sertürner isolated the psychoactive agent morphine from the opium plant. His accomplishment is especially important because not only was it the first such agent extracted from opium, but also it was the first alkaloid obtained from any plant. Sertürner named his new discovery after the Greek god of dreams, Morpheus, for its powerful analgesic and sedative properties.

Friedrich Wilhelm Adam Ferdinand Sertürner was born in Neuhaus, Prussia, on June 19, 1783. His parents were in service to Prince Friedrich Wilhelm, who was also his godfather. When both his father and the prince died in 1794, he was left without means of support and, therefore, was apprenticed to a court apothecary by the name of Cramer. One of the topics in which he became interested in his new job was the chemical composition of opium, a plant that had long been known for its powerful analgesic and sedative properties. By 1803, he had extracted from opium seeds a white crystalline powder clearly responsible for the pharmacological properties of the plant. He named the new substance *morphine* and proceeded to test its properties, first on stray animals available at the castle, and later on his friends and himself. His friends soon withdrew from the experiments because, while pleasurable enough in its initial moderate doses, the compound ultimately caused unpleasant physical effects, including nausea and vomiting. Sertürner continued, however, to test the drug on himself, unaware of its ultimate addictive properties.

Sertürner was awarded his apothecary license in 1806 and established his own pharmacy in the Prussian town of Einbeck. In addition to operating his business, he continued to study the chemical and pharmacological properties of morphine for a number of years. His work drew little attention from professional scientists, however, and he eventually turned his attention to other topics, including the development of improved firearms and ammunition. During the last few years of his life, he became increasingly depressed about his failure to interest the scientific community in his research on opium. He withdrew into his own world and turned to morphine for comfort against his disillusionment with what he saw as the failure of his life. He did receive some comfort in 1831 when he was awarded a Montyon Prize by the Académie Française, sometimes described as the forerunner of the Nobel Prizes, with its cash award of 2,000 francs. By the time of his death in Hamelin, Prussia, on February 20, 1841, however, the scientific world in general had still not appreciated the enormous significance of his research on morphine.

Alexander "Sasha" Shulgin (1925–2014)

Shulgin was arguably the best known and most highly regarded advocates of so-called designer drugs within the scientific community. He is thought to have synthesized and tested more than 200 psychoactive compounds in his life, and wrote a number of important books and articles on the properties and potential benefits of such substances.

Alexander Shulgin, widely known as "Sasha," was born in Berkeley, California, on June 17, 1925. He graduated from high school at the age of 16 and received a full scholarship to Harvard University. His tenure at Harvard was cut short, however, with the beginning of World War II, during which he served with the U.S. Navy in both the North Atlantic and the Pacific campaigns. After the war, he returned to Berkeley, where he eventually earned his BA in chemistry at the University of California in 1949 and his PhD in biochemistry at 1954. He completed his postdoctoral studies at the University of California at San Francisco (UCSF) in pharmacology and psychiatry. After working for a year at the BioRad Laboratories company, he took a position with Dow Chemical, where he was a research scientist from 1955 to 1961 and senior research chemist from 1961 to 1966.

Shulgin's most significant accomplishment at Dow was to develop a pesticide known as *physostigmine*, a substance that was to become one of Dow's best-selling products. In appreciation of Shulgin's work, Dow provided him with a laboratory of his own where he was allowed to work on projects that were of special interest to him. One of those projects turned out to be the synthesis and study of psychedelic compounds. Shulgin later reported that his interest in psychedelics was prompted by his first experience in taking mescaline in 1960. As a result of that experience, he told an interviewer from *Playboy* magazine in 2004, he had found his "learning path," the direction he wanted the rest of his career to go.

In 1965, Shulgin decided to leave Dow in order to enter medical school at UCSF. He left that program after only two years, however, to pursue his interest in psychedelics. That decision posed a problem for both Shulgin and the U.S. Drug Enforcement Administration (DEA), the federal agency responsible for control of illegal drug use in the United States. Although its primary function is to discourage the development and use of illegal drugs, the DEA apparently saw some benefit in Shulgin's work, and they agreed to a special dispensation that allowed him to synthesize and study a number of otherwise illegal substances. That relationship eventually worked out well for both partners, as it permitted Shulgin to pursue the studies in which he was most interested and provided the DEA with invaluable information on substances about which it might otherwise have little or no information. In 1988, for example, he wrote *Controlled Substances: Chemical & Legal Guide to Federal Drug Laws*, a book that has become a standard reference for DEA employees.

Shulgin's special relationship with the DEA ended in 1994 when the agency raided his Berkeley laboratory and withdrew his license to conduct research on illegal substances, claiming that he had failed to keep proper records. Some observers believe, however, that the agency's actions were prompted by a book that Shulgin and his wife Ann had written a few years earlier, *PiHKAL: A Chemical Love Story*. (The PiHKAL of the title stands for "phenethylamines I have known and loved.")

The Shulgins later wrote a second book about another group of psychedelic substances, *TiHKAL: The Continuation*. In this case, the title word TiHKAL stands for "tryptamines I have known and loved." Another of Shulgin's books, *The Simple Plant Isoquinolines* (2002; with Wendy E. Perry), is somewhat more technically oriented. In 2008, his first two laboratory books were scanned and placed online.

During the last years of his life, Shulgin suffered from a variety of medical problems, including cardiac issues, a stroke, dementia, and liver cancer. He died at his home in Lafayette, California, on June 2, 2014.

Substance Abuse and Mental Health Services Administration

The Substance Abuse and Mental Health Services Administration (SAMHSA) was created in 1992 during the reorganization of the federal government's agencies responsible for mental health services. It assumed most of the responsibilities of the Alcohol, Drug Abuse, and Mental Health Administration, which was disbanded in the reorganization. The organization is charged with developing and supporting programs that improve the quality and availability of prevention, treatment, and rehabilitation for abusers of both legal and illegal drugs. Its work is divided among four major divisions, the Center for Mental Health Service, Center for Substance Abuse Prevention, Center for Substance Abuse Treatment, and Office of Applied Studies. Some of the programs the agency has recently funded include conferences for the dissemination of new knowledge about substance abuse, campus suicide prevention programs, community mental health services programs for children and their parents, jail diversion and trauma recovery programs (with special preference for veterans), supportive housing services, drug-free community programs, offender reentry programs, and state and community prevention programs.

SAMHSA has available a wealth of publications on all aspects of substance abuse, including reports such as Characteristics of

Substance Abuse Treatment Facilities Offering Acupuncture and Treatment for Substance Abuse and Depression among Adults by Race/Ethnicity; Fiscal Year 2008 Annual SYNAR Reports: Youth Tobacco Sales; SAMHSA Newsletter; informational brochures, pamphlets, flyers, and posters, such as those in the "Tips for Teens" series (about marijuana, methamphetamines, inhalants, heroin, steroids, club drugs, etc.) as well as "Keeping Your Teens Drug-Free: A Family Guide," "Get the Facts on Drugs," and "Good Mental Health Is Ageless."

Substance Abuse Librarians and Information Specialists

Substance Abuse Librarians and Information Specialists (SALIS) was formed in 1978 with the assistance of the U.S. National Institute on Drug Abuse and the National Institute on Alcohol Abuse and Alcoholism. SALIS merged with its Canadian counterpart, Librarians and Information Specialists in Addictions, in 1986. The organization's goals are to disseminate accurate information about the use and misuse of drugs; to provide a communications network for specialists working in the field of alcohol, tobacco, and other drug use and abuse; to serve as an advocate for members on issues of common interest; and to support programs for professional development. SALIS sponsors an annual national convention and provides a small number of scholarships for students in the field. The organization's main publications include *SALIS News,* a quarterly newsletter; ATOD Serials Database, an online database; *How to Organize and Operate an ATOD Information Center: A Guide,* an instruction manual; New Books List, an online database; and Alcohol, Tobacco and Other Drug Databases, online databases.

Luther L. Terry (1911–1985)

Terry was the ninth surgeon general of the United States. He was appointed to the office by President John F. Kennedy, and he served through Kennedy's incomplete first term in office and the first year of Lyndon B. Johnson's first term. He is probably best known today for the first report issued by the U.S. Public Health Service on the health effects of smoking, *Smoking and Health: Report of the Advisory Committee to the Surgeon General*, released in 1964. Among the many findings in that report, some of the most outstanding were that the mortality rate was 70 percent higher for smokers than for nonsmokers of a comparable age, that moderate smokers were 9 to 10 times more likely (and heavy smokers 20 times more likely) to develop cancer than nonsmokers, and that health risks rose and fell consistently with increases and decreases, respectively, in the amount of smoking.

Luther Leonidas Terry was born in Red Level, Alabama, on September 15, 1911, to James Edward and Lula M. (Durham) Terry. He attended Birmingham Southern College, from which he received his BA degree in 1931, and the Tulane Medical School, which awarded his MD in 1935. Terry completed his internship at the Hillman Hospital in Birmingham and his residency at City Hospitals in Cleveland. In 1938, he served an additional internship in pathology at Washington University, in St. Louis. In 1940, he accepted an appointment as instructor at the University of Texas, Galveston, where he remained for four years. He then moved to the Johns Hopkins University Medical School in Baltimore, while also holding an appointment at the Public Health Service Hospital in Baltimore. In 1950, he accepted an appointment as chief of General Medicine and Experimental Therapeutics at the National Heart Institute in Bethesda in 1950. The position was, at first, a part-time appointment, but it became a full-time post three years later when his division was transferred to the newly established National Institutes of Health Clinical Center. In 1958, Terry was appointed assistant director of the National Heart Institute and, three years later, became surgeon general of the United States.

Shortly after assuming his post as surgeon general, Terry appointed a committee to study the health effects of smoking.

His action was motivated to a large extent by a similar study that had just been completed and announced by the Royal College of Physicians in Great Britain, in which strong evidence for somewhat dramatic health effects as a result of smoking had been reported. Terry decided that a similar report for the United States was needed, although it would almost certainly be controversial and economically risky. The final report, issued on January 11, 1964, summarized the findings of more than 7,000 scientific articles and the expert testimony of more than 130 witnesses before Terry's committee.

After his retirement as surgeon general in 1965, Terry took a post as vice president for medical affairs and professor of medicine and community medicine at the University of Pennsylvania. He maintained his affiliation with Pennsylvania until 1982, and then accepted a position as corporate vice president for medical affairs and, later, as consultant to ARA Services, Inc. Terry died in Philadelphia on April 29, 1985.

United Nations Office on Drugs and Crime

The United Nations Office on Drugs and Crime (UNODC) was established in 1997 through the merger of the United Nations Drug Control Programme and the Centre for International Crime Prevention. The agency's mission is to assist member states in their battles against illegal substance abuse, crime, and terrorism. The three primary components of UNODC's work are providing technical assistance to member states in dealing with drug abuse, crime, and terrorism; conducting research to collect up-to-date information on these topics; and assisting member states in the ratification and implementation of various regional and international treaties dealing with drug use and crime. The agency currently conducts four major campaigns dealing with illegal substance abuse and crime: World Drug Day, International Anti-Corruption Day, World AIDS Day, and the Blue Heart Campaign against human trafficking. Much of the agency's work is carried out through two commissions. The Commission on Narcotic Drugs is the primary policy-making agency for the United Nations in the area of illegal substance abuse. The Commission on Crime Prevention and Criminal Justice provides the United Nations with guidance on policies and practices in these two fields.

Arguably the organization's most important single publication is the World Drug Report, an annual survey of the status of substance abuse throughout the world. UNODC also produces periodic reports on the status of drug abuse and crime worldwide, such as United Nations Surveys on Crime Trends and the Operations of Criminal Justice Systems and International Homicide Statistics. Its regular publications include the journal *Bulletin on Narcotics*, a popular magazine, *Perspectives*, an annual report of the agency's activities in the preceding year, and reports on a variety of specific topics, such as "Addiction Crime and Insurgency" (the threat posed by opium from Afghanistan), "Colombia Coca Survey," "Handbook for Parliamentarians on Combating Trafficking in Persons," "Handbook on Prisoners with Special Needs," and "HIV and AIDS in Places of Detention."

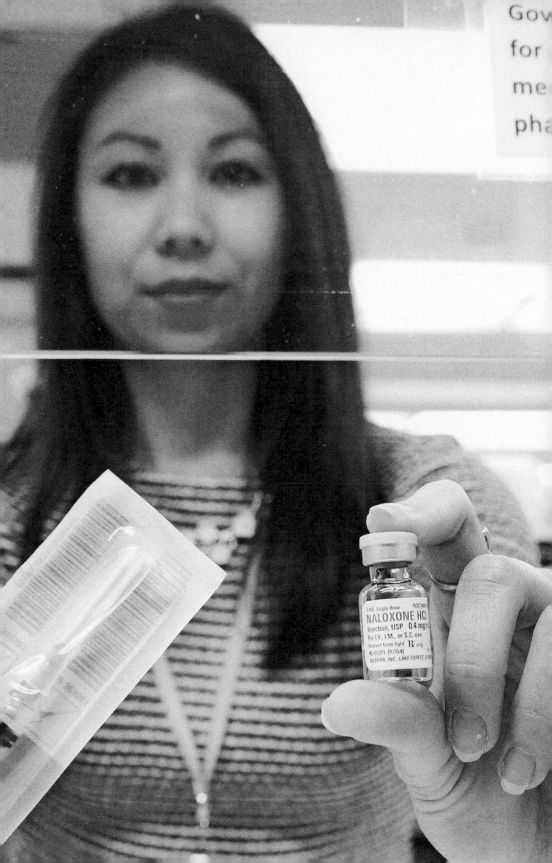

Introduction

An overview of the way in which the United States and other nations have tried to deal with substance abuse problems can be found by reviewing important documents related to the issue. This chapter contains examples of laws, treaties, reports, court cases, and other documents associated with one or another aspect of substance abuse. The chapter also provides data and statistics on the extent and effects of substance abuse.

Data

Table 5.1 Drug-Induced Deaths, 1999–2013

Year	Total	Male	Female	White	Black	Indian[1]	Asian[2]
1999	19,128	12,885	6,243	15,714	3,100	164	150
2000	19,720	13,137	6,583	16,388	3,034	160	138
2001	21,705	14,253	7,452	18,195	3,165	184	161
2002	26,040	16,734	9,306	22,146	3,463	230	201
2003	28,723	18,426	10,297	24,683	3,527	295	218
2004	30,711	19,362	11,349	26,474	3,633	354	250
2005	33,541	21,208	12,333	28,804	4,098	362	277

(Continued)

Tess Nishida, a pain pharmacist at the University of Washington, holds a vial of Naloxone, which can be used to block the potentially fatal effects of an opioid overdose, at an outpatient pharmacy at the university on October 7, 2016. (AP Photo/Ted S. Warren)

Table 5.1   (Continued)

Year	Total	Male	Female	White	Black	Indian[1]	Asian[2]
2006	38,396	24,507	13,889	32,866	4,790	407	333
2007	38,371	23,883	14,488	33,480	4,194	388	309
2008	38,649	23,928	14,721	34,237	3,662	451	299
2009	39,147	24,015	15,132	34,633	3,660	405	359
2010	40,393	24,376	16,017	36,020	3,561	458	354
2011	43,544	26,444	17,100	38,719	3,852	519	454
2012	43,819	26,594	17,225	38,890	3,940	562	427
2013	46,471	28,381	18,090	41,053	4,376	559	483

[1]American Indian or Alaska Native.
[2]Asian or Pacific Islander.

Source: "Number of Deaths, Death Rates, and Age-Adjusted Death Rates for Drug-Induced Causes, by Race and Sex: United States, 1999–2013." *National Vital Statistics Reports*, Vol. 64 No. 2, February 16, 2016, Table 1–3, page 6. http://www.cdc.gov/nchs/data/nvsr/nvsr64/nvsr64_02_tables.pdf#I03. Accessed on July 6, 2016.

Table 5.2   Schedules of Drugs, as Defined by the Controlled Substances Act of 1970

Schedule	Examples
I	Heroin, lysergic acid diethylamide (LSD), marijuana, mescaline, methaqualone, morphine, peyote, psilocybin
II	Amphetamine, cocaine, codeine, fentanyl, hydrocodone, meperidine, methadone, methamphetamine, morphine, opium and its extracts, phencyclidine (PCP)
III	Anabolic steroids (including testosterone and derivatives), barbituric acid derivatives ("barbiturates"), some codeine and hydrocodone products, ketamine, lysergic acid
IV	Alprazolam (Xanax), Chlordiazepoxide (e.g., Librium), chloral hydrate, diazepam (e.g., Valium), meprobamate (e.g., Miltown), phenobarbital (e.g., Luminal), zolpidem (e.g., Ambien), zopiclone (e.g., Lunesta)
V	Codeine and derivatives preparations, diphenoxylate preparations (e.g., Lomotil), opium preparations (e.g., Parapectolin)

Source: "Controlled Substances Schedule." 2016. Office of Diversion Control. Drug Enforcement Administration. U.S. Department of Justice. http://www.deadiversion.usdoj.gov/schedules/. Accessed on July 6, 2016.

Table 5.3 Treatment Admissions for Substance Abuse (2013)*

Substance	1997	1999	2001	2003	2005	2007	2009	2011	2013
Total	1,607,957	1,725,885	1,780,239	1,867,796	1,885,507	1,817,577	2,047,041	1,928,792	1,683,451
Alcohol	796,674	824,641	788,259	776,091	741,987	732,925	852,714	756,829	631,578
Alcohol only	455,699	461,532	433,620	430,990	408,422	406,038	477,963	416,918	355,366
Alcohol with secondary drug	350,975	363,109	354,639	345,101	333,565	326,887	374,751	339,911	276,212
Opiates	251,417	280,145	315,869	326,836	329,730	337,387	433,516	478,056	471,575
Heroin	235,143	257,508	277,653	273,996	259,462	246,871	287,388	282,459	316,797
Other opiates/ synthetics	16,274	22,637	38,216	52,840	70,268	90,516	146,128	195,597	154,778
Non-R$_X$ methadone	1,209	1,606	2,050	2,719	4,070	5,094	6,349	6,814	4,915
Other opiates/ synthetics	15,065	21,031	36,166	50,121	66,198	85,422	139,779	188,783	149,863
Cocaine	236,770	242,143	230,870	254,687	266,420	234,772	192,827	152,038	102,387
Smoked cocaine	174,900	176,507	168,890	184,846	191,973	167,914	138,362	105,166	69,629
Non-smoked cocaine	61,870	65,636	61,980	69,841	74,447	66,858	54,465	46,872	32,758
Marijuana/hashish	197,840	232,105	265,975	291,470	301,263	287,933	372,245	352,397	281,991
Stimulants	68,166	73,568	97,358	135,063	173,081	143,921	120,115	117,598	139,345
Methamphetamine	53,694	58,801	78,390	114,451	154,447	137,154	111,839	107,430	130,033
Other amphetamines	13,737	13,890	17,527	19,327	17,667	5,870	7,251	8,611	8,481

(Continued)

Table 5.3 (Continued)

Substance	1997	1999	2001	2003	2005	2007	2009	2011	2013
Other stimulants	735	877	1,441	1,285	967	897	1,025	1,557	831
Other drugs	18,942	26,702	33,324	29,821	28,167	25,823	43,415	46,629	36,498
Tranquilizers	4,796	5,913	7,447	8,164	8,458	9,949	15,538	19,234	15,384
Benzodiazepine	3,835	5,048	6,497	7,402	7,928	9,491	14,974	18,798	15,077
Other tranquilizers	961	865	950	762	530	458	564	436	307
Sedatives/hypnotics	3,240	3,459	3,998	4,277	4,456	4,210	5,293	3,985	3,307
Barbiturates	1,278	1,148	1,274	1,337	1,380	1,013	1,342	946	982
Other sedatives/ hypnotics	1,962	2,311	2,724	2,940	3,076	3,197	3,951	3,039	2,325
Hallucinogens	2,672	2,789	3,149	2,236	2,006	1,502	1,867	1,995	2,088
PCP	1,896	2,321	3,193	4,177	2,861	3,124	4,435	5,756	5,109
Inhalants	1,819	1,423	1,259	1,217	1,372	992	1,603	1,252	913
Over-the-counter	506	1,091	624	708	768	802	1,723	1,314	1,020
Other	4,013	9,706	13,654	9,042	8,246	5,244	12,956	13,093	8,677
None reported	38,148	46,581	48,584	53,828	44,859	54,816	32,209	25,245	20,077

*Latest year for which data are available, as of July 5, 2016.

Sources: Table 1a. Admissions by primary substance of abuse: TEDS 1997–2007. Number. Treatment Episode Data Set (TEDS) Highlights—2007. Rockville, MD: Substance Abuse and Mental Health Services Administration, February 2009. http://wwwdasis.samhsa.gov/dasis2/teds_pubs/2007_teds_highlights_rpt.pdf. Accessed on July 5, 2016, and Table 1.1a. Admissions aged 12 and older, by primary substance of abuse: Number, 2003–2013. http://www.samhsa.gov/data/sites/default/files/2013_Treatment_Episode_Data_Set_National/2013_Treatment_Episode_Data_Set_National_Tables.html. Accessed on July 5, 2016.

Table 5.4   Past Month Illicit Drug Use among People Aged 12 or Older, by Age Group and by Drug: Percentages, 2002–2014

Any illicit drug

Age	2002	2003	2004	2005	2006	2007	2008	2009	2010	2011	2012	2013	2014
>12	8.3	8.2	7.9	8.1	8.3	8.0	8.1	8.7	8.9	8.7	9.2	9.5	10.2
12 to 17	11.6	11.2	10.6	9.9	9.8	9.6	9.3	10.1	10.1	10.1	9.5	8.8	9.4
18 to 25	20.2	20.3	19.4	20.1	19.8	19.8	19.7	21.4	21.6	21.4	21.3	21.5	22.0
26 or older	5.8	5.6	5.5	5.8	6.1	5.8	5.9	6.3	6.6	6.3	7.0	7.3	8.3

Marijuana

Age	2002	2003	2004	2005	2006	2007	2008	2009	2010	2011	2012	2013	2014
>12	6.2	6.2	6.1	6.0	6.0	5.8	6.1	6.7	6.9	7.0	7.3	7.5	8.4
12 to 17	8.2	7.9	7.6	6.8	6.7	6.7	6.7	7.4	7.4	7.9	7.2	7.1	7.2
18 to 25	17.3	17.0	16.1	16.6	16.3	16.5	16.6	18.2	18.5	19.0	18.7	19.1	19.6
26 or older	4.0	4.0	4.1	4.1	4.2	3.9	4.2	4.6	4.8	4.8	5.3	5.6	6.6

Any prescription drug

Age	2002	2003	2004	2005	2006	2007	2008	2009	2010	2011	2012	2013	2014
>12	2.7	2.7	2.5	2.7	2.9	2.8	2.5	2.8	2.7	2.4	2.6	2.5	2.5
12 to 17	4.0	4.0	3.6	3.3	3.3	3.3	2.9	3.1	3.0	2.8	2.8	2.2	2.6
18 to 25	5.5	6.1	6.1	6.3	6.5	5.9	5.9	6.4	5.9	5.0	5.3	4.8	4.4
26 or older	2.0	2.0	1.8	1.9	2.2	2.2	1.9	2.1	2.2	1.9	2.1	2.1	2.1

(Continued)

231

Table 5.4 (Continued)

Cocaine

Age	2002	2003	2004	2005	2006	2007	2008	2009	2010	2011	2012	2013	2014
>12	0.9	1.0	0.8	1.0	1.0	0.8	0.7	0.7	0.6	0.5	0.6	0.6	0.6
12 to 17	0.6	0.6	0.5	0.6	0.4	0.4	0.4	0.3	0.2	0.3	0.1	0.2	0.2
18 to 25	2.0	2.2	2.1	2.6	2.2	1.7	1.6_	1.4	1.5	1.4	1.1	1.1	1.4
26 or Older	0.7	0.8	0.7	0.8	0.8	0.7	0.7	0.6	0.5	0.4	0.6	0.5	0.5

Heroin

Age	2002	2003	2004	2005	2006	2007	2008	2009	2010	2011	2012	2013	2014
>12	0.1	0.1	0.1	0.1	0.1	0.1	0.1	0.1	0.1	0.1	0.1	0.1	0.2
12 to 17	0	0.1	0.1	0.1	0.1	0.0	0.1	0.1	0.0	0.1	*_	0.1	0.1
18 to 25	0.1	0.1	0.1	0.2	0.2	0.1	0.2	0.2	0.3	0.3	0.4	0.3	0.2
26 or older	0.1	0.0	0.1	0.0	0.1	0.1	0.1	0.1	0.1	0.1	0.1	0.1	0.2

Any stimulant

Age	2002	2003	2004	2005	2006	2007	2008	2009	2010	2011	2012	2013	2014
>12	0.6	0.6	0.5	0.5	0.6	0.4	0.4	0.5	0.4	0.4	0.5	0.5	0.6
12 to 17	0.8	0.9	0.7	0.7	0.7	0.5	0.5	0.5	0.4	0.4	0.5	0.3	0.7
18 to 25	1.3	1.3	1.5	1.4	1.4	1.1	1.1	1.3	1.2	1.0	1.2	1.3	1.2
26 or older	0.4	0.4	0.4	0.3	0.4	0.3	0.2	0.4	0.3	0.3	0.3	0.4	0.5

Any tranquilizer

Age	2002	2003	2004	2005	2006	2007	2008	2009	2010	2011	2012	2013	2014
>12	0.8	0.8	0.7	0.7	0.7	0.7	0.7	0.8	0.9	0.7	0.8	0.6	0.7
12 to 17	0.8	0.9	0.6	0.6	0.5	0.7	0.6	0.6	0.5	0.6	0.6	0.4	0.4
18 to 25	1.6	1.7	1.8	1.9	2.0	1.7	1.7	1.9	1.7	1.6	1.6	1.2	1.2
26 or Older	0.6	0.6	0.5	0.6	0.5	0.6	0.6	0.7	0.7	0.6	0.7	0.6	0.7

*Low precision; no estimate reported.

Source: Hedden, Sarra L., et al. 2015. "Behavioral Health Trends in the United States: Results from the 2014 National Survey on Drug Use and Health." HHS Publication No. SMA 15-4927, NSDUH Series H-50, Tables for Figures 2, 3, 4, 7, 9, 11, 12, pages 5–11. http://www.samhsa.gov/data/sites/default/files/NSDUH-FRR1-2014/NSDUH-FRR1-2014.pdf. Accessed on July 5, 2016.

Table 5.5 Cigarette Consumption, in Billions, in the United States, 1900–2007

Year	1900	1901	1902	1903	1904	1905	1906	1907	1908	1909
Total cigarettes	2.5	2.5	2.8	3.1	3.3	3.6	4.5	5.3	5.7	7.0
Cigarettes per capita	54	53	60	64	66	70	86	99	105	125
Year	**1910**	**1911**	**1912**	**1913**	**1914**	**1915**	**1916**	**1917**	**1918**	**1919**
Total cigarettes	8.6	10.1	13.2	15.8	16.5	17.9	25.2	35.7	45.6	48.0
Cigarettes per capita	151	173	223	260	267	285	395	551	697	727
Year	**1920**	**1921**	**1922**	**1923**	**1924**	**1925**	**1926**	**1927**	**1928**	**1929**
Total cigarettes	44.6	50.7	53.4	64.4	71.0	79.8	89.1	97.5	106.0	118.6
Cigarettes per capita	665	742	770	911	982	1,085	1,191	1,279	1,366	1,504
Year	**1930**	**1931**	**1932**	**1933**	**1934**	**1935**	**1936**	**1937**	**1938**	**1939**
Total cigarettes	119.3	114.0	102.8	111.6	125.7	134.4	152.7	162.8	163.4	172.1
Cigarettes per capita	1,485	1,399	1,245	1,334	1,483	1,564	1,754	1,847	1,830	1,900
Year	**1940**	**1941**	**1942**	**1943**	**1944**	**1945**	**1946**	**1947**	**1948**	**1949**
Total cigarettes	181.9	208.9	245.0	284.3	296.3	340.6	344.3	345.4	358.9	360.9
Cigarettes per capita	1,976	2,236	2,585	2,956	3,039	3,449	3,446	3,416	3,505	3,480
Year	**1950**	**1951**	**1952**	**1953**	**1954**	**1955**	**1956**	**1957**	**1958**	**1959**
Total cigarettes	369.8	397.1	416.0	408.2	387.0	396.4	406.5	422.5	448.9	467.5
Cigarettes per capita	3,552	3,744	3,886	3,778	3,546	3,597	3,650	3,755	3,953	4,073

Year	1960	1961	1962	1963	1964	1965	1966	1967	1968	1969
Total cigarettes	484.4	502.5	508.4	523.9	511.3	528.8	541.3	549.3	545.6	528.9
Cigarettes per capita	4,171	4,266	4,266	4,345	4,194	4,258	4,287	4,280	4,186	3,993

Year	1970	1971	1972	1973	1974	1975	1976	1977	1978	1979
Total cigarettes	536.5	555.1	566.8	589.7	599.0	607.2	613.5	617.0	616.0	621.5
Cigarettes per capita	3,985	4,037	4,043	4,148	4,141	4,122	4,091	4,043	3,970	3,861

Year	1980	1981	1982	1983	1984	1985	1986	1987	1988	1989
Total cigarettes	631.5	640.0	634.0	600.0	600.4	594.0	583.8	575.0	562.5	540.0
Cigarettes per capita	3,849	3,836	3,739	3,488	3,446	3,370	3,274	3,197	3,096	2,926

Year	1990	1991	1992	1993	1994	1995	1996	1997	1998	1999
Total cigarettes	525.0	510.0	500.0	485.0	486.0	487.0	487.0	480.0	465.0	435.0
Cigarettes per capita	2,834	2,727	2,647	2,543	2,524	2,474	2,445	2,422	2,275	2,101

Year	2000	2001	2002	2003	2004	2005	2006	2007	2008	2009
Total cigarettes	435.6	426.7	415.7	400.3	397.6	381.1	380.6	361.6	346.4	317.7
Cigarettes per capita	2,076	2,010	1,936	1,844	1,811	1,717	1,695	1,591	1,507	1,367

Year	2010	2011
Total cigarettes	300.4	292.8
Cigarettes per capita	1,278	1,232

Source: 1900–1999: "Trends in Tobacco Use." 2011. American Lung Association. http://www.lung.org/assets/documents/research/tobacco-trend-report.pdf. Accessed on July 6, 2016. 2000–2011: "Consumption of Cigarettes and Combustible Tobacco—United States, 2000–2011."

Table 5.6   Alcohol-Related Vehicular Accident Fatalities, United States, 1982–2004

Year	Traffic Crashes	Traffic Fatalities	Alcohol-Related Traffic Crash Fatalities	Percentage of Alcohol-Related Traffic Crash Fatalities
1982	39,092	43,945	26,172	59.6
1983	37,976	42,589	24,634	57.8
1984	39,631	44,257	24,761	55.9
1985	39,195	43,825	23,166	52.9
1986	41,090	46,087	25,017	54.3
1987	41,438	46,390	24,093	51.9
1988	42,130	47,087	23,833	50.6
1989	40,741	45,582	22,423	49.2
1990	39,836	44,599	22,587	50.6
1991	36,937	41,508	20,159	48.6
1992	34,942	39,250	18,290	46.6
1993	35,780	40,150	17,908	44.6
1994	36,254	40,716	17,308	42.5
1995	37,241	41,817	17,732	42.4
1996	37,494	42,065	17,749	42.2
1997	37,324	42,013	16,711	39.8
1998	37,107	41,501	16,673	40.2
1999	37,140	41,717	16,572	39.7
2000	37,526	41,945	17,380	41.4
2001	37,862	42,196	17,400	41.2
2002	38,491	43,005	17,524	40.7
2003	38,477	42,884	17,105	39.9
2004	38,444	42,836	16,919	39.5
2005	—	43,443	16,885	39
2006	—	42,532	15,829	37
2007	—	41,059	15,387	37
2008	—	37,261	13,846	37
2009	—	33,808	12,744	38
2010	—	32,885	10,228	31
2011	—	32,367	9,878	38

A crash is considered as alcohol-related if either a driver or a nonoccupant (pedestrian or pedal cyclist) had a blood alcohol concentration (BAC) of 0.01 g/dl or greater. When alcohol tests were not done or test results are unknown, imputed BAC data provided by NHTSA are used. (*Footnote from original table.*)

Source: 1982–2004: Yi, Hsiao-ye Yi, Chiung M. Chen, and Gerald D. Williams. *Surveillance Report #76: Trends in Alcohol-Related Fatal Traffic Crashes, United States, 1982–2004.* Washington, DC: National Institute on Alcohol Abuse and Alcoholism. Division of Epidemiology and Prevention Research. Alcohol Epidemiologic Data System, August 2006, 30, Table 8. 2005–2011: "2011 Drunk Driving Statistics." 2016. Alcohol Alert. http://www.alcoholalert.com/drunk-driving-statistics.html. Accessed on July 6, 2016.

Documents

Harrison Narcotic Act (1914)

Probably the first effort by the U.S. government to exert some control over the production, distribution, and consumption of recreational drugs was the Harrison Narcotic Act of 1914. Although this act did not make the drugs with which it dealt—opiates—illegal, it did place a tax on their production, distribution, and sale. In retrospect, the Harrison Act was a weak effort to control substance abuse, but it is historically significant because of its being the first attempt to interrupt substance abuse in any way whatsoever by the federal government. The core of the act is expressed in its first section, reproduced here.

Be it enacted by the Senate and House of Representatives of the United States of America in Congress assembled, that on and after the first day of March, nineteen hundred and fifteen, every person who produces, imports, manufactures, compounds, deals in, dispenses, distributes, or gives away opium or coca leaves or any compound, manufacture, salt, derivative, or preparation thereof, shall register with the collector of internal revenue of the district, his name or style, place of business, and place or places where such business is to be carried on: Provided, that the office, or if none, then the residence of any person shall be considered for purposes of this Act to be his place of business. At the time of such registry and on or before the first of July annually thereafter, every person who produces, imports, manufactures, compounds, deals in, dispenses, distributes, or gives away any of the aforesaid drugs shall pay to the said collector a special tax at the rate of $1 per annum: Provided, that no employee of any person who produces, imports, manufactures, compounds, deals in, dispenses, distributes, or gives away any of the aforesaid drugs, acting within the scope of his employment, shall be required to register or to pay the special tax provided by this section: Provided further, That officers of the United States Government who are lawfully engaged in making purchases of the above-named drugs for the various departments of the Army and Navy, the Public Health Service, and for Government hospitals and prisons, and officers of State governments or any municipality therein, who are lawfully engaged in making purchases of the above-named drugs for State, county, or municipal hospitals or prisons, and officials of any Territory or insular possession, or the District of Columbia or of the United States who are lawfully engaged in making purchases of the above-named drugs for hospitals or prisons therein shall not be required to register and pay the special tax as herein required.

Source: Public Law No. 223, 63rd Cong. Available at Schaffer Library of Drug Policy. http://druglibrary.org/schaffer/history/e1910/harrisonact.htm. Accessed on July 3, 2016.

Eighteenth Amendment to the U.S. Constitution (1919)

On December 17, 1917, the U.S. House of Representatives took the first step in amending the U.S. Constitution to prohibit the use of alcoholic beverages in the United States. The U.S. Senate approved the same act the following day. The proposed amendment was then submitted to the separate states, where it was finally approved by the required number of states (36) on January 16, 1919. Ultimately, only two states defeated the proposed amendment: Connecticut and Rhode Island. On January 26, 1919, Acting Secretary of State Frank L. Polk certified adoption of the amendment. The amendment did not specifically prohibit the use of alcoholic beverages in the United States, although it made it very difficult to obtain such beverages legally. The text of the amendment is as follows.

Amendment XVIII

> Section 1. After one year from the ratification of this article the manufacture, sale, or transportation of intoxicating liquors within, the importation thereof into, or the exportation thereof from the United States and all territory subject to the jurisdiction thereof for beverage purposes is hereby prohibited.
>
> Section 2. The Congress and the several states shall have concurrent power to enforce this article by appropriate legislation.
>
> Section 3. This article shall be inoperative unless it shall have been ratified as an amendment to the Constitution by the legislatures of the several states, as provided in the Constitution, within seven years from the date of the submission hereof to the states by the Congress.

Source: Charters of Freedom, National Archives.

Twenty-First Amendment to the U.S. Constitution (1933)

After more than a decade of Prohibition in the United States, many people were convinced that the great experiment to control the use of alcohol in this country was a failure. In response to that feeling, the U.S. Congress on February 20, 1933, adopted an act initiating the repeal of the Eighteenth Amendment by the adoption of a new amendment to the Constitution, the Twenty-First Amendment, which abrogated the earlier amendment. On December 5, 1933, the 36th state, Utah, ratified the amendment, and it was certified on the same date. Only one state, South Carolina, rejected the proposed amendment, although eight other states never took action on the amendment. The text of the amendment is as follows.

Amendment XXI

Section 1. The eighteenth article of amendment to the Constitution of the United States is hereby repealed.

Section 2. The transportation or importation into any state, territory, or possession of the United States for delivery or use therein of intoxicating liquors, in violation of the laws thereof, is hereby prohibited.

Section 3. This article shall be inoperative unless it shall have been ratified as an amendment to the Constitution by conventions in the several states, as provided in the Constitution, within seven years from the date of the submission hereof to the states by the Congress.

Source: Charters of Freedom, National Archives.

Federal Cigarette Labeling and Advertising Act (1965)

The first significant government report on the health effects of smoking—Smoking and Health: Report of the Advisory Committee to the Surgeon General of the Public Health Service—was issued in 1965. The report had a significant impact on the general public, on advocacy groups opposed to smoking, and on lawmakers. One direct result of the report was the Federal Cigarette Labeling and Advertising Act of 1965, which was later amended a number of times. The provisions of the original law and later amendments are now part of the U.S. Code, at Title 15, Chapter 36. A note about the 1984 amendment is included in the following excerpt.

§ 1331. Congressional Declaration of Policy and Purpose

It is the policy of the Congress, and the purpose of this chapter, to establish a comprehensive Federal Program to deal with cigarette labeling and advertising with respect to any relationship between smoking and health, whereby—

(1) the public may be adequately informed about any adverse health effects of cigarette smoking by inclusion of warning notices on each package of cigarettes and in each advertisement of cigarettes; and

(2) commerce and the national economy may be

   (A) protected to the maximum extent consistent with this declared policy and

   (B) not impeded by diverse, nonuniform, and confusing cigarette labeling and advertising regulations with respect to any relationship between smoking and health.

Section 1332 provides definitions for a number of terms used in the act.

The core of the bill is found in Section 1333, which provides, in part, that:

§ 1333. Labeling; Requirements; Conspicuous Statement

(a) Required warnings; packages; advertisements; billboards

   (1) It shall be unlawful for any person to manufacture, package, or import for sale or distribution within the United States any cigarettes the package of which fails to bear, in accordance with the requirements of this section, one of the following labels:

   SURGEON GENERAL'S WARNING: Smoking Causes Lung Cancer, Heart Disease, Emphysema, And May Complicate Pregnancy.

   SURGEON GENERAL'S WARNING: Cigarette Smoke Contains Carbon Monoxide.

   (2) It shall be unlawful for any manufacturer or importer of cigarettes to advertise or cause to be advertised (other than through the use of outdoor billboards) within the United States any cigarette unless the advertising bears,

in accordance with the requirements of this section, one of the following labels:

SURGEON GENERAL'S WARNING: Smoking Causes Lung Cancer, Heart Disease, Emphysema, And May Complicate Pregnancy.

SURGEON GENERAL'S WARNING: Cigarette Smoke Contains Carbon Monoxide.

(3) It shall be unlawful for any manufacturer or importer of cigarettes to advertise or cause to be advertised within the United States through the use of outdoor billboards any cigarette unless the advertising bears, in accordance with the requirements of this section, one of the following labels: SURGEON GENERAL'S WARNING: Cigarette Smoke Contains Carbon Monoxide.

SURGEON GENERAL'S WARNING: Smoking Causes Lung Cancer, Heart Disease, And Emphysema.

(b) Conspicuous statement; label statement format; outdoor billboard statement format

(1) Each label statement required by paragraph (1) of subsection (a) of this section shall be located in the place label statements were placed on cigarette packages as of October 12, 1984. The phrase "Surgeon General's Warning" shall appear in capital letters and the size of all other letters in the label shall be the same as the size of such letters as of October 12, 1984. All the letters in the label shall appear in conspicuous and legible type in contrast by typography, layout, or color with all other printed material on the package.

This section continues with more detailed instructions about the precise nature of the labeling to be used.

In 1984, the original act was amended to change the wording required on all cigarette packages. The new ruling required the use of one of the four following statements:

- SURGEON GENERAL'S WARNING: Smoking Causes Lung Cancer, Heart Disease, Emphysema, And May Complicate Pregnancy.
- SURGEON GENERAL'S WARNING: Quitting Smoking Now Greatly Reduces Serious Risks to Your Health.
- SURGEON GENERAL'S WARNING: Smoking by Pregnant Women May Result in Fetal Injury, Premature Birth, and Low Birth Weight.
- SURGEON GENERAL'S WARNING: Cigarette Smoke Contains Carbon Monoxide.

Source: U.S. Code, Title 15, Chapter 36, Sections 1331 and 1333.

Controlled Substances Act (1970)

The cornerstone of the U.S. government's efforts to control substance abuse is the Controlled Substances Act of 1970, now a part of the U.S. Code, Title 21, Chapter 13. That act established the system of "schedules" for various categories of drugs that is still used by agencies of the U.S. government today. It also provides extensive background information about the domestic and international status of drug abuse efforts. Some of the most relevant sections for the domestic portion of the act are reprinted here.

Section 801 of the act presents Congress's findings and declarations about controlled substances, with special mention in Section 801a of psychotropic drugs.

§ 801. Congressional Findings and Declarations:

Controlled Substances

The Congress makes the following findings and declarations:

(1) Many of the drugs included within this subchapter have a useful and legitimate medical purpose and are necessary to maintain the health and general welfare of the American people.

(2) The illegal importation, manufacture, distribution, and possession and improper use of controlled substances have a substantial and detrimental effect on the health and general welfare of the American people.

. . .

(7) The United States is a party to the Single Convention on Narcotic Drugs, 1961, and other international conventions designed to establish effective control over international and domestic traffic in controlled substances.

§ 801a. Congressional Findings and Declarations:

Psychotropic Substances

The Congress makes the following findings and declarations:

(1) The Congress has long recognized the danger involved in the manufacture, distribution, and use of certain psychotropic substances for nonscientific and nonmedical purposes, and has provided strong and effective legislation to control illicit trafficking and to regulate legitimate uses of psychotropic substances in this country. Abuse of psychotropic substances has become a phenomenon common to many countries, however, and is not confined to national borders. It is, therefore, essential that the United States cooperate with other nations in establishing effective controls over international traffic in such substances.

(2) The United States has joined with other countries in executing an international treaty, entitled the Convention on Psycho-tropic Substances and signed at Vienna, Austria, on February 21, 1971, which is designed to establish suitable controls over the manufacture, distribution, transfer, and use of certain psychotropic substances. The Convention is not self-executing, and the obligations of the United States thereunder may only be performed pursuant to appropriate legislation. It is the intent of the Congress that the

amendments made by this Act, together with existing law, will enable the United States to meet all of its obligations under the Convention and that no further legislation will be necessary for that purpose.

. . .

Section 802 deals with definitions used in the act, and section 803 deals with a minor housekeeping issue of financing for the act. Section 811 deals with the attorney general's authority for classifying and declassifying drugs and the manner in which these steps are to be taken. In general:

§ 811. Authority and criteria for classification of substances

(a) Rules and regulations of Attorney General; hearing

The Attorney General shall apply the provisions of this subchapter to the controlled substances listed in the schedules established by section 812 of this title and to any other drug or other substance added to such schedules under this subchapter. Except as provided in subsections (d) and (e) of this section, the Attorney General may by rule—

(1) add to such a schedule or transfer between such schedules any drug or other substance if he—

    (A) finds that such drug or other substance has a potential for abuse, and

    (B) makes with respect to such drug or other substance the findings prescribed by subsection (b) of section 812 of this title for the schedule in which such drug is to be placed; or

(2) remove any drug or other substance from the schedules if he finds that the drug or other substance does not meet the requirements for inclusion in any schedule.

. . .

Section (b) provides guidelines for the evaluation of drugs and other substances. The next section, (c), is a key element of the act.

(c) Factors determinative of control or removal from schedules

In making any finding under subsection (a) of this section or under subsection (b) of section 812 of this title, the Attorney General shall consider the following factors with respect to each drug or other substance proposed to be controlled or removed from the schedules:

(1) Its actual or relative potential for abuse.

(2) Scientific evidence of its pharmacological effect, if known.

(3) The state of current scientific knowledge regarding the drug or other substance.

(4) Its history and current pattern of abuse.

(5) The scope, duration, and significance of abuse.

(6) What, if any, risk there is to the public health.

(7) Its psychic or physiological dependence liability.

(8) Whether the substance is an immediate precursor of a substance already controlled under this subchapter.

Section (d) is a lengthy discussion of international aspects of the nation's efforts to control substance abuse. Sections (e) through (h) deal with related, but less important, issues of the control of substance abuse. Section 812 is perhaps of greatest interest to the general reader in that it establishes the system of classifying drugs still used in the United States, along with the criteria for classification and the original list of drugs to be included in each schedule (since greatly expanded):

§ 812. Schedules of Controlled Substances

(a) Establishment

There are established five schedules of controlled substances, to be known as schedules I, II, III, IV, and V. Such schedules shall initially consist of the substances listed in this section. The schedules established by this section shall be updated and republished on a semiannual basis during the two-year period beginning one year after October 27, 1970, and shall be updated and republished on an annual basis thereafter.

(b) Placement on schedules; findings required

Except where control is required by United States obligations under an international treaty, convention, or protocol, in effect on October 27, 1970, and except in the case of an immediate precursor, a drug or other substance may not be placed in any schedule unless the findings required for such schedule are made with respect to such drug or other substance. The findings required for each of the schedules are as follows:

(1) Schedule I.—

    (A) The drug or other substance has a high potential for abuse.

    (B) The drug or other substance has no currently accepted medical use in treatment in the United States.

    (C) There is a lack of accepted safety for use of the drug or other substance under medical supervision.

(2) Schedule II.—

    (A) The drug or other substance has a high potential for abuse.

    (B) The drug or other substance has a currently accepted medical use in treatment in the United States or a currently accepted medical use with severe restrictions.

    (C) Abuse of the drug or other substances may lead to severe psychological or physical dependence.

(3) Schedule III.—

    (A) The drug or other substance has a potential for abuse less than the drugs or other substances in schedules I and II.

    (B) The drug or other substance has a currently accepted medical use in treatment in the United States.

    (C) Abuse of the drug or other substance may lead to moderate or low physical dependence or high psychological dependence.

(4) Schedule IV.—

   (A) The drug or other substance has a low potential for abuse relative to the drugs or other substances in schedule III.

   (B) The drug or other substance has a currently accepted medical use in treatment in the United States.

   (C) Abuse of the drug or other substance may lead to limited physical dependence or psychological dependence relative to the drugs or other substances in schedule III.

(5) Schedule V.—

   (A) The drug or other substance has a low potential for abuse relative to the drugs or other substances in schedule IV.

   (B) The drug or other substance has a currently accepted medical use in treatment in the United States.

   (C) Abuse of the drug or other substance may lead to limited physical dependence or psychological dependence relative to the drugs or other substances in schedule IV.

(c) Initial schedules of controlled substances

Schedules I, II, III, IV, and V shall, unless and until amended [1] pursuant to section 811 of this title, consist of the following drugs or other substances, by whatever official name, common or usual name, chemical name, or brand name designated: *The initial list of drugs under each schedule follows.*

Source: U.S. Code, Title 21, Chapter 13.

Vernonia v. Acton, 515 U.S. 646 (1995)

The U.S. Supreme Court has acted on a number of cases involving drug testing in a variety of situations. Its first decision in a school-related setting came in 1995 in the case of Vernonia School District 47J, Petitioner V. Wayne Acton, et ux. *In that case, the school board of the Vernonia (Oregon) school district decided that any student wishing to participate in athletics at the school had to sign an agreement to take a drug test. One student who declined to do so, James Acton, chose not to take the test, and was prohibited from joining the school's seventh-grade football team. Ultimately, his parents brought suit against the school district on his behalf, claiming that suspicionless drug testing was unconstitutional. The case worked its way through the courts, with each side recording at least one favorable ruling along the way, until it reached the U.S. Supreme Court in 1995, at which time the Court ruled for the school district by a vote of 6 to 3. The main arguments of the Court, as provided in Justice Scalia's decision, were as follows (citations omitted, as indicated by ellipsis, . . .).*

The Fourth Amendment to the United States Constitution provides that the Federal Government shall not violate "[t]he right of the people to be secure in their persons, houses, papers, and effects, against unreasonable searches and seizures . . . . "We have held that the Fourteenth Amendment extends this constitutional guarantee to searches and seizures by state officers, . . . including public school officials. . . . In Skinner v. Railway Labor Executives' Assn., . . . we held that state compelled collection and testing of urine, such as that required by the Student Athlete Drug Policy, constitutes a "search" subject to the demands of the Fourth Amendment. . . .

As the text of the Fourth Amendment indicates, the ultimate measure of the constitutionality of a governmental search is "reasonableness." At least in a case such as this, where there was no clear practice, either approving or disapproving the type of search at issue, at the time the constitutional provision was enacted, . . . whether a particular search meets the reasonableness standard" 'is judged by balancing its intrusion on the individual's Fourth Amendment interests against its promotion of legitimate governmental interests.' ". . . Where a search is undertaken by law enforcement officials to discover evidence of criminal wrongdoing, this Court has said that reasonableness generally requires the obtaining of a judicial warrant. . . . Warrants cannot be issued, of course, without the showing of probable cause required by the Warrant Clause. But a warrant is not required to establish the reasonableness of all government searches; and when a warrant is not required (and the Warrant Clause therefore not applicable), probable cause is not invariably required either. A search unsupported by probable cause can be constitutional, we have said, "when special needs, beyond the normal need for law enforcement, make the warrant and probable cause requirement impracticable." . . .

We have found such "special needs" to exist in the public school context. There, the warrant requirement "would unduly interfere with the maintenance of the swift and informal disciplinary procedures [that are] needed," and "strict adherence to the requirement that searches be based upon probable cause" would undercut "the substantial need of teachers and administrators for freedom to maintain order in the schools." . . . The school search we approved in T. L. O., while not based on probable cause, was based on individualized suspicion of wrongdoing. As we explicitly acknowledged, however, " 'the Fourth Amendment imposes no irreducible requirement of such suspicion,' " . . . We have upheld suspicionless searches and seizures to conduct drug testing of railroad personnel involved in train accidents, . . . ; to conduct random drug testing of federal customs officers who carry arms or are involved in drug interdiction. . . .

. . .

Fourth Amendment rights, no less than First and Fourteenth Amendment rights, are different in public schools than elsewhere; the "reasonableness" inquiry cannot disregard the schools' custodial and tutelary responsibility for children. For their own good and that of their classmates, public school children are routinely required to submit to various physical examinations, and to be vaccinated against various diseases. . .

Legitimate privacy expectations are even less with regard to student athletes. School sports are not for the bashful. They require "suiting up" before each practice or event, and showering and changing afterwards. . . .

There is an additional respect in which school athletes have a reduced expectation of privacy. By choosing to "go out for the team," they voluntarily subject themselves to a degree of regulation even higher than that imposed on students generally. In Vernonia's public schools, they must submit to a preseason physical exam (James testified that his included the giving of a urine sample, App. 17), they must acquire adequate insurance coverage or sign an insurance waiver, maintain a minimum grade point average, and comply with any "rules of conduct, dress, training hours and related matters as may be established for each sport by the head coach and athletic director with the principal's approval." . . . Somewhat like adults who choose to participate in a "closely regulated industry," students who voluntarily participate in school athletics have reason to expect intrusions upon normal rights and privileges, including privacy.

Having considered the scope of the legitimate expectation of privacy at issue here, we turn next to the character of the intrusion that is complained of. We recognized in Skinner that collecting the samples for urinalysis intrudes upon "an excretory function traditionally shielded by great privacy." . . . We noted, however, that the degree of intrusion depends upon the manner in which production of the urine sample is monitored. . . . Under the District's Policy, male students produce samples at a urinal along a wall. They remain fully clothed and are only observed from behind, if at all. Female students produce samples in an enclosed stall, with a female monitor standing outside listening only for sounds of tampering. These conditions are nearly identical to those typically encountered in public restrooms, which men, women, and especially school children use daily. Under such conditions, the privacy interests compromised by the process of obtaining the urine sample are in our view negligible.

Finally, we turn to consider the nature and immediacy of the governmental concern at issue here, and the efficacy of this means for meeting it. In both Skinner and Von Raab, we characterized the government interest motivating the search as "compelling." . . .

That the nature of the concern is important-indeed, perhaps compelling can hardly be doubted. Deterring drug use by our Nation's schoolchildren is at least as important as enhancing efficient enforcement of the Nation's laws against the importation of drugs, which was the governmental concern in Von Raab, . . ., or deterring drug use by engineers and trainmen, which was the governmental concern in Skinner. . . .

Taking into account all the factors we have considered above-the decreased expectation of privacy, the relative unobtrusiveness of the search, and the severity of the need met by the search we conclude Vernonia's Policy is reasonable and hence constitutional.

Source: *Vernonia School District 47J, Petitioner v. Wayne Acton, et ux., etc.* 515 U.S. 646 (1995).

Gonzales v. Raich, **545 U.S. 1 (2005)**

One of the most contentious issues related to the use of illegal drugs concerns the use of marijuana to treat a wide variety of medical conditions, such as alcohol abuse, attention deficit hyperactivity disorder (ADHD or AD/HD), various forms of arthritis, asthma, atherosclerosis, autism, bipolar disorder, colorectal cancer, depression, epilepsy, digestive diseases, hepatitis C, hypertension, leukemia, and skin tumors, to name just a few. The drug has also been recommended for the treatment of side effects of various diseases and of treatments used against those diseases, side effects such as nausea, vomiting, loss of appetite, and weight loss. While many medical professionals, laypersons, and government officials support the legalization of marijuana for use in such situations, many others argue that marijuana is still an illegal drug in the United States, and its use should be prohibited even for such "compassionate" situations as those listed here. Local, state, and federal courts have had to decide a number of cases with regard to the "compassionate use" versus "illegal drug" controversy over the past two decades. More and more of these cases have arisen as individual states have adopted laws that permit the use of marijuana in certain medical situations. As of early 2017, 25 states in the United States have adopted such laws. A decision in the most recent medical marijuana case by the U.S. Supreme Court was announced on June 6, 2005. In that case, the Court was asked to decide whether the federal government had the authority under the U.S. Constitution to prohibit the local cultivation and use of marijuana that was approved by the state of California. The Court decided in favor of the U.S. government in this case by a vote of 6 to 3. That decision did not end the controversy over the medical use of marijuana, however, as four years later the Court, in an unsigned statement, rejected appeals from San Bernardino and San Diego Counties in California to have the California state medical marijuana law overturned because it violated federal restrictions on the use of the drug for any purpose whatsoever. The main points in the Gonzales v. Raich *case are cited here (citations omitted, as indicated by ellipsis).*

In the introduction to his ruling for the majority, Justice John Paul Stevens lays out the fundamental constitutional issue and the basis for the Court's decision:

The case is made difficult by respondents' strong arguments that they will suffer irreparable harm because, despite a congressional finding to the contrary, marijuana does have valid therapeutic purposes. The question before us, however, is not whether it is wise to enforce the statute in these circumstances; rather, it is whether Congress' power to regulate interstate markets for medicinal substances encompasses the portions of those markets that are supplied with drugs produced and consumed locally. Well-settled law controls our answer. The CSA [Controlled Substances Act] is a valid exercise of federal power, even as applied to the troubling facts of this case. We accordingly vacate the judgment of the Court of Appeals.

Later in his statement, Justice Stevens highlights two essential points about the case:

First, the fact that marijuana is used "for personal medical purposes on the advice of a physician" cannot itself serve as a distinguishing factor. . . . The CSA designates marijuana as contraband for any purpose; in fact, by characterizing marijuana as a Schedule I drug, Congress expressly found that the drug has no acceptable medical uses. Moreover, the CSA is a comprehensive regulatory regime specifically designed to regulate which controlled substances can be utilized for medicinal purposes, and in what manner. Indeed, most of the substances classified in the CSA "have a useful and legitimate medical purpose." . . . Thus, even if respondents are correct that marijuana does have accepted medical uses and thus should be redesignated as a lesser schedule drug, the CSA would still impose controls beyond what is required by California law. The CSA requires manufacturers, physicians, pharmacies, and other handlers of controlled substances to comply with statutory and regulatory provisions mandating registration with the DEA, compliance with specific production quotas, security controls to guard against diversion, recordkeeping and reporting obligations, and prescription requirements. . . . Furthermore, the dispensing of new drugs, even when doctors approve their use, must await federal approval. . . . Accordingly, the mere fact that marijuana— like virtually every other controlled substance regulated by the CSA—is used for medicinal purposes cannot possibly serve to distinguish it from the core activities regulated by the CSA.

. . .

Second, limiting the activity to marijuana possession and cultivation "in accordance with state law" cannot serve to place respondents' activities beyond congressional reach. The Supremacy Clause unambiguously provides that if there is any conflict between federal and state law, federal law shall prevail. It is beyond peradventure that federal power over commerce is " 'superior to that of the States to provide for the welfare or necessities of their inhabitants,' "however legitimate or dire those necessities may be. . . . Just as state acquiescence to federal regulation cannot expand the bounds of the Commerce Clause, . . . so too state action cannot circumscribe Congress' plenary commerce power.

Justice Stevens concludes with a brief statement about one way in which those in favor of medical marijuana can achieve their objectives:

We do note, however, the presence of another avenue of relief. As the Solicitor General confirmed during oral argument, the statute authorizes procedures for the reclassification of Schedule I drugs. But perhaps even more important than these legal avenues is the democratic process, in which the voices of voters allied with these respondents may one day be heard in the halls of Congress.

Source: *Gonzales v. Raich* 545 U.S. 1 (2005).

Family Smoking Prevention and Tobacco Control and Federal Retirement Reform (2009)

The question as to whether the federal government should have any control over the use of tobacco has been an issue in the United States for many years. Since tobacco use is not prohibited by any federal law, some people have argued that the federal government has no authority, legal or moral, to control the use of tobacco products. Other observers disagree. They point out that tobacco products contain substances that are harmful to a person's health and that some agency in the U.S. government—presumably the Food and Drug Administration (FDA)—should have some authority to regulate the use of tobacco products. In 2009, that issue was resolved to some extent when the U.S. Congress passed legislation to give the FDA authority to regulate the use of tobacco products. The legislation was originally introduced in the House of Representatives by Rep. Henry Waxman (D–CA) on March 22, 2009, as H.R.1256, while matching legislation was introduced in the U.S. Senate by Sen. Edward Kennedy (D–MA) on May 5, 2009. In a somewhat surprising turn of events, the bills moved quickly through the Congress, were approved on June 12, 2009, and signed by President Barack Obama on June 22, 2009. The bill is 84 pages in length in the U.S. Code, but the fundamental rationale of the act is expressed in its first few sections, which are reprinted here.

Public Law 111-31

111th Congress

The act consists of four main sections: Table of Contents, Authority of the Food and Drug Administration, Tobacco Product Warnings, Constituent and Smoke Constituent Disclosure, and Prevention of Illicit Trade in Tobacco Products. The first part of the act outlines its rationale in its "Findings" section, which consists of 49 statements about tobacco, its health effects, its marketing, and other related issues. Among these findings are the following:

(1) The use of tobacco products by the Nation's children is a pediatric disease of considerable proportions that results in new generations of tobacco-dependent children and adults.

(2) A consensus exists within the scientific and medical communities that tobacco products are inherently dangerous and cause cancer, heart disease, and other serious adverse health effects.

(3) Nicotine is an addictive drug.

(4) Virtually all new users of tobacco products are under the minimum legal age to purchase such products.

(5) Tobacco advertising and marketing contribute significantly to the use of nicotine-containing tobacco products by adolescents.

(6) Because past efforts to restrict advertising and marketing of tobacco products have failed adequately to curb tobacco use by adolescents, comprehensive restrictions on the sale, promotion, and distribution of such products are needed.

(7) Federal and State governments have lacked the legal and regulatory authority and resources they need to address comprehensively the public health and societal problems caused by the use of tobacco products.

(8) Federal and State public health officials, the public health community, and the public at large recognize that the tobacco industry should be subject to ongoing oversight.

. . .

(12) It is in the public interest for Congress to enact legislation that provides the Food and Drug Administration with the authority to regulate tobacco products and the advertising and promotion of such products. The benefits to the American people from enacting such legislation would be significant in human and economic terms.

. . .

(15) Advertising, marketing, and promotion of tobacco products have been especially directed to attract young persons to use tobacco products, and these efforts have resulted in increased use of such products by youth. Past efforts to oversee these activities have not been successful in adequately preventing such increased use.

. . .

(26) Restrictions on advertising are necessary to prevent unrestricted tobacco advertising from undermining legislation prohibiting access to young people and providing for education about tobacco use.

. . .

(30) The final regulations promulgated by the Secretary of Health and Human Services in the August 28, 1996, issue of the Federal Register (61 Fed. Reg. 44615–44618) for inclusion as part 897 of title 21, Code of Federal Regulations, are consistent with the first amendment to the United States Constitution and with the standards set forth in the amendments made by this subtitle for the regulation of tobacco products by the Food and Drug Administration, and the restriction on the sale and distribution of, including access to and the advertising and

promotion of, tobacco products contained in such regulations are substantially related to accomplishing the public health goals of this division.

(31) The regulations described in paragraph (30) will directly and materially advance the Federal Government's substantial interest in reducing the number of children and adolescents who use cigarettes and smokeless tobacco and in preventing the life-threatening health consequences associated with tobacco use. . . .

(32) The regulations described in paragraph (30) impose no more extensive restrictions on communication by tobacco manufacturers and sellers than are necessary to reduce the number of children and adolescents who use cigarettes and smokeless tobacco and to prevent the life-threatening health consequences associated with tobacco use. Such regulations are narrowly tailored to restrict those advertising and promotional practices which are most likely to be seen or heard by youth and most likely to entice them into tobacco use, while affording tobacco manufacturers and sellers ample opportunity to convey information about their products to adult consumers.

. . .

(36) It is essential that the Food and Drug Administration review products sold or distributed for use to reduce risks or exposures associated with tobacco products and that it be empowered to review any advertising and labeling for such products. It is also essential that manufacturers, prior to marketing such products, be required to demonstrate that such products will meet a series of rigorous criteria, and will benefit the health of the population as a whole, taking into account both users of tobacco products and persons who do not currently use tobacco products.

. . .

(44) The Food and Drug Administration is a regulatory
    agency with the scientific expertise to identify harmful
    substances in products to which consumers are exposed,
    to design standards to limit exposure to those substances,
    to evaluate scientific studies supporting claims about the
    safety of products, and to evaluate the impact of labels,
    labeling, and advertising on consumer behavior in order
    to reduce the risk of harm and promote understanding
    of the impact of the product on health. In connection
    with its mandate to promote health and reduce the risk
    of harm, the Food and Drug Administration routinely
    makes decisions about whether and how products may be
    marketed in the United States.

Source: Public Law 111–31, June 22, 2009.

Sottera, Inc. v. Food and Drug Administration (No. 10-5032; 627 F.3d 891) (2010)

*One of the most significant changes in the use of substances for
recreational purposes in recent history has been the development
of electronic cigarettes (e-cigarettes), devices for the delivery of
tobacco-like products (especially nicotine) by means of a battery-
operated vaporizer. Considerable dispute has developed over the
safety and usefulness of e-cigarettes, producing, as expected, a number of court cases dealing with their manufacture, distribution,
and use. One of the most important of those cases arose out of a
decision by the U.S. Food and Drug Administration (FDA) to
begin regulating e-cigarettes under the authority granted to it by
the Federal Food, Drug, and Cosmetic Act of 1938 (FDCA). Some
e-cigarette makers argued that the appropriate regulatory power
was not the FDCA, but the Tobacco Control Act of 2009 (TCA),
which provided different standards for the tobacco products that
the FDA could regulate. A district court agreed with the e-cigarette
companies and, when the FDA appealed to the U.S. Circuit Court
of Appeals for the District of Columbia, that court agreed with the*

lower court's decision. As a consequence, e-cigarettes are currently not regulated by any federal statute or regulation. The appeal court's ruling was as follows. (Asterisks [*] represent omitted citations.)

Under the FDCA, the FDA has authority to regulate articles that are "drugs," "devices," or drug/device combinations. 21 U.S.C. § 321(g)(1) defines drugs to include (B) articles intended for use in the diagnosis, cure, mitigation, treatment, or prevention of disease in man or other animals; and (C) articles (other than food) intended to affect the structure or any function of the body of man or other animals.

*

Until 1996, the FDA had never attempted to regulate tobacco products under the FDCA (with one exception, irrelevant for reasons discussed below) unless they were sold for therapeutic uses, that is, for use in the "diagnosis, cure, mitigation, treatment, or prevention of disease" under § 321(g)(1) (B). *But in that year, the FDA changed its long-held position, promulgating regulations affecting tobacco products as customarily marketed, i.e., ones sold without therapeutic claims. *The agency asserted that nicotine is a drug that affects the structure or function of the body under § 321(g)(1)(C) and that cigarettes and smokeless tobacco were therefore drug/device combinations falling under the FDA's regulatory purview, even absent therapeutic claims.*

In *FDA v. Brown & Williamson*, the Supreme Court rejected the FDA's claimed FDCA authority to regulate tobacco products as customarily marketed. Looking to the FDCA's "overall regulatory scheme," the "tobacco-specific legislation" enacted since the FDCA, and the FDA's own frequently asserted position, it held that Congress had "ratified . . . the FDA's plain and resolute position that the FDCA gives the agency no authority to regulate tobacco products as customarily marketed."*

To fill the regulatory gap identified in To fill the regulatory gap identified in *Brown & Williamson*, Congress in 2009 passed the Tobacco Act, Pub. L. No. 111-31, 123 Stat. 1776, 21 U.S.C. §§ 387 et seq., providing the FDA with authority to regulate tobacco products. The act defines tobacco products so as to include all consumption products derived from tobacco except articles that qualify as drugs, devices, or drug-device combinations under the FDCA:

(rr) (1) The term "tobacco product" means any product made or derived from tobacco that is intended for human consumption, including any component, part, or accessory of a tobacco product. . . .

(2) The term "tobacco product" does not mean an article that is a drug under [the FDCA's drug provision], a device under [the FDCA's device provision], or a combination product described in [the FDCA's combination product provision]

[The court then discusses in detail the history of tobacco legislation and its implications for this particular case. They conclude that:]

. . . *Brown & Williamson* interprets the six statutes [passed by Congress] not as a particular carve-out from the FDCA for cigarettes and smokeless tobacco (plus any additional products covered in the six statutes, which the FDA briefs make no effort to itemize), but rather as "a distinct regulatory scheme to address the problem of tobacco and health"—one that Congress intended would "preclude[] any role for the FDA" with respect to "tobacco absent claims of therapeutic benefit by the manufacturer." *In doing so, Congress also "persistently acted to preclude a meaningful role for any administrative agency in making policy on the subject of tobacco and health." *As customarily marketed, tobacco products were to remain the province of Congress.

[The court's opinion then concludes with:]

As we have already noted, the FDA has authority to regulate customarily marketed tobacco products—including ecigarettes—under the Tobacco Act. It has authority to regulate therapeutically marketed tobacco products under the FDCA's drug/device provisions. And, as this decision is limited to tobacco products, it does not affect the FDA's ability to regulate other products under the "structure or any function" prong defining drugs and devices in 21 U.S.C.§ 321 (g) and (h), as to the scope of which—tobacco products aside—we express no opinion. Of course, in the event that Congress prefers that the FDA regulate e-cigarettes under the FDCA's drug/device provisions, it can always so decree.

The judgment of the district court is
Affirmed.

Source: *Sottera, Inc., Doing Business as Njoy, Appellee v. Food & Drug Administration, et al.,* Appellants (No. 10 5032; 627 F.3d 891) (2010).

Memorandum for All United States Attorneys (2013)

The decision by many states to approve the use of marijuana for medical purposes has created a problem for the federal government. Since marijuana is still a Schedule I drug under the Controlled Substances Act of 1970, should or must federal law enforcement agencies follow federal law or state law in dealing with individuals who use the drug in states where it has been approved for medical use? The administration of President Barack Obama made up its mind on this issue early on in his term of office, deciding essentially not to prosecute people who were using marijuana for medical purposes in states that had adopted laws permitting such use. Perhaps the most famous statement on the issue was announced to U.S. attorneys in a memorandum from Deputy Attorney General James M. Cole in August 2013, a portion of which is reprinted here.

As the Department noted in its previous guidance, Congress has determined that marijuana is a dangerous drug and that the illegal distribution and sale of marijuana is a serious crime that provides a significant source of revenue to large-scale criminal enterprises, gangs, and cartels. The Department of Justice is committed to enforcement of the CSA consistent with those determinations. The Department is also committed to using its limited investigative and prosecutorial resources to address the most significant threats in the most effective, consistent, and rational way. In furtherance of those objectives, as several states enacted laws relating to the use of marijuana for medical purposes, the Department in recent years has focused its efforts on certain enforcement priorities that are particularly important to the federal government:

- Preventing the distribution of marijuana to minors;
- Preventing revenue from the sale of marijuana from going to criminal enterprises, gangs, and cartels;
- Preventing the diversion of marijuana from states where it is legal under state law in some form to other states;
- Preventing state-authorized marijuana activity from being used as a cover or pretext for the trafficking of other illegal drugs or other illegal activity;
- Preventing violence and the use of firearms in the cultivation and distribution of marijuana;
- Preventing drugged driving and the exacerbation of other adverse public health consequences associated with marijuana use;
- Preventing the growing of marijuana on public lands and the attendant public safety and environmental dangers posed by marijuana production on public lands; and
- Preventing marijuana possession or use on federal property.

These priorities will continue to guide the Department's enforcement of the CSA against marijuana-related conduct. Thus, this memorandum serves as guidance to Department attorneys and law enforcement to focus their enforcement resources and efforts, including prosecution, on persons or organizations whose conduct interferes with any one or more of these priorities, regardless of state law. *[Footnote omitted here.]*

Outside of these enforcement priorities, the federal government has traditionally relied on states and local law enforcement agencies to address marijuana activity through enforcement of their own narcotics laws. For example, the Department of Justice has not historically devoted resources to prosecuting individuals whose conduct is limited to possession of small amounts of marijuana for personal use on private property. Instead, the Department has left such lower-level or localized activity to state and local authorities and has stepped in to enforce the CSA only when the use, possession, cultivation, or distribution of marijuana has threatened to cause one of the harms identified above.

The enactment of state laws that endeavor to authorize marijuana production, distribution, and possession by establishing a regulatory scheme for these purposes affects this traditional joint federal-state approach to narcotics enforcement. The Department's guidance in this memorandum rests on its expectation that states and local governments that have enacted laws authorizing marijuana-related conduct will implement strong and effective regulatory and enforcement systems that will address the threat those state laws could pose to public safety, public health, and other law enforcement interests. A system adequate to that task must not only contain robust controls and procedures on paper; it must also be effective in practice. Jurisdictions that have implemented systems that provide for regulation of marijuana activity must provide the necessary resources and demonstrate the willingness to enforce their laws and regulations in a manner that ensures they do not undermine federal enforcement priorities.

Source: Memorandum for All United States Attorneys. 2013. U.S. Department of Justice. https://www.justice.gov/iso/opa/resources/3052013829132756857467.pdf. Accessed on May 7, 2016.

Coats v. Dish Network (Colorado Supreme Court Case No. 13SC394) (2015)

Brandon Coats was a customer service representative for Dish Network. Coats is a quadriplegic who has been in a wheelchair since he was a teenager. He obtained a license in Colorado in 2009 for the use of marijuana for medical purposes. In 2010, Coats failed a test for THC conducted by Dish, the result of his having used marijuana during his off hours. He sued the company on the basis of Colorado law that prohibits a company from firing a person for carrying on legal activities while not on the job. Coats noted that medical marijuana was legal in Colorado at the time of his firing, so the company's action violated state law. The district court, appeals court, and supreme court all disagreed with Coats, as the following decision indicates. Ellipses indicate omitted text.

We review de novo the question of whether medical marijuana use prohibited by federal law is a "lawful activity" protected under section 24-34-402.5 *[the relevant state law on which Coats bases his claim]*. . . .

We still must determine, however, whether medical marijuana use that is licensed by the State of Colorado but prohibited under federal law is "lawful" for purposes of section 24-34-402.5. Coats contends that the General Assembly intended the term "lawful" here to mean "lawful under Colorado state law," which, he asserts, recognizes medical marijuana use as "lawful." . . . We do not read the term "lawful" to be so restrictive. Nothing in the language of the statute limits the term "lawful" to state law. Instead, the term is used in its general, unrestricted sense, indicating that a "lawful" activity is that which complies with applicable "law," including state and federal law. We therefore decline Coats's invitation to engraft a state law limitation onto the statutory language. . . .

Echoing *[appeals court]* Judge Webb's dissent, Coats argues that because the General Assembly intended section 24-34-402.5 to broadly protect employees from discharge for outside-of-work activities, we must construe the term "lawful" to mean "lawful under Colorado law." . . . In this case, however, we find nothing to indicate that the General Assembly intended to extend section 24-34-402.5's protection for "lawful" activities to activities that are unlawful under federal law. In sum, because Coats's marijuana use was unlawful under federal law, it does not fall within section 24-34-402.5's protection for "lawful" activities.

Source: *Coats v. Dish Network.* Colorado Supreme Court. Case No. 13SC394.

United States of America, Plaintiff, v. Marin Alliance for Medical Marijuana, and Lynette Shaw (2015)

The Rohrabacher-Farr Amendment adopted by the U.S. Congress in 2015 appeared to be fairly straightforward: It forbade the U.S. Drug Enforcement Administration (DEA) from pursuing individuals for the use of medical marijuana in states where the practice was legal. The DEA, however, had a different view of the amendment; It believed that the agency was prohibited from acting only against states in which medical marijuana was legal, not against individuals in those states. The question as to which interpretation was correct was first resolved later in 2015 when a case arose between a medical marijuana group in Marin County, California, and the DEA. The court concluded that "the Government's contrary reading so tortures the plain meaning of the statute" that it had to be rejected virtually out of hand. Specifically, it explained that:

The plain reading of the text of Section 538 forbids the Department of Justice from enforcing this injunction against MAMM to the extent that MAMM operates in compliance with California law.

    . . .

    . . . this Court is not in a position to "override Congress' policy choice, articulated in a statute, as to what behavior should be prohibited." . . . On the contrary: This Court's only task is to interpret and apply Congress's policy choices, as articulated in its legislation. And in this instance, Congress dictated in Section 538 that it intended to prohibit the Department of Justice from expending any funds in connection with the enforcement of any law that interferes with California's ability to "implement [its] own State law[] that authorize[s] the use, distribution, possession, or cultivation of medical marijuana."

. . .

[The court then noted that the sponsors of the amendment had addressed this very issue in offering it to the House:]

In fact, the members of Congress who drafted Section 538 had the opportunity to respond to the very same argument that the DOJ advances here. In a letter to Attorney General Eric Holder on April 8, 2015, Congressmen Dana Rohrabacher and Sam Farr responded as follows to "recent statements indicating that the [DOJ] does not believe a spending restriction designed to protect [the medical marijuana laws of 35 states] applies to specific ongoing cases against individuals and businesses engaged in medical marijuana activity":

As the authors of the provision in question, we write to inform you that this interpretation of our amendment is emphatically wrong. Rest assured, the purpose of our amendment was to prevent the Department from wasting its limited law enforcement resources on prosecutions and asset forfeiture actions against medical marijuana patients and providers, including businesses that operate legally under state law. In fact, a close look at the Congressional Record of the floor debate of the amendment clearly illustrates the intent of those who sponsored and supported this measure. Even those who argued against the amendment agreed with the proponents' interpretation of their amendment.

Conclusion

For the foregoing reasons, as long as Congress precludes the Department of Justice from expending funds in the manner proscribed by Section 538, the permanent injunction will only be enforced against MAMM insofar as that organization is in violation of California "State laws that authorize the use, distribution, possession, or cultivation of medical marijuana."

Source: *United States of America, Plaintiff, v. Marin Alliance for Medical Marijuana, and Lynette Shaw.* United States District Court for the Northern District of California. https://cases.justia.com/federal/district-courts/california/candce/3:19 98cv00086/116898/277/0.pdf?ts=1445324671. Accessed on July 4, 2016.

State Doctor Shopping Laws (2016)

One of the most serious substance abuse problems of the early twenty-first century is prescription drug abuse, in which individuals obtain, in one way or another, prescriptions drugs (such as opioids) that can then be used for recreational or other nonmedical purposes. A common method by which such drugs are obtained is by going from physician to physician (a procedure known as "doctor shopping") having the same prescription refilled over and over again. Although the federal government has no specific law prohibiting such practices, every state has enacted some form of legislation to prevent doctor shopping. These laws differ substantially from state to state. The two selections provided here are examples of the types of laws that exist.

South Dakota

22-42-17. Controlled substances obtained concurrently from different medical practitioners—Misdemeanor. Any person who knowingly obtains a controlled substance from a medical practitioner and who knowingly withholds information from that medical practitioner that he has obtained a controlled substance of similar therapeutic use in a concurrent time period from another medical practitioner is guilty of a Class 1 misdemeanor.

Source: SL 1990, ch 168. http://legis.sd.gov/Statutes/Codified_Laws/DisplayStatute.aspx?Type=Statute&Statute=22-42-17. Accessed on July 4, 2016.

Connecticut

Sec. 21a-266. (Formerly Sec. 19-472). Prohibited acts. (a) No person shall obtain or attempt to obtain a controlled substance or procure or attempt to procure the administration of a controlled substance (1) by fraud, deceit, misrepresentation or subterfuge, or (2) by the forgery or alteration of a prescription or of any written order, or (3) by the concealment of a material fact, or (4) by the use of a false name or the giving of a false address.

(b) Information communicated to a practitioner in an effort unlawfully to procure a controlled substance, or unlawfully to procure the administration of any such substance, shall not be deemed a privileged communication.

(c) No person shall wilfully make a false statement in any prescription, order, report or record required by this part.

(d) No person shall, for the purpose of obtaining a controlled substance, falsely assume the title of, or claim to be, a manufacturer, wholesaler, pharmacist, physician, dentist, veterinarian, podiatrist or other authorized person.

(e) No person shall make or utter any false or forged prescription or false or forged written order.

(f) No person shall affix any false or forged label to a package or receptacle containing controlled substances.

(g) No person shall alter an otherwise valid written order or prescription except upon express authorization of the issuing practitioner.

(h) No person who, in the course of treatment, is supplied with controlled substances or a prescription therefor by one practitioner shall, knowingly, without disclosing such fact, accept during such treatment controlled substances or a prescription therefor from another practitioner with intent to obtain a quantity of controlled substances for abuse of such substances.

(i) The provisions of subsections (a), (d) and (e) shall not apply to manufacturers of controlled substances, or their agents or employees, when such manufacturers or their authorized agents or employees are actually engaged in investigative activities directed toward safeguarding of the manufacturer's trademark, provided prior written approval for such investigative activities is obtained from the Commissioner of Consumer Protection.

Source: Chapter 420b. Dependency-Producing Drugs. https:// www.cga.ct.gov/current/pub/chap_420b.htm#sec_21a-266. Accessed on July 4, 2016.

Comprehensive Addiction and Recovery Act of 2016

In July 2016, the U.S. Congress passed and President Barack Obama signed the Comprehensive Addiction and Recovery Act of 2016, a piece of legislation called by some observers "the most consequential piece of drug legislation adopted in the United States in forty years." The bill was 130 pages long and covered a vast array of issues relating to opioid use and misuse. The rage of topics can be appreciated from the Table of Contents at the beginning of the bill, which reads as follows:

TITLE I—PREVENTION AND EDUCATION

Sec. 101. Task force on pain management.

Sec. 102. Awareness campaigns.

Sec. 103. Community-based coalition enhancement grants to address local drug crises.

Sec. 104. Information materials and resources to prevent addiction related to youth sports injuries.

Sec. 105. Assisting veterans with military emergency medical training to meet requirement for becoming civilian health care professionals.

Sec. 106. FDA opioid action plan.

Sec. 107. Improving access to overdose treatment.

Sec. 108. NIH opioid research.

Sec. 109. National All Schedules Prescription Electronic Reporting Reauthorization.

Sec. 110. Opioid overdose reversal medication access and education grant programs.

TITLE II—LAW ENFORCEMENT AND TREATMENT

Sec. 201. Comprehensive Opioid Abuse Grant Program.

Sec. 202. First responder training.

Sec. 203. Prescription drug take back expansion.

TITLE III—TREATMENT AND RECOVERY

Sec. 301. Evidence-based prescription opioid and heroin treatment and interventions demonstration.

Sec. 302. Building communities of recovery.

Sec. 303. Medication-assisted treatment for recovery from addiction.

TITLE IV—ADDRESSING COLLATERAL CONSEQUENCES

Sec. 401. GAO report on recovery and collateral consequences.

TITLE V—ADDICTION AND TREATMENT SERVICES FOR WOMEN, FAMILIES, AND VETERANS

Sec. 501. Improving treatment for pregnant and postpartum women.

Sec. 502. Veterans treatment courts.

Sec. 503. Infant plan of safe care.

Sec. 504. GAO report on neonatal abstinence syndrome (NAS).

TITLE VI—INCENTIVIZING STATE COMPREHENSIVE INITIATIVES TO ADDRESS PRESCRIPTION OPIOID ABUSE

TITLE VII—MISCELLANEOUS

TITLE VIII—KINGPIN DESIGNATION IMPROVEMENT

TITLE IX—DEPARTMENT OF VETERANS AFFAIRS

Subtitle A—Opioid Therapy and Pain Management

Sec. 911. Improvement of opioid safety measures by Department of Veterans Affairs.

Sec. 912. Strengthening of joint working group on pain management of the Department of Veterans Affairs and the Department of Defense.

Sec. 913. Review, investigation, and report on use of opioids in treatment by Department of Veterans Affairs.

Sec. 914. Mandatory disclosure of certain veteran information to State controlled substance monitoring programs.

Sec. 915. Elimination of copayment requirement for veterans receiving opioid antagonists or education on use of opioid antagonists.

Subtitle B—Patient Advocacy

Sec. 921. Community meetings on improving care furnished by Department of Veterans Affairs.

Sec. 922. Improvement of awareness of patient advocacy program and patient bill of rights of Department of Veterans Affairs.

Sec. 923. Comptroller General report on patient advocacy program of Department of Veterans Affairs.

Sec. 924. Establishment of Office of Patient Advocacy of the Department of Veterans Affairs.

Subtitle C—Complementary and Integrative Health

Sec. 931. Expansion of research and education on and delivery of complementary and integrative health to veterans.

Sec. 932. Expansion of research and education on and delivery of complementary and integrative health to veterans.

Sec. 933. Pilot program on integration of complementary and integrative health and related issues for veterans and family members of veterans.

Subtitle D—Fitness of Health Care Providers

Sec. 941. Additional requirements for hiring of health care providers by Department of Veterans Affairs.

Sec. 942. Provision of information on health care providers of Department of Veterans Affairs to State medical boards.

Sec. 943. Report on compliance by Department of Veterans Affairs with reviews of health care providers leaving the Department or transferring to other facilities.

Source: S.524—Comprehensive Addiction and Recovery Act of 2016. Congress.Gov. https://www.congress.gov/bill/114th-congress/senate-bill/524/text. Accessed on December 26, 2016.

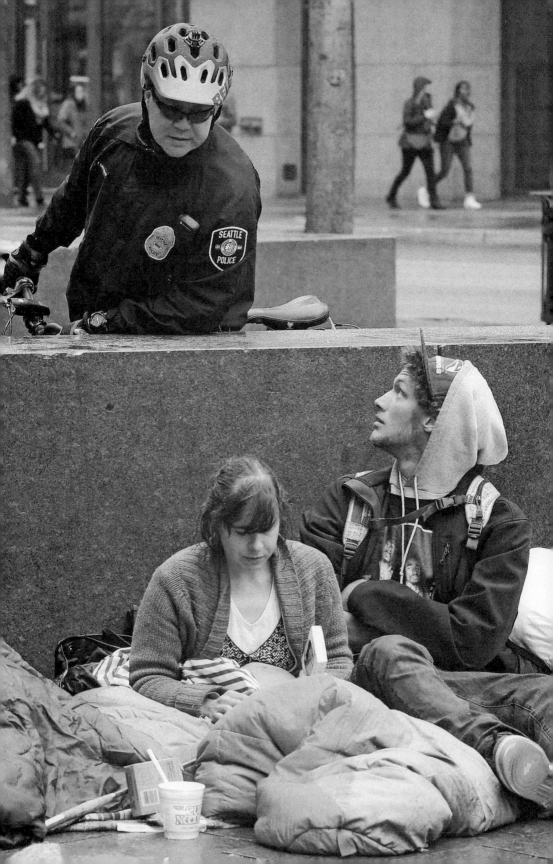

The legal and illegal use of psychoactive substances has been an issue of greater or lesser concern to human societies for thousands of years. Endless numbers of stories have been told and written about the salubrious and dangerous effects of these substances on the human body, as well as on the cultures in which they have been used for a variety of purposes. This chapter lists a sample of the many books, articles, reports, and other essays that have been written on the subject. Of course, they represent only a small sample of the many items that could be listed. Today, many items that were once available only in print form are now also available in electronic format, most commonly on the Internet. When an item listed here is available in more than one format, that fact is so indicated in the annotation. The reader is also referred to the references at the end of Chapters 1 and 2 for a number of other items used in the preparation of this book and of interest to those who wish to pursue their studies of the topic in more detail.

Gailen Lopton, seated, talks with Seattle police officer Tom Christenson in downtown Seattle on April 7, 2015. When Lopton was caught injecting heroin in a downtown alley in March, police officers offered him a chance to enroll in a first-of-its-kind program called Law Enforcement Assisted Diversion, aimed at keeping low-level drug offenders and prostitutes out of jail and providing services for housing, counseling, and job training. (AP Photo/ Ted S. Warren)

Books

Abadinsky, Howard. 2014. *Drug Use and Abuse: A Comprehensive Introduction*, 8th ed. Belmont, OH: Wadsworth/Cengage Learning.

The author, an expert in criminology, discusses the issue of substance abuse from the standpoint of law enforcement, with chapters on the impact of drugs on society, the history of drug use and abuse, the pharmacological impact of drugs on the human body, drug policy considerations, drug abuse as a law enforcement issue, the treatment and prevention of drug abuse, theories of substance abuse, and the drug business.

Agnew, Jeremy. 2014. *Alcohol and Opium in the Old West: Use, Abuse, and Influence.* Jefferson, NC: McFarland & Company, Inc.

This book provides fascinating information about a period in America's history about which little has been written concerning alcohol and drug abuse. The book covers the period from about 1840 to about 1900.

Benavie, Arthur. 2016. *How the Drug War Ruins American Lives.* Santa Barbara, CA: Praeger.

The author explains how the battle against drugs has damaged personal and property rights in the United States without achieving much—if any—of its major goals.

Bennett, William J. 2016. *Going to Pot: Why the Rush to Legalize Marijuana Is Harming America.* New York: Center Street.

Bennett is the former director of National Drug Control policy under President George H. W. Bush. He explains why he believes that the legalization of marijuana poses a serious threat to fundamental values of American society.

Booth, Martin. 1998. *Opium: A History.* New York: St. Martin's Press.

Booth, Martin. 2005. *Cannabis: A History.* New York: Picador Press.

Booth has written two of the standard books on the history of psychoactive substances that provide detailed and extensive histories of each substance.

Caulkins, Jonathan P., Beau Kilmer, and Mark Kleiman. 2016. *Marijuana Legalization: What Everyone Needs to Know*. New York: Oxford University Press.

> This book contains almost everything a person might want to know about the legalization of marijuana, from a description of the plant itself and the people who use it to the medical and nonmedical effects of using marijuana to current trends in legalization, along with specific examples of actions that have been taken.

Chasin, Alexandra. 2016. *Assassin of Youth: A Kaleidoscopic History of Harry J. Anslinger's War on Drugs*. Chicago: The University of Chicago Press.

> This book is both a biography of one of the most important figures in the history of drug legislation in the United States and a review of the events taking place around him during that period of history.

De Micheli, Denise, et al., eds. 2016. *Drug Abuse in Adolescence: Neurobiological, Cognitive, and Psychological Issues*. Cham, Switzerland: Springer.

> The essays in this collection deal with a number of issues relating to development of the central nervous system during adolescence and the effects of a variety of substances on that process. Although the presentations are quite technical, they provide some valuable information about the effects of substance abuse during adolescence.

Escohotado, Antonio. 1999. *A Brief History of Drugs: From the Stone Age to the Stoned Age*. Rochester, VT: Park Street Press.

> A very interesting history of the role of psychoactive substances from the earliest periods of human history to the modern day. The book was first published in Spain and then translated to English and published in the United States only in 2012.

Estren, Mark J., and Beverly A. Potter. 2013. *Prescription Drug Abuse*. Oakland, CA: Ronin Publishing.

> The authors discuss the problem of pain medicine in the United States today and explain how the nation's prescription drug epidemic is related to that problem. It provides further information on the epidemic and suggests ways of dealing with it.

Fisher, Gary L., and Thomas C. Harrison. 2013. *Substance Abuse: Information for School Counselors, Social Workers, Therapists, and Counselors*, 4th ed. Boston: Pearson.

> This book is designed for the general reader as well as for use in educational settings. It covers the complete range of substance abuse issues with which professionals named in the title are likely to deal. It presents useful background information, as well as suggestions for diagnosis, prevention, and treatment of substance abuse issues.

Gahlinger, Paul. 2004. *Illegal Drugs: A Complete Guide to Their History, Chemistry, Use, and Abuse*. New York: Plume, 2004.

> This superb overview of virtually all aspects of substance abuse includes chapters on the history of specific drugs, such as opium, marijuana, and heroin; a history of legal efforts to control substance abuse; drug testing; the pharmacological effects of drugs; the business of illegal drugs; and a review of legal psychoactive drugs.

Gately, Iain. 2003. *Tobacco: A Cultural History of How an Exotic Plant Seduced Civilization*. New York: Grove Press.

> This and the following book provide very nice summaries of the role of alcohol and smoking in human society over the centuries.

Gately, Iain. 2008. *Drink: A Cultural History of Alcohol*. New York: Gotham Books.

Hamidi, Mehrdad, Mohammad-Ali Shahbazi, and Hajar Ashrafi, eds. 2012. *Drug Abuse in Sport: Doping*. New York Nova Science Publishers.

The papers in this anthology provide a general overview of issues relating to doping in sports, but the greatest emphasis is on detailed discussions of individual agents used for doping purposes.

Hanson, Glen, Peter Venturelli, and Annette Fleckenstein. 2015. *Drugs and Society*, 12th ed. Boston: Jones and Bartlett.
This widely used textbook opens with a general discussion of substance abuse issues, along with an explanation of the way drugs affect the central nervous system. The main body of the book is then devoted to detailed discussions of the major drugs of concern, including alcohol, narcotics, stimulants, hallucinogens, inhalants, marijuana, and over-the-counter and prescription drugs.

Hari, Johann. 2015. *Chasing the Scream: The First and Last Days of the War on Drugs*. London: Bloomsbury Publishing.
A work of investigative reporting, this book provides a fresh and intriguing view as to what the war on drugs is really all about, how it started, and how it is likely to end.

Hillman, D.C.A. 2008. *The Chemical Muse: Drug Use and the Roots of Western Civilization*. New York: Thomas Dunne Books/ St. Martin's Press.
The author reports on his research on the use of psychoactive substances in ancient Greece and Rome and their role in the early history of modern civilization.

Howard, Sherrel G. 2014. *Drugs of Abuse: Pharmacology and Molecular Mechanisms*. Ames, IA: John Wiley & Son.
For a number of psychoactive substances that are commonly misused, Howard offers a moderately detailed explanation of the molecular mechanisms by which they affect the human body, along with an extensive review of their physiological and psychological effects and other relevant data for the substances.

Inaba, Darryl, and William E. Cohen. 2014. *Uppers, Downers, All Arounders: Physical and Mental Effects of Psychoactive Drugs.* 8th ed. Medford, OR: CNS Publications.

> This book covers in detail almost every legal and illegal drug of interest to the general public, from whom it receives generally very positive reviews. Chapters deal with topics such as the history of drug use and abuse, classification of drugs, the pharmacology of drugs, stimulants, depressants, alcohol, hallucinogens, drug treatment, and drug use and mental health.

Julien, Robert M., Claire D. Advokat, and Joseph E. Comaty. 2014. *A Primer of Drug Action: A Concise, Non-Technical Guide to the Actions, Uses, and Side Effects of Psychoactive Drugs.* New York: Worth Publishers.

> This book is designed for the general reader. It provides a technical and detailed description of the biochemistry and pharmacology of drug action, beginning with a description of the nervous system and its response to psychoactive substances, followed by detailed explanations of the actions of specific drugs and drug classes, including alcohol and inhalants of abuse; barbiturates; benzodiazepines; cocaine, amphetamines, and other stimulants; caffeine and nicotine; opioids; and hallucinogenics.

Kaelin, Christopher J., and Meredith Nutting. 2013. *Prescription Drug Monitoring.* Hauppauge, NY: Nova Science.

> This book provides a broad, general introduction to the types of prescription drug monitoring programs that states have developed as one way of dealing with the U.S. epidemic of prescription drug abuse.

Kuhn, Cynthia, Scott Swartzwelder, and Wilkie Wilson. 2014. *Buzzed: The Straight Facts about the Most Used and Abused Drugs from Alcohol to Ecstasy,* 4th ed. New York: W.W. Norton, 2008.

> The title somewhat misrepresents the content of the book, which is less "streetwise" than it is technical and academic,

although still easily accessible to the general reader. Part I of the book contains chapters on individual drugs and drug groups, ranging from herbal concoctions and coffee and tea to ecstasy and hallucinogens of all types. Part II of the book deals with more general topics, such as the nature of addiction, the neurological effects of drugs, legal issues, and drug treatment and recovery.

Levinthal, Charles F. 2016. *Drugs, Society, and Criminal Justice*. Boston: Pearson.

This book provides a view of the nation and the world's substance abuse problems, largely from the standpoint of law enforcement and the legal system.

Loddenkemper, Robert, and Michael Kreuter, eds. 2015. *The Tobacco Epidemic*. Basel; New York: Karger.

The essays in this book cover a wide range of tobacco-related subjects, such as the history of tobacco production and use, the global tobacco epidemic, chemistry and toxicity of tobacco and tobacco smoke, nicotine dependence, the tobacco smoker, electronic cigarettes, smokeless tobacco, and water pipe smoking.

Lovering, Rob. 2015. *A Moral Defense of Recreational Drug Use*. Houndmills, Basingstoke, Hampshire; New York: Palgrave Macmillan.

The author reviews four major arguments against the use of psychoactive substances for recreational purposes and concludes for all that "they do not succeed."

Madras, Bertha, and Michael J. Kuhar, eds. 2013. *The Effects of Drug Abuse on the Human Nervous System*. Oxford, UK: Academic Press.

The articles in this collection provide an excellent review of current knowledge about some fundamental questions with regard to the effects of psychoactive substances on the human nervous system, including chapters on the consequences of drug use, in general; genetic factors; the etiology of substance abuse; neurobiological consequences of various types of drug use, such as cocaine, alcohol, and methamphetamine; and emerging designer drugs.

Maisto, Stephen A., Mark Galizio, and Gerard J. Connors. 2015. *Drug Use and Abuse*, 7th ed. Belmont, CA: Wadsworth Publishing, 2007.

This textbook takes a broad-range view of the issue of drug use and abuse, drawing on information from biology, medicine, history, psychology, and sociology. Introductory chapters deal with pharmacology and psychopharmacology, while middle chapters focus on specific drugs, such as heroin, cocaine, caffeine, alcohol, and opiates. The final two chapters discuss prevention and treatment of substance abuse.

Marion, Nancy E., and Joshua B. Hill, eds. 2016. *Legalizing Marijuana: A Shift in Policies across America.* Durham, NC: Carolina Academic Press.

This collection of papers deal with topics such as the conflict between federal and state laws on marijuana; decriminalization of marijuana in Portugal, the Netherlands, and Uruguay; legalization of recreational marijuana in Colorado and Washington; cannabis-impaired driving; and the use of marijuana on college campuses as a result of new legalization laws.

Miller, Peter M., et al., eds. 2013. *Principles of Addiction.* Amsterdam; Boston: Elsevier Academic Press.

This book covers essentially all of the basic principles related to substance addiction, including the nature and characteristics of addiction in general, specific types of addiction (alcoholism, marijuana use, and dependence on other drugs), with a section on prevention and treatment of addiction among college students and young adults.

Murphy, Jennifer. 2015. *Illness or Deviance?: Drug Courts, Drug Treatment, and the Ambiguity of Addiction.* Philadelphia, PA: Temple University Press.

> Murphy reviews the arguments as to whether and/or to what extent addiction is a disease and to what extent a criminal behavior. She then outlines some of the current practices for preventing and treating addiction that reflect these generally opposing views.

Musto, David. 2002. *Drugs in America: A Documentary History.* New York: New York University Press, 2002.

> This fascinating book collects speeches, sermons, policy statements, laws, personal letters, and other documents that describe all facets of the use and abuse of drugs in the United States.

Robinson, Matthew B., and Renee G. Scherien. 2014. *Lies, Damned Lies, and Drug War Statistics: A Critical Analysis of Claims Made by the Office of National Drug Control Policy,* 2nd ed. Albany: State University of New York Press.

> The authors analyze annual reports from the Office of National Drug Control Policy and claim to find extensive evidence of ways in which the office has "massaged" data and statistics to project an unrealistic view of the nation's drug problems and national efforts to solve those problems.

Ruck, Carl A. P., and Mark A. Hofmann. 2013. *Entheogens, Myth & Human Consciousness.* Berkeley, CA: Ronin Publishing.

> The authors point out that psychoactive substances have played a far more extensive and complex role in the development of human civilization than has previously been acknowledged. They provide examples of that role in religion, mythology, art, and other fields of culture.

Rush, John A, ed. 2013. *Entheogens and the Development of Culture: The Anthropology and Neurobiology of Ecstatic Experience: Essays.* Berkeley, CA: North Atlantic Books.

The essays in this book speak to the many ways in which the use of psychoactive substances by early cultures has influenced the evolution of the human brain and human culture itself.

Steiker, Lori Holleran. 2016. *Youth and Substance Use: Prevention, Intervention, and Recovery*. Chicago: Lyceum Books.
　　Steiker discusses the etiology and epidemiology of drug addiction and reviews a variety of programs and approaches for preventing and treating the condition.

Sullum, Jacob. 2014. "How Is Marijuana Legalization Going? The Price of Pot Peace Looks Like a Bargain." *Forbes*. http://www.forbes.com/sites/jacobsullum/2014/07/10/how-is-marijuana-legalization-going-so-far-the-price-of-pot-peace-looks-like-a-bargain/#42327659167c. Accessed on July 11, 2016.
　　The writer reviews public opinion and studies on the effects of marijuana legalization in Colorado and finds that the results are less harmful than critics had predicted before the November 2012 referendum.

Winograd, Rachel P., and Kenneth J. Sher. 2015. *Binge Drinking and Alcohol Misuse among College Students and Young Adults*. Boston: Hogrefe Publishing.
　　This short book begins by reviewing the data on binge drinking among college students and young adults, and then focuses primarily on diagnosis and treatment of the disorder.

Articles

Some of the academic journals that focus specifically on substance abuse–related issues are the following:

Addiction. ISSN: 0965–2140.
　　Addiction has published continuously since its first edition in 1884. It currently has the highest impact factor

(number of citations) of any journal in the field of substance abuse.

Addiction Biology. ISSN: 1355–6215.
Addiction Biology has the second highest impact factor among substance abuse journals, following its sister publication, *Addiction.*

American Journal of Drug and Alcohol Abuse. ISSN: 0095–2990.
Published six times a year, this journal reports on advances in neurobiology, pathophysiology, and treatment of drug abuse and alcoholism.

Journal of Drug Issues. ISSN: 0022–0426.
This quarterly publication focuses on national and international issues relating to (primarily illicit) drug use.

Journal of Substance Abuse Treatment. ISSN: 0740–5472.
Published eight times a year, this journal is concerned with substance abuse treatment specifically.

Research Journal of Drug Abuse. ISSN 2057–3111.
The primary focus of this journal is on "mood-altering or psycho-active drugs, steroids for performance enhancement in sports, illicit drugs and problems with impulse control and impulsive behaviour."

Substance Abuse. ISSN: 0889–7077.
This quarterly journal is one of the premier publications for the most recent research and opinion on substance abuse issues.

Substance Abuse and Rehabilitation. ISSN: 1179–8467.
This journal publishes results of research, case reports, commentaries, and reviews on all areas of addiction and substance abuse.

Substance Abuse: Research and Treatment. ISSN: 1178–2218.

This open-access, peer-reviewed journal publishes papers dealing with medical treatment and screening, mental health services, research, and evaluation of substance abuse programs.

Substance Abuse Treatment, Prevention, and Policy. ISSN: 1747–597X.

This journal is especially important to students of substance abuse issues because many of its articles are available through its open-access policy, which allows readers the right to copy, distribute, and display articles; to make derivative works from an article; and to use an article for commercial purposes.

Ahuja, S. C., and U. Ahuja. 2011. "Betel Leaf and Betel Nut in India: History and Uses." *Asian Agri-History.* 15(1): 13–35.

The author provides a fascinating history of the use of the betel plant in India, where it has long been used as a mild stimulant for medicinal, religious, cultural, and recreational purposes.

Albertson, Timothy E., et al. 2016. "The Changing Drug Culture: Emerging Drugs of Abuse and Legal Highs." *FP Essentials.* 441: 18–24.

This article takes note of a significant number of legal substances that are now being used for recreational purposes because of their psychoactive properties, along with the special problems posed for health professionals by these substances.

Backett-Milburn, Kathryn, et al. 2008. "Challenging Childhoods: Young People's Accounts of 'Getting By' in Families with Substance Use Problems." *Childhood.* 15(4): 461–479.

A number of studies have attempted to discover and interpret the health, social, and other issues faced by substance abusers. Much less attention has been paid to the children of adult substance abusers. In this review, researchers explore the methods that such individuals develop to survive in the real world with parents who are often incapable of taking care of themselves, let alone their children. They discuss a number of survival strategies that those children develop and use in their everyday lives.

Bao, Yuhua, et al. 2016. "Prescription Drug Monitoring Programs Are Associated with Sustained Reductions in Opioid Prescribing by Physicians." *Health Affairs*. 35(6): 1045–1051.

In the study reported here, researchers attempted to determine the effect of prescription drug monitoring programs in four states between the years 2001 and 2010. They found that such programs were responsible for a decrease of more than 30 percent in the number of Schedule II opioids prescribed by health care providers in those states.

Blanke, D. Douglas, and Kerry Cork. 2008. "Exploring the Limits of Smoking Regulation." *William Mitchell Law Review*. 34(4): 1587–1593.

This paper reviews a discussion held at the William Mitchell Law School on October 23, 2007, with regard to recent regulation on smoking in a number of venues. The question raised at this meeting was whether and to what extent recent laws had "crossed the line" in attempting to restrict the use of a legal product by the general product. The meeting was sponsored by the Tobacco Control Legal Consortium.

Brecher, Edward M. 1988(?). *Licit and Illicit Drugs: The Consumers Union Report on Narcotics, Stimulants, Depressants, Inhalants, Hallucinogens, and Marijuana—Including Caffeine, Nicotine, and Alcohol*, 16th printing. Boston; Toronto: Little, Brown. http://www.druglibrary.org/schaffer/library/studies/cu/cumenu.htm. Accessed on July 11, 2016.

Obviously a very dated publication, this book, originally released in 1972, remains one of the best general introductions to the topic of psychoactive substances, their nature, and attempts to bring them under control. A superb introduction for the general reader, even with recognition of its limited factual information.

Bretteville-Jensen, Anne Line. 2006. "To Legalize or Not to Legalize? Economic Approaches to the Decriminalization of Drugs." *Substance Use and Misuse.* 41(4): 555–565.
Discussions about decriminalizing the use of certain currently illegal substances often focuses on ethical and social issues. In this paper, the author considers the economic implications of legalizing drugs such as marijuana, cocaine, and heroin, the first and primary effect probably being a significant decrease in prices. In this event, the number of drug users may increase.

Brown, Lawrence S. 1981. "Substance Abuse and America: Historical Perspective on the Federal Response to a Social Phenomenon." *Journal of the National Medical Association.* 73(6): 497–506.
This article points out that substance abuse has been a characteristic feature of American history from its earliest history, but that society has responded in a variety of ways to that phenomenon. He explores U.S. policy and practices with regard to substance abuse from the colonial period through the 1960s.

Caulkins, Jonathan P., et al. 2015. "Cocaine's Fall and Marijuana's Rise: Questions and Insights Based on New Estimates of Consumption and Expenditures in US Drug Markets." *Addiction.* 110(5): 728–736.
This article explores the interesting phenomenon of illicit drug popularity and how one explains the significant increase in marijuana use and decrease in cocaine use in the United States during the early 2000s.

Cobaugh, Daniel J., et al. 2014. "The Opioid Abuse and Misuse Epidemic: Implications for Pharmacists in Hospitals and Health

Systems." *American Journal of Health System Pharmacy.* 71(18): 1539–1554.

This article provides an excellent general overview of the opioid abuse epidemic that swept through the United States beginning at the turn of the twenty-first century, although with suggestions as to how pharmacists can help in dealing with that problem.

Coyle, Sue. 2015. "Recovery High Schools: Getting an Education and Learning to Stay Clean and Sober." *Social Work Today.* 15(3): 18. Full text online at http://www.socialworktoday.com/archive/051815p18.shtml. Accessed on July 14, 2016.

This excellent article provides an overview of recovery schools, the way they operate, and their benefits and drawbacks.

Degenhardt, Louisa, et al. 2016. "The Increasing Global Health Priority of Substance Use in Young People." *The Lancet. Psychiatry.* 3(3): 251–264.

The authors review the biological reasons that substance abuse is an issue of special importance for young adults and then discuss reasons that substance abuse among adolescents is likely to become a major health issue worldwide in the near future.

Hall, Wayne, and Mega Weier. 2015. "Assessing the Public Health Impacts of Legalizing Recreational Cannabis Use in the USA." *Clinical Pharmacology & Therapeutics.* 97(6): 607–615.

The authors note that there is little research available to predict the effects of legalizing marijuana for recreational use on public health, but they attempt to make some educated guesses as to what some likely outcomes might be.

Herring, Rachel, Virginia Berridge, and Betsy Thom. 2008. "Binge Drinking Today: Learning Lessons from the Past." *Drugs: Education, Prevention, and Policy.* 15(5): 475–486.

The authors point out that binge drinking is a serious social problem in the United States, but that it is not a new problem. They review the literature on binge drinking in the past and explore possible lessons for the present epidemic of binge drinking.

Herzberg, David, et al. 2016. "Recurring Epidemics of Pharmaceutical Drug Abuse in America: Time for an All-Drug Strategy." *American Journal of Public Health*. 106(3): 408–410.

The authors suggest that the current prescription drug epidemic is only the most recent of three such epidemics in U.S. history, and much is to be learned from what happened in the first two of those epidemics. A major reason for society's inability to deal with such events, they say, has been the fact that "policy has been shaped by the racially charged division of drug users into deserving and morally salvageable victims, or fearsome and morally repugnant criminals."

Hornik, Robert, et al. 2008. "Effects of the National Youth Anti-Drug Media Campaign on Youths." *American Journal of Public Health*. 98(12): 2229–2236.

In 1998, U.S. Congress created the National Youth Anti-Drug Media Campaign in an effort to reduce drug abuse by young Americans. This study attempted to determine the effect of that campaign on the target audience in the period between 1999 and 2004. Researchers concluded that "[m]ost analyses showed no effects from the campaign."

Ibrahim, Jennifer K., and Stanton A. Glantz. 2007. "The Rise and Fall of Tobacco Control Media Campaigns, 1967–2006." *American Journal of Public Health*. 97(8): 1383–1396.

Research has shown that public media campaigns to limit smoking have been very successful. The tobacco industry, however, has contested these campaigns in a number of ways, by preventing their creation, limiting or eliminating their funding, contesting their content, or preventing their existence by legal action. The authors have documented the existence of these efforts and have pointed out their effectiveness in the continuation of public media campaigns against smoking. They conclude that "[t]obacco control advocates must learn from the past and continue to confront the tobacco industry and its third-party allies to defend antitobacco media campaigns or, despite evidence of their effectiveness, they will be eliminated."

Jager, Justin, Katherine M. Keyes, and John E. Schulenberg. 2015. "Historical Variation in Young Adult Binge Drinking Trajectories and Its Link to Historical Variation in Social Roles and Minimum Legal Drinking Age." *Developmental Psychology*. 51(7): 962–974.

Using long-term data from the Monitoring the Future study, the authors study trends in binge drinking over a 30-year period, compared to present-day patterns and search for factors that may explain the trends they discover, such as changes in drinking age and evolution of social expectations of young adults in the United States.

Kenkel, Donald S. 2016. "Healthy innovation: Vaping, Smoking, and Public Policy." *Journal of Policy Analysis and Management*. 35(2): 473–479.

The author provides an excellent history of and general introduction to the subject of electronic cigarettes and vaping, along with a review of what is currently known about the health effects of the practice and the policy decisions that need to be made about vaping.

King, Ryan S., and Marc Mauer. 2006. "The War on Marijuana: The Transformation of the War on Drugs in the 1990s." *Harm Reduction Journal*. 3(6): 3–6.

The authors review U.S. policy and practices with regard to marijuana use in the 1990s and find that 82 percent of the increase of 450,000 drug arrests made between 1900 and 2002 were for marijuana use, and, of that number, 79 percent were for possession alone. They also found that an estimated $4 billion is spent annually for the arrest, prosecution, and incarceration of marijuana offenders. They argue that the effort and expense devoted to the control of marijuana could be more efficiently spent on other types of drug enforcement.

Kritikos, P.G., and S.P. Papadaki. 1967. "The History of the Poppy and of Opium and Their Expansion in Antiquity in the Eastern Mediterranean Area." *Bulletin on Narcotics.* 19(3): 17–38.

This article provides a detailed history of the use of opium from the earliest known times (about 3500 BCE) to the first century AD. It is nicely illustrated with a number of depictions of the way the poppy and opium were included in the arts and crafts of ancient peoples. The article originally appeared in Greek in the *Journal of the Archaeological Society of Athens*, but was later reprinted in the *UN Bulletin on Narcotics*. It is also available on the Internet in English at https://www.unodc.org/unodc/en/data-and-analysis/bulletin/bulletin_1967-01-01_3_page004.html.

Mays, Darren, et al. 2016. "Openness to Using Non-Cigarette Tobacco Products among U.S. Young Adults." *American Journal of Preventive Medicine.* 50(4): 528–534.

The researchers ask young adults which non-cigarette tobacco devices they are open to trying and finding that hookahs (28.2%) and electronic cigarettes (25.5%) are the most popular choices. They suggest ways in which this information can be used in tobacco prevention programs.

Moberg, D. Paul, and Andrew Finch. 2007. "Recovery High Schools: A Descriptive Study of School Programs and Students." *Journal of Groups in Addiction & Recovery.* 2(2/3/4): 128–161.

http://www.ncbi.nlm.nih.gov/pmc/articles/PMC2629137/. Accessed on July 11, 2016.

The authors provide an excellent general introduction to the concept of recovery schools and report on a study of 17 such institutions operating on this principle. They found that the programs "appeared to be successful" in achieving their objective of helping students maintain their sobriety while completing their secondary education.

Nadelman, Ethan A., and David T. Courtwright. 1993. "Should We Legalize Drugs? History Answers." *American Heritage*. 44(1): 41–56.

Nadelman and Courtwright debate one of the oldest and most fundamental questions in the field of substance abuse: how and to what extent would legalization of drugs affect this social problem? Although somewhat dated, the arguments presented on both sides are still cogent and relevant to the present day.

Passie, Torsten, and Udo Benzenhöfer. 2016. "The History of MDMA as an Underground Drug in the United States, 1960–1979." *Journal of Psychoactive Drugs*. 48(2): 67–75.

This article provides a fascinating introduction to the rise of MDMA (ecstasy) as a drug of abuse during the 1960s and 1970s in the United States and around the world.

Rasmussen, Nicolas. 2008. "America's First Amphetamine Epidemic 1929–1971: A Quantitative and Qualitative Retrospective with Implications for the Present." *American Journal of Public Health*. 98(6): 974–985.

The author reviews an amphetamine epidemic that swept the United States in the 1940s through the 1960s and concludes that current amphetamine abuse patterns are similar to those of the earlier period. He suggests that lessons can be learned about the control of the present-day epidemic from the earlier experience.

Rowe, C. L., 2012. "Family Therapy for Drug Abuse: Review and Updates 2003–2010." *Journal of Marital and Family Therapy.* 38(1): 59–81.

> This review of research over the indicated period of time suggests that family therapy is "among the most effective approaches for treating both adults and adolescents with drug problems."

Saah, Tammy. 2005. "The Evolutionary Origins and Significance of Drug Addiction." *Harm Reduction Journal.* 2(1): 1–7.

> The author explores the association between the use of psychoactive substances by early humans and in early civilizations and evolutionary changes that were occurring at the time.

Shanon, Benny. 2002. "Entheogens, Reflections on Psychoactive Sacramentals." *Journal of Consciousness Studies.* 9(4): 85–94.

> This essay provides a very nice general introduction to the topic of entheogens, psychoactive substances that have traditionally been used primarily for spiritual and religious purposes.

Stein, David M., Kendra J. Homan, and Scott DeBerard. 2015. "The Effectiveness of Juvenile Treatment Drug Courts: A Meta-Analytic Review of Literature." *Journal of Child & Adolescent Substance Abuse.* 24(2): 80–93.

> The authors review 31 studies on the rate of recidivism of adolescents with substance abuse problems who have been exposed to a variety of treatments and find that drug courts "had slightly more gains" than other forms of treatment. Other measures of success and failure are also discussed.

Stolberg, Victor B. 2006. "A Review of Perspectives on Alcohol and Alcoholism in the History of American Health and Medicine." *Journal of Ethnicity in Substance Abuse.* 5(4): 39–106.

The author provides an extended review of the way Americans have viewed alcohol—in both positive and negative terms, as it turns out—throughout the nation's history. He pays special attention to the conflicted attitudes of the medical profession toward alcohol and alcohol abuse.

Sung, Hung-En, and Alana Henninger. 2014. "History of Substance Abuse Treatment." In Gerben Bruinsma and David Weisburd, eds. *Encyclopedia of Criminology and Criminal Justice*. New York: Springer, 2257–2269. http://www.academia.edu/5187736/History_of_substance_abuse_treatment. Accessed on July 8, 2016.

This encyclopedia entry provides an excellent history overview of the approach to the treatment of substance abuse dating to colonial America.

Tamburro, Lauren P., Jenan H. Al-Hadidi, and Ljubis Jovan Dragovic. 2016. "Resurgence of Fentanyl as a Drug of Abuse." *Journal of Forensic Science and Medicine*. 2(2): 111–114.

The use of fentanyl for nonmedical purposes spiked in about 2006, before dropping off in popularity after the turn of the century. This article notes that its illicit use has begun to rise again. It explores this trend and comments on its potential implications.

Tupper, Kenneth W. 2009. "Ayahuasca Healing beyond the Amazon: The Globalization of a Traditional Indigenous Entheogenic Practice." *Global Networks*. 9(1): 117–136.

This paper discusses the worldwide spread of the use of ayahuasca, a psychoactive brew traditionally used by Amazonian peoples for spiritual and healing uses. The author discusses not only the tradition of ayahuasca use itself, but also a number of issues that have arisen as a much broader selection of individuals around the globe have taken to using the brew for a variety of purposes.

Wackowski, Olivia A., and Christine D. Delnevo. 2016. "Young Adults' Risk Perceptions of Various Tobacco Products Relative to Cigarettes: Results from the National Young Adult Health Survey." *Health Education and Behavior*. 43(3): 328–336.

> The authors asked a sample of young adults about their perceived risk of using a variety of tobacco products and found that subjects rated e-cigarettes as less risky than traditional cigarettes and smoke products less risky than noncombustible products (such as snus).

Wittchen, H. U., et al. 2008. "What Are the High Risk Periods for Incident Substance Use and Transitions to Abuse and Dependence? Implications for Early Intervention and Prevention." *International Journal of Methods in Psychiatric Research*. 17(Special Issue 1): S16–S29.

> This team of researchers attempted to discover the time period during which individuals transitioned from first exposure to a drug to becoming addicted to that drug for a number of substances, including alcohol, nicotine, cannabis, and other illicit drugs. They found that, except for alcohol, that transition occurs quite rapidly and, as a result, "the time windows for targeted intervention to prevent progression to malignant patterns in adolescence are critically small, leaving little time for targeted intervention to prevent transition."

Zuzek, Crystal. 2013. "Pill Mills." *Texas Medicine*. 109(4): 18–24. https://www.texmed.org/Template.aspx?id=26765. Accessed on July 14, 2016.

> This well-written article describes the practice of providing prescription medications for individuals who use those drugs for recreational purposes in the state of Texas. The description of the practice is vivid and down-to-earth, with a review of actions taken by the state to reduce the existence of pill mills.

Reports

"Addressing Prescription Drug Abuse in the United States: Current Activities and Future Opportunities." [2013]. Washington, DC: Behavioral Health Coordinating Committee. Prescription Drug Abuse Subcommittee. U.S. Department of Health and Human Services. https://www.cdc.gov/drugoverdose/pdf/hhs_prescription_drug_abuse_report_09.2013.pdf. Accessed on July 9, 2016.

This report was issued in response to a congressional directive for the department to "improve the understanding of current prescription drug abuse activities and produce a report which provides a review of current initiatives and identifies opportunities to ensure the safe use of prescription drugs with the potential for abuse and the treatment of prescription drug dependence."

"Adolescent Substance Abuse." 2011. National Center on Addiction and Substance Abuse. Columbia University. http://www.casacolumbia.org/addiction-research/reports/adolescent-substance-use. Accessed on July 9, 2016.

This report summarizes the result of an extensive study that involved interviews with 1,000 high school students, 1,000 parents of high school students, and 500 school personnel, we well as an exhaustive review of the literature on teenage substance abuse. The authors conclude that substance abuse by adolescents is the largest preventable and most costly health problem in the United States today. The report provides a wealth of data about the topic and is a "must-read" for anyone interested in the subject.

"Behavioral Health Trends in the United States: Results from the 2014 National Survey on Drug Use and Health." 2015. Washington, DC: Center for Behavioral Health Statistics and Quality. Substance Abuse and Mental Health Services Administration.

This annual study collects basic information about the use of legal and illegal substances in the United States and analyzes those data on the basis of a number of demographic characteristics, such as age, gender, ethnicity and race, and previous experiences with substances. It is one of the most important sources of demographic data about substance use in the United States.

"The CBHSQ Report: A Day in the Life of American Adolescents: Substance Use Facts Update." 2013. Center for Behavioral Health Statistics and Quality. http://archive.samhsa.gov/data/2k13/CBHSQ128/sr128-typical-day-adolescents-2013.htm. Accessed on July 9, 2016.

This collection of data comes from a variety of national surveys and provides statistics on tobacco and alcohol use, along with data on substance use and abuse by adolescents.

"A Century of International Drug Control." [2009]. United Nations Office on Drugs and Crime. http://www.unodc.org/documents/data-and-analysis/Studies/100_Years_of_Drug_Control.pdf. Accessed on July 9, 2016.

This report provides a detailed description of the state of drug use prior to the installation of international drug controls, a summary of the most important of those regulations, and the changes produced by their implementation beginning in the early twentieth century.

"Dextromethorphan. Pre-Review Report." 2012. World Health Organization. http://www.who.int/medicines/areas/quality_safety/5.1Dextromethorphan_pre-review.pdf. Accessed on July 9, 2016.

This document is one in a WHO series on specific substances of abuse. It includes detailed information about a range of aspect for the substance, such as its physical and chemical properties, pharmacology, toxicology, adverse reactions in humans, dependence potential, abuse potential, industrial uses, therapeutic applications, and marketing authorizations as a medicine.

European Drug Report. 2016. European Monitoring Centre for Drugs and Drug Addiction. Luxembourg: Publications Office of the European Union.

This report is published annually and includes information on topics such as the market for illicit drugs in the European Union, the sources of supply, the arrival of new drugs on the market, and the physiological effects of such drugs on the human body.

"Guide for Policymakers: Prevention, Early Intervention and Treatment of Risky Substance Use and Addiction." 2015. [Washington, DC]: National Center on Addiction and Substance Abuse. file:///C:/Users/David/Downloads/Guide-for-policymakers .pdf. Accessed on July 9, 2016.

This report brings together information and research evidence on the best current methods for prevention and treatment of substance abuse and addiction.

Hibell, Björn, et al. 2012. "The 2011 ESPAD Report: Substance Abuse among Students in 36 European Countries." http://www .espad.org/Uploads/ESPAD_reports/2011/The_2011_ESPAD_ Report_FULL_2012_10_29.pdf. Accessed on July 9, 2016.

This report provides a detailed overview of the state of substance abuse by adolescents in 36 European nations, with statistics for each nation, an overview for all 36 nations, special trends from 1995 through 2011, and special sections on cannabis screening tests and polydrug use on the continent.

Kacir, Christopher D. 2010. "The Evolutionary Bases of Substance Use and Abuse." Forum on Public Policy. http://forumon publicpolicy.com/spring2010.vol2010/spring2010archive/kacir .pdf. Accessed on July 11, 2016.

This article reviews research and thought on the argument that substance abuse has evolved over time for adaptive reasons in ways that have changed the structure and function of the human brain in response to such substances.

Perhaps the most valuable part of the article, beyond its explication of the theory itself, is the extended collection of references to other works on the same topic.

Kann, Laura, et al. 2013. "Youth Risk Behavior Surveillance—United States. 2013." *MMWR*. 63(4): all. http://www.cdc.gov/mmwr/pdf/ss/ss6304.pdf. Accessed on July 9, 2016.
This publication is one of the most complete and detailed summaries of the statistics and data related to the abuse and misuse of substances by teenagers in the United States as of the publication date.

Kilmer, Beau, et al. 2014. "What America's Users Spend on Illegal Drugs: 2000–2010: Technical Report." Washington, DC: Executive Office of the President of the United States.
This report on the cost of substance abuse in the United States was prepared for the Office of National Drug Control Policy by the Rand Corporation.

"The Legalization of Marijuana in Colorado: The Impact." 2015. Rocky Mountain High Intensity Drug Trafficking Area. http://www.rmhidta.org/html/2015%20PREVIEW%20Legalization%20of%20MJ%20in%20Colorado%20the%20Impact.pdf. Accessed on July 11, 2016.
This report is volume 3 of a three-part report summarizing the effects that have been measured since the legalization of marijuana for recreational use in Colorado in 2012. It covers topics such as drugged driving, use of marijuana in the general population and by those under the age of 18, emergency room and hospital admissions related to marijuana-related causes, and business and economic data.

Levi, Jeffrey, Laura M. Segal, and Amanda Fuchs Miller. 2013. "Prescription Drug Abuse: Strategies to Stop the Epidemic." Washington, DC: Trust for America's Health. http://healthyamericans.org/assets/files/TFAH2013RxDrugAbuseRpt16.pdf. Accessed on July 9, 2016.

This report consists of two parts, the first of which is a summary and evaluation of state laws on prescription drug abuse. The second section provides a review of federal actions on the issue and offers a number of recommendations for dealing with the epidemic.

"Monitoring the Future: A Continuing Study of American Youth. Ann Arbor: Institute for Social Research. University of Michigan. http://www.monitoringthefuture.org/. Accessed on July 9, 2016.

The Monitoring the Future (MTF) research project is far and away the most important single resource on substance abuse patterns among American eighth, tenth, and twelfth graders, along with information about their attitudes about substance use and abuse. MTF researchers have produced a huge number of documents on specific aspects of American youth substance use and abuse over the 40 years of the project's existence.

O'Brien, Charles P., Maryjo Oster, and Emily Morden, eds. 2013. *Substance Abuse Disorders in the U.S. Armed Forces*. Washington, DC: The National Academies Press.

This report provides a summary of existing knowledge about the nature and extent of substance abuse in the U.S. armed forces and reviews methods and systems that are currently available or that could be developed for preventing and treating this problem.

"Office of National Drug Control Policy. Office Could Better Identify Opportunities to Increase Program Coordination." 2013. United States Government Accountability Office. http://www.gao.gov/assets/660/653354.pdf. Accessed on July 9, 2016.

In 2010, the Office of National Drug Control Policy (ONDCP) developed a five-year plan to reduce illicit drug use in the United States. This report assesses the office's success in achieving those goals. It concludes that ONDCP "has not made progress toward achieving most of the goals articulated in the 2010 National Drug Control Strategy."

"The Partnership Attitude Tracking Study." 2014. Partnership for Drug-Free Kids and MetLife Foundation. http://drug free.scdn1.secure.raxcdn.com/wp-content/uploads/2014/07/PATS-2013-FULL-REPORT.pdf. Accessed on July 9, 2016.

This study is the 22nd version of research that has been conducted since 1987 to measure attitudes and behaviors associated with substance use and abuse among children and adolescents and their parents. Data for the most recent study were collected from existing literature as well as interviews with 1,000 young adults, 1,000 parents, and 500 school officials.

Stagman, Shannon, Susan Wile Schwarz, and Danielle Powers. 2011. "Adolescent Substance Use in the U.S.: Facts for Policymakers." National Center for Children in Poverty. http://www .nccp.org/publications/pdf/text_1008.pdf. Accessed on July 9, 2016.

This report presents some basic facts about substance abuse among adolescents from the special perspective of the sponsoring agency, the National Center for Children in Poverty. It also provides some very specific recommendations for dealing with this problem for its target population.

"Understanding and Addressing Nicotine Addiction." 2015. [Washington, DC]: National Center on Addiction and Substance Abuse. file:///C:/Users/David/Downloads/Understanding-and-addressing-nicotine-addiction.pdf. Accessed on July 9, 2016.

This report reviews the best available current information on nicotine dependence and addiction and uses that information to develop a number of recommendations for programs to prevent and treat nicotine-related problems.

"World Drug Report." [issued annually]. Vienna: United Nations Office on Drugs and Crime.

This report is one of the most important summaries of the state of substance abuse worldwide, issued annually by the United Nations Office on Drugs and Crime. It provides statistics and data, along with commentaries, on drug issues that the office has selected as among the most important of the preceding year. The 2015 report is available online at https://www.unodc.org/documents/wdr2015/World_Drug_Report_2015.pdf.

"Youth Risk Behavior Surveillance—United States 2015." 2016. Centers for Disease Control and Prevention. http://www.cdc.gov/healthyyouth/data/yrbs/pdf/2015/ss6506_updated.pdf. Accessed on July 11, 2016.

YRBS is an annual surveillance of risky behavior attributable to youth in the United States in six categories: behaviors that contribute to unintentional injuries and violence; tobacco use; alcohol and other drug use; sexual behaviors related to unintended pregnancy and sexually transmitted infections, including human immunodeficiency virus infection; unhealthy dietary behaviors; and physical inactivity. It is one of the most complete data sets available on these health characteristics.

Internet

Above the Influence. 2016. [Office of National Drug Control Policy]. http://abovetheinfluence.com/. Accessed on July 11, 2016.

Above the Influence is a federal drug abuse prevention program aimed at young adults that evolved out of the National Youth Anti-Drug Media Campaign. Its goal is to increase the awareness of both adults and young people of the dangers of substance abuse. The program is carried out by the organization Partnership for Drug-Free Kids.

"Addiction Treatment Forum." 2016. Clinco Communications, Inc. http://www.atforum.com. Accessed on July 10, 2016.

This website is produced by Clinco Communications, Inc., an independent medical communications agency, and is supported by a grant from Mallinckrodt Pharmaceuticals. It provides a variety of sources of information, including a quarterly newsletter, *Addiction Treatment Forum*; news and updates; links to a number of resources with information on substance abuse; special information on methadone (manufactured by Mallinckrodt); frequently asked questions about substance abuse; patient brochures on a number of topics, available for downloading from the website; a list of conferences, meetings, and other events; and a locator for methadone clinics.

"Alcohol and Your Health." 2016. National Institute on Alcohol Abuse and Alcoholism. http://www.niaaa.nih.gov/alcohol-health. Accessed on July 10, 2016.

This website provides a comprehensive overview of the effects of alcohol on the human body, with separate sections on alcohol facts and statistics, binge drinking, alcohol use disorder, fetal alcohol syndrome, and underage drinking.

"Anabolic Steroids." 2013. Center for Substance Abuse Research. http://www.cesar.umd.edu/cesar/drugs/steroids.asp. Accessed on July 12, 2016.

Anabolic steroids are common substances of abuse among professional, college, and high school students who wish to improve their performance in one or another sport. This page provides extensive detail on the anabolic steroids and their effects—both good and bad—on the human body.

Anderson, Brian T., et al. "Statement on Ayahuasca." 2012. *International Journal of Drug Policy.* http://canadianharmreduction. com/sites/default/files/Statement%20on%20Ayahuasca%20 -%20IJDP%202012%20in%20press.pdf. Accessed on July 12, 2016.

This editorial provides a broad general introduction to a psychoactive substance that has a long history of use in Brazil and whose use as a recreational drug has spread throughout South and North America in the last few years.

"Assessment of Khat (Catha Edulis Forsk)." 2006. World Health Organization. http://www.who.int/medicines/areas/quality_safety/4.4KhatCritReview.pdf. Accessed on January 13, 2016.

Khat is a psychoactive substance that is widely and legally used for recreational purposes in large regions of the Middle East and Africa. It has also become popular as a recreational, but illegal, drug of use in other parts of the world. This WHO document provides a very detailed description of the chemistry, pharmacology, toxicology, dependence potential, epidemiology, and other characteristics of this psychoactive substance.

Borio, Gene. 2001. "The Tobacco Timeline." http://archive.tobacco.org/History/Tobacco_History.html. Accessed on July 10, 2016.

This outstanding review of the history of the use and regulation of tobacco products begins in the prehistory era and continues through 2002. It is a superb review of the role of tobacco in human society.

Buck, Jordan M., and Jessica A. Siegel. 2015. "The Effects of Adolescent Methamphetamine Exposure." *Frontiers in Neuroscience*. http://journal.frontiersin.org/article/10.3389/fnins.2015.00151/full. Accessed on July 12, 2016.

The authors provide a summary of current research information on the effects of methamphetamine use in both clinical settings and in animal models. They conclude that methamphetamine use during adolescence "results in increased risky sexual behaviors and psychiatric problems in humans."

Chaudry, Bilal. 2014. "Caught in a Rundown: The Need for a Zero-Tolerance Drug Policy to Bring Integrity Back into Professional Sports and Stop the Spread of Performance Enhancing Drugs into Society." *Hofstra Law Review*. 43(2): 563–600.

>This article provides an excellent general review of the history and nature of drug policies and drug testing in professional sports and, to a lesser extent, some fields of amateur sports, with the observation that the use of performance-enhancing drugs "remains rampant among all professional sports."

"A Comprehensive Historical Timeline of the Relationship between Psychedelic Substances and Mammalian Brains." 2012. The Cosmic LOL. https://cl.nfshost.com/psychedelics-chronology.html. Accessed on July 13, 2016.

>This web page is an extraordinary accomplishment, listing hundreds of specific events in history relating to the use of psychoactive substances, with a very useful list of references with which to follow up on each event.

Drug Abuse/Addiction Videos. 2016. https://www.google.com/#q=drug+abuse+videos+youtube. Accessed on July 14, 2016.

>The web has been flooded with videos discussing one aspect or another of substance abuse and addiction. This address leads to some of those videos available through YouTube. For other suggestions, see "The Film."

"Drugs, Brains, and Behavior: The Science of Addiction." 2014. National Institute on Drug Abuse. https://www.drugabuse.gov/sites/default/files/soa_2014.pdf. Accessed on July 12, 2016.

>This publication provides an easily understandable introduction to the basics of what scientists know about the way in which psychoactive substances affect the human brain along with a review of prevention and treatment methods.

Engber, Daniel. 2015. "Why Do Employers Still Routinely Drug-Test Workers?" Slate. http://www.slate.com/articles/health_and_

science/cover_story/2015/12/workplace_drug_testing_is_wide-spread_but_ineffective.html. Accessed on July 12, 2016.

> Engber reviews the history of workplace drug testing, concludes that it's a holdover from the Reagan era and that "there's very little evidence that it's worth the cost or hassle."

Erbentraut, Joseph. 2015. "Recovery Schools Save Teen Addicts, So Why Aren't They Everywhere?" *Huffington Post*. http://www.huffingtonpost.com/entry/recovery-high-schools-teen-addicts_us_561eb212e4b050c6c4a408ee. Accessed on July 11, 2016.

> Erbentraut suggests that an important part of the answer to his question is that society tends to view teenagers who abuse substances are "throw-away" kids who don't deserve the special form of education provided by recovery schools.

"50 Years of Tobacco Control." 2015. Robert Wood Johnson Foundation. http://www.rwjf.org/maketobaccohistory. Accessed on July 13, 2016.

> This primarily visual presentation demonstrates the role that smoking has played in American culture since about the beginning of World War II and how efforts to reduce smoking have affected the number of people who use tobacco.

"The Film." 2016. http://www.hbo.com/addiction/thefilm/index.html. Accessed on July 14, 2016.

> In association with the Robert Wood Johnson Foundation, the National Institute on Drug Abuse, and the National Institute on Alcohol Abuse and Alcoholism, HBO has produced a documentary film titled "Addiction" that consists of nine segments and is supplemented by a variety of additional print and electronic materials. A list of and link to the segments that make up the documentary is provided on this page.

"Frequently Asked Questions about Drug Testing." 2016. NCAA. http://www.ncaa.org/health-and-safety/policy/frequently-asked-questions-about-drug-testing. Accessed on July 12, 2016.

This website provides answers to most of the commonly asked questions about the National Collegiate Athletic Association's drug testing policies for individuals who compete in sports controlled by the body. For more information on this topic, see also the NCAA drug testing home page at http://www.ncaa.org/themes-topics/drug-testing.

Hanson, David J. 2014. "Drug Abuse Resistance Education: The Effectiveness of DARE." Alcohol Abuse Prevention. http://www.alcoholfacts.org/DARE.html. Accessed on July 11, 2016.

The author reviews the extensive evidence about the effectiveness of one of the U.S. oldest and largest substance abuse prevention programs, Drug Abuse Resistance Education, or D.A.R.E. He concludes that "the estimated cost of DARE annually is already $1 to 1.3 billion. That's a lot for a completely ineffective, often counterproductive, program."

Hudak, John, and Jonathan Rauch. 2016. "Worry about Bad Marijuana—Not Big Marijuana." Washington, DC: Brookings Institution.

Concern has been expressed about the possibility that companies dealing in the sale of marijuana will, under new legalization decisions in some states, grow into a giant industry similar to Big Tobacco. The authors explain why such an event is unlikely to occur, and that concern should be directed instead at the development of unethical business practices in the advertising and sale of the product.

Huetteman, Emmarie. 2016. "Senate Approves Bill to Combat Opioid Addiction Crisis." *The New York Times.* http://www.nytimes.com/2016/07/14/us/politics/senate-opioid-addiction-bill.html. Accessed July 15, 2016.

The adoption of this bill drew considerable comment partly because it passed the House and Senate with large bipartisan majorities, and partly because it was the first bill of its kind ever approved by the U.S. Congress. Unfortunately, the legislation included no financing for the policies adopted.

"Inhalant Abuse Information." 2016. National Inhalant Prevention Coalition. http://www.inhalants.org/. Accessed on July 10, 2016.

This website is an excellent source of information on all aspects of the abuse of inhalants, with sections on general information on inhalants, frequently asked questions about inhalants, the Inhalant Prevention Campaign, and news about inhalant abuse.

Kamenetz, Anya. 2014. "The History of Campus Sexual Assault." NPREd. http://www.npr.org/sections/ed/2014/11/30/366348383/the-history-of-campus-sexual-assault. Accessed on July 15, 2016.

This article provides an excellent introduction to the history, nature, and consequences of date rape. It generated a rather long list of responses and comments that are of considerable interest in exposing individual viewpoints on the topic.

"Lesson 3: Biology, Physiology, and Pharmacology of Psychoactive Drugs." 2016. University of Idaho. http://www.webpages.uidaho.edu/psyc470www/lessons/lesson03/lesson3.htm. Accessed on July 13, 2016.

This lesson is part of a course, Introduction to Chemical Addictions," offered in the Department of Psychology at the University of Idaho. It is one of the best single sources of information on how drugs work within and on the brain, with great detail provided for every aspect of the processes involved.

"Lessons from Prevention Research." 2014. National Institute on Drug Abuse. https://www.drugabuse.gov/sites/default/files/drugfacts_lessonsfromprevention.pdf. Accessed on July 12, 2016.

Although it is difficult to find examples of effective drug abuse prevention programs, a number of agencies have developed list of basic principles that should be used in developing such programs. This list contains 16 principles that the agency claims have been verified by research as forming the basis of an effective drug abuse prevention program.

"Library Resources." 2016. Schaffer Library of Drug Policy. http://www.druglibrary.org/schaffer/. Accessed on July 10, 2016. The documents in this web page originally appeared in an exhibit at the Pelletier Library of Allegheny College, Pennsylvania, from October 15, 1999 through March 1, 2000. They deal with virtually every issue related to the use and abuse of all kinds of drugs. It may well be the largest single source of articles of substance abuse available to the general public.

Liecht, Matthias E. 2015. "Novel Psychoactive Substances (Designer Drugs): Overview and Pharmacology of Modulators of Monoamine Signalling." *Swiss Medical Weekly*. 145:w14043. doi:10.4414/smw.2015.14043. http://www.smw.ch/content/smw-2015-14043/. Accessed on July 13, 2016. This paper provides a detailed overview of a number of new synthetic psychoactive substances with explanations of their biological functions in the human body. Parts of the paper are fairly technical, but it is well worth reading for the general themes presented.

"Management of Substance Abuse." 2016. World Health Organization. http://www.who.int/substance_abuse/en/. Accessed on July 10, 2016. The World Health Organization (WHO) is a division of the United Nations, with responsibility for collecting information about substance abuse in nations around the world and to provide information to individuals and groups wishing to know more about this issue. WHO has three primary responsibilities in this field: (1) preventing and reducing the negative health and social consequences of substance abuse, (2) reducing the demand for non-medical uses of psychoactive substances, and (3) assessing psychoactive substances so as to be able to advise the United Nations on regulation of these substances. This website includes a list of current WHO programs related to substance abuse, terminology and classification used in discussions of substance abuse, facts and figures, publications, latest research results, and links to other sites dealing with substance abuse.

McMurtrie, Beth. 2014. "Why Colleges Haven't Stopped Binge Drinking." *The New York Times.* http://www.nytimes.com/2014/12/15/us/why-colleges-havent-stopped-binge-drinking.html. Accessed on July 15, 2016.

This article provides a nice historical perspective on binge drinking in college and reviews some of the reasons that colleges have been unsuccessful in reducing the rate at which binge drinking occurs on their campuses.

Medina, Johnna. 2015. "Symptoms of Substance Use Disorders (Revised for DSM-5)." PsychCentral. http://psychcentral.com/disorders/revised-alcoholsubstance-use-disorder/. Accessed on July 13, 2016.

This web page provides a "2-minute read" review of the diagnostic criteria for substance abuse disorder, as provided in the latest edition of the *Diagnostic and Statistical Manual of Mental Disorders* (DSM-V).

"Mescaline." 2010. Science in Context. http://ic.galegroup.com/ic/scic/ReferenceDetailsPage/DocumentToolsPortletWindow?displayGroupName=Reference&jsid=6136ddee7859183bb7f3594c8cdef566&action=2&catId=&documentId=GALE%7CCCV2645000032&u=gotitans&zid=af1c2c1b5c6309cb697cd501a797bd69. Accessed on July 12, 2016.

This web page provides a good general introduction to the psychoactive substance mescaline, along with its potential effects on the human body and current use among adolescents and adults.

"The National Institute on Drug Abuse Media Guide: How to Find What You Need to Know about Drug Abuse and Addiction." 2014. National Institute on Drug Abuse. https://www.drugabuse.gov/sites/default/files/mediaguide_web_3_0.pdf. Accessed on July 14, 2016.

Although this publication is intended for journalists, it contains a great deal of information that will be useful to anyone interested in the topic of substance abuse.

"NIDA for Teens." 2016. National Institute on Drug Abuse. https://teens.drugabuse.gov/. Accessed on July 10, 2016.

This website contains a wealth of materials on substance use and abuse from the National Institute on Drug Abuse. The information is arranged in six major categories: drug facts, drugs and health blog, interactives and videos, information for teachers, teen prescription drug abuse, and National Drug and Alcohol facts week.

"NREPP: SAMHSA's National Registry of Evidence-Based Programs and Practices." 2016. Substance Abuse and Mental Health Services Administration. http://www.nrepp.samhsa.gov/AdvancedSearch.aspx. Accessed on July 11, 2016.

This website provides a searchable database of more than 300 programs that have been found to be effective by one definition or another in the area of substance abuse and mental health services. One of the interesting features of the database is the paucity of programs that have been found to be effective in the prevention or treatment of substance abuse (none for heroin or cocaine and two for marijuana abuse).

"Pathology of Drug Abuse." 2016. The Internet Pathology Laboratory for Medical Education. http://library.med.utah.edu/Web Path/TUTORIAL/DRUG/DRUG.html. Accessed on July 20, 2016.

> This tutorial from the University of Utah Medical School contains many photographs of the effects of tobacco, alcohol, and other drugs on the human body.

PDMP Center of Excellence. 2016. Brandeis University. http:// pdmpexcellence.org/. Accessed on July 14, 2016.

> The Center of Excellence is the U.S. foremost program for analyzing and contributing to the development of prescription drug monitoring programs. Its website contains a wealth of information about the current prescription drug epidemic and efforts that are being made to deal with that problem.

Project CORK. 2014. Dartmouth Medical School. http://www .projectcork.org/search/. Accessed on July 10, 2016.

> Project CORK was founded at the Dartmouth Medical School in 1977 through a grant from Operation Cork, an arm of the Kroc Foundation. The purpose of the project is to provide up-to-date information on a host of drug-related issues for users of the Internet. The project's database currently contains more than 120,000 items in a searchable format on its website. It is very user-friendly, with an extensive listing of more than 200 topics that are updated on a regular basis.

Provini, Celine. 2011. "Your Drug Prevention Program Probably Isn't Working." Education World. http://www.educationworld .com/a_curr/school_climate/drug_prevention_program_isnt_ working.shtml. Accessed on July 11, 2016.

> The author points out that research suggests that only a relatively small fraction of drug abuse prevention programs that have been carefully evaluated have been shown

to be effective, about 35% of such programs in public schools and 13% in private schools.

"Psilocybin." 2016. Hallucinogens. http://hallucinogens.com/psilocybin/. Accessed on January 12, 2016.

Psilocybin is a psychedelic compound present in a number of species of mushroom. This article provides a general introduction to the substance and the "magic mushrooms" in which it occurs. It provides links to a number of other online articles that also discuss this psychoactive compound.

"Psychoactive Drugs Tobacco, Alcohol, and Illicit Substances." 2016. Green Facts. http://www.greenfacts.org/en/psychoactive-drugs/psychoactive-drugs-greenfacts-level2.pdf. Accessed on July 13, 2016.

This website is designed to provide information on scientific topics of current interest in a way that can be understand by the average individual. This page contains an excellent general overview of the nature of psychoactive substances and the way they work on the human brain.

"Risk & Protective Factors." 2016. Commonwealth of Massachusetts. http://www.mass.gov/eohhs/gov/departments/dph/programs/substance-abuse/providers/prevention/risk-and-pro tective-factors.html. Accessed on July 12, 2016.

One focus of research on substance abuse is the search for factors that may predispose a person toward (a "risk factor") or help to avoid developing (a "protective factor") substance abuse. This concise summary lists a number of the factors that appear to be supported by rigorous research.

Roberts, Thomas B. 2016. "Psychedelic Drugs Can Deepen Religious Experiences." Religion News Service. http://religionnews.com/2016/04/29/psychedelic-drugs-can-deepen-religious-expe riences-commentary/. Accessed on July 15, 2016.

The author claims that certain types of psychoactive substances have been shown to increase the impact of religious experiences, and society should be more open to allowing the use of such drugs for those experiences. He concludes by asking, "Will a country that prides itself in religious liberty stop persecuting entheogenists?"

Roland, Takeesha. 2016. "Rohypnol Addiction and Recovery Facts." Recovery.org. http://www.recovery.org/topics/rohypnol-facts/. Accessed on January 14, 2016.

Rohypnol (flunitrazepam) is a central nervous system depressant that is used for the treatment of insomnia, anxiety, and sleep disorders, as well as used as a sedative, in some countries of the world. It is not approved for medical use in the United States. This article provides a good general overview of Rohypnol, with special emphasis on its use as a "date rape" drug.

"The Salvia Divinorum Research and Information Center." 2015. http://www.sagewisdom.org/. Accessed on July 12, 2016.

Salvia divinorum is a plant native to Mexico that has been used for centuries for inducing mystical visions. It remains popular today for such purposes. This website provides detailed information on virtually every aspect that can be imagined of the substance, including its legal status worldwide, instructions for growing the plant, a user's guide in many languages, its use in religious and ceremonial events, and reports from those who have used the drug for a variety of purposes.

"Substance Abuse Problems." 2015. http://www.nlm.nih.gov/medlineplus/substanceabuseproblems.html. Accessed on July 10, 2016.

This web page is a service of the U.S. National Library of Medicine and the National Institutes of Health. It provides an index to more than 50 topics in the general area of substance abuse, such as alcohol, anabolic steroids, cocaine, drug abuse, inhalants, marijuana, methamphetamine, prescription drug abuse, and prescription drug abuse.

Substance.com. 2016. http://www.substance.com/. Accessed on July 14, 2016.

This website is run by a fairly large group of individuals who are interested in substance abuse and its prevention and treatment. The purpose of the group's effort is to "report, investigate and analyze developments in the areas of addiction, addiction treatment, harm reduction, recovery, problem and nonproblem use, and the associated politics and cultures."

"Synthetic Cathinones (Bath Salts): An Emerging Domestic Threat." 2011. National Drug Intelligence Center. https://www .justice.gov/archive/ndic/pubs44/44571/44571p.pdf. Accessed on July 12, 2016.

This brochure provides a detailed explanation of the nature of synthetic cathinones (bath salts), their rise as a drug of concern, and somewhat dated statistics on their use, especially among pre-adult individuals.

Szalavitz, Maia. 2014. "Recovery High Schools' Is Their Strength." Substance.com. http://www.substance.com/recovery-high-schools-flexibility-strength/5873/. Accessed on July 14, 2016.

This blog article provides a very personal view of recovery schools, how they operate, and what they can contribute to young people who are attempting to recover from substance abuse and/or addiction.

"Teen Drug Abuse." 2015. MedicineNet.com. http://www.medi cinenet.com/teen_drug_abuse/article.htm. Accessed on July 12, 2016.

This excellent website provides detailed information about a range of topics related to substance abuse, including basic facts, data and statistics, effects of drug use by teens, symptoms and warning signs of drug abuse, causes of substance abuse, and programs for prevention and treatment.

"Topics." 2016. Substance Abuse and Mental Health Services Administration. http://www.samhsa.gov/topics. Accessed on July 10, 2016.

SAMHSA is the federal government's primary agency for information about and action programs on all types of substance abuse issues. This web page provides leads to individual topics for which more detailed information is available.

Wallach, Philip A., and Jonathan Rauch. 2016. "Bootleggers, Baptists, Bureaucrats, and Bongs: How Special Interests Will Shape Marijuana Legalization." Washington, DC: Brookings Institution.

The authors point out that the legalization of marijuana for medical and/or recreational uses is affected by and affects a variety of stakeholders, each of whom has some special interest in decisions made about such an action.

"What Are Drug Courts?" 2016. National Association of Drug Court Professionals. http://www.nadcp.org/learn/what-are-drug-courts. Accessed on July 14, 2016.

This web page is sponsored by an organization of professionals who are associated with drug courts. It explains what drug courts are, how they operate, who is eligible to use a drug court, and other relevant information about the institution.

"What Is Date Rape? 2016. Teens Health. http://kidshealth.org/teen/your_mind/problems/date_rape.html. Accessed on July 12, 2016.

This web page points out that date rape is different from what most people think of when they hear the term *rape*. It explains the ways in which date rape is different and provides a number of very specific and practical actions one can take to reduce the risk of being involved in a date rape.

"Workplace Drug Testing." 2016. U.S. Department of Labor. https://webapps.dol.gov/elaws/asp/drugfree/drugs/dt.asp. Accessed on July 12, 2016.

This web page is based on the assumption that workplace drug testing is an important and worthwhile activity for most business operations and provides an excellent general introduction to programs of this type that can be implemented in U.S. businesses.

"World Alcohol and Drinking History Timeline." 2016. Alcohol: Problems and Solutions. http://www.alcoholproblemsand solutions.org/timeline/Alcoholic-Beverages-from-Antiq uity-through-the-Ancient-Greeks.html. Accessed on July 12, 2016.

This website provides a detailed and very complete timeline of important events in the history of alcohol and drinking from 10000 BCE to the present day. It includes a bibliography of more than 70 additional resources.

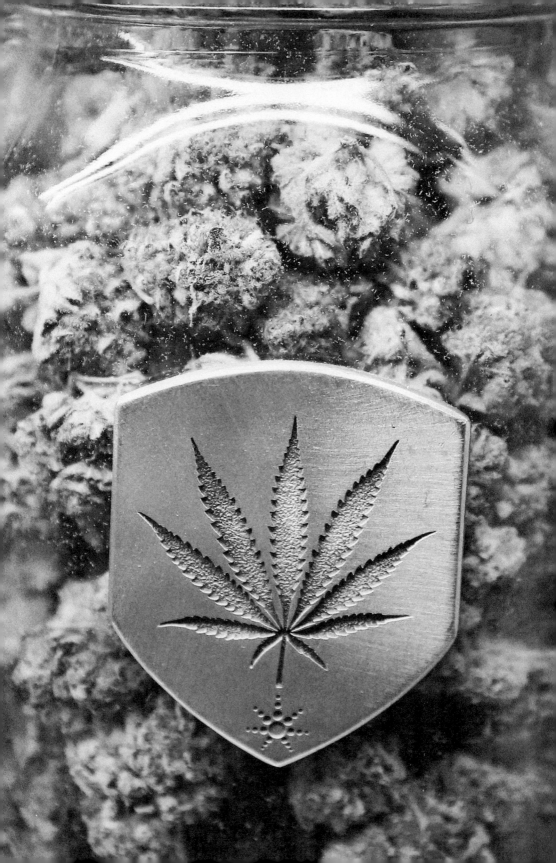

Introduction

The use of natural plant products to produce altered states of consciousness dates to the earliest years of human history. There has hardly been a period since then when substances such as cocaine, opiates, marijuana and other cannabis products, and a host of other natural and synthetic materials, have not been used for such effects. This chapter lists a number of important events in the history of the use of psychoactive substances in human cultures, along with a number of efforts to control the use of such products.

ca. Archaeologists discover remains of the herbal stimulant ephedra

50,000 BCE   at a burial site in Iraq dated to about 50,000 years ago.

ca. Among products discovered at the earliest agricultural sites,

10,000 BCE   dating to about 10,000 years ago, are cannabis, tobacco, and mandrake, which contains hallucinogenic alkaloids.

One of many different strains of pot on display at a marijuana dispensary in Denver, Colorado. The state of Colorado released a report on April 18, 2016, detailing changes in everything from pot arrests to tax collections to calls to poison control. The most striking statistic wasn't a change at all, but the fact that surveys indicate marijuana use by people under 18 didn't rise significantly in the years after the 2012 vote to legalize recreational pot sales. (AP Photo/Brennan Linsley)

ca. 9000–   Prehistoric rock art suggests the use of psychedelic mushrooms

7000 BCE   by early humans.

ca. 7000 BCE   Seeds of the betel nut, still chewed today for their stimulant effects in many parts of the world, are found at sites dating to 7,000 years ago.

ca. 7000 BCE   Clay vessels containing remnants of wine dating to about 7000 BCE are found at the site of a Neolithic village in Iran.

ca. 6000 BCE   The first cultivation of tobacco in the New World (South America) dates to about 6000 BCE.

ca. 4300 BCE   The first recipes for making beer, recorded on clay tablets from Babylonia, date to about 4300 BCE.

ca. 3300 BCE   The earliest written records of the use of opium date to about 3300 BCE, although evidence for its cultivation dates to about 1,000 years earlier.

ca. 3000 BCE   Charred seeds of the cannabis plant found in a ritual brazier at a burial site in modern-day Romania, suggesting that they were used in a religious ceremony, date to about 3000 BCE.

2500–   The earliest evidence for the cultivation of the coca plant in

1800 BCE   northern Peru dates to 2500–1800 BCE.

5th century AD   In his book *The Persian Wars*, Greek historian Herodotus records the use of cannabis as a recreational drug by the Scythians.

620 AD   In one of the earliest (perhaps the earliest) attempts at regulating drinking, the prophet Muhammed prohibits the consumption of alcohol by Muslims (Qur'an 2:219 and 5:91).

1484   Pope Innocent VIII bans the use of cannabis. His action was part of the Church's program against heretics because common belief at the time was that witches used cannabis as an "antisacrament" in place of wine at their "black masses."

1493   Christopher Columbus and his crew, returning from America, introduce the use of tobacco products to Europe.

ca. 1525   The Swiss-Austrian physician and alchemist Phillip von Hohenheim (better known as Paracelsus) introduces the use of a tincture of opium called *laudanum* to medical practice in Europe.

1590   A Japanese law makes possession of tobacco illegal. Anyone found with the substance is subject to imprisonment and/or loss of property.

1613–1614   John Rolfe, husband of the Indian princess Pocahontas, sends the first shipment of tobacco from the New World to Europe.

1619   The Jamestown Colony adopts the first so-called "must grow" law for hemp, noting that the product has many useful applications. Other colonies soon adopt similar laws as a way of improving the supply of an essential raw material in difficult economic times.

1633   The Sultan Murad IV of Turkey declares the use of tobacco a capital offense, punished by hanging, beheading, or starvation.

1638   A Chinese law declares use of tobacco a capital offense, to be punished by beheading.

1690   The British Parliament passes an Act for the Encouraging of the Distillation of Brandy and Spirits from Corn, which results in the production of about a million gallons of alcoholic beverages, primarily gin, only four years later.

1736   Concerned about the widespread popularity of gin among all classes, the British Parliament passes the Gin Act, which raises taxes on the drink to 20 shillings per gallon, a point at which only members of the upper classes can afford the substance.

1751   The British Parliament passes a new Gin Act. After the Gin Act of 1736 resulted in riots in the streets, it was revoked for a few years, before being reimposed by this act, which imposes a tax of five shillings per gallon on gin.

1785   In his book *An Inquiry into the Effects of Ardent Spirits upon the Human Body and Mind,* American physician Benjamin Rush calls the intemperate use of alcohol a disease and lists a number of symptoms, such as unusual garrulity, unusual silence, profane swearing and cursing, a clipping of words, fighting, and certain extravagant acts that indicate a temporary fit of madness, such as singing, roaring, and imitating the noises of brute animals. He estimates the annual death rate from alcoholism at about 4,000 in a population of about 6 million.

1789   An estimated 200 farmers living in the vicinity of Litchfield, Connecticut, meet to form the nation's first temperance society.

1791   The U.S. Congress enacts the nation's first tax on whiskey, the so-called whiskey tax.

1793–1797   Opposition to the whiskey tax of 1791 leads to outbreaks of violence in various parts of Pennsylvania, all of which are eventually put down by federal forces.

ca. 1800   Members of Napoleon's army, returning from the war in Egypt, bring with them information about the use of cannabis (in the form of hashish and marijuana) to France. Medical personnel are impressed by the painkilling properties of the drug, and some members of the general public are more interested in its use as a recreational drug.

1802   The whiskey tax of 1791 is repealed.

1805   German chemist Friedrich Sertürner extracts morphine from opium. He names the substance after Morpheus, the Greek god of dreams.

1819   German chemist Friedrich Ferdinand Runge isolates caffeine from coffee.

1848   President James Polk signs the Drug Importation Act, which establishes standards for the purity of drugs imported to the United States. The act is necessitated primarily by the fact that the United States is the last major nation in the world without legislation of this kind. The act does not, however, establish standards for drugs manufactured domestically.

1859 As a doctoral student, German chemist Albert Niemann obtains pure cocaine from coca leaves.

1868 In one of the first efforts to regulate the sale and use of drugs, the British Parliament passes the Pharmacy Act, which makes it illegal to sell opium and other drugs without a license.

1870 In New York City, a group of "scientific and medical gentlemen" found the American Association for the Cure of Inebriates, with the goals of studying the condition of "inebriety," discussing its proper treatment, and bringing about a "co-operative public sentiment and jurisprudence." The action was significant because it was one of the first times that the medical profession acknowledged that alcoholism might be a hereditary disease that could be treated like other medical conditions.

1875 The city of San Francisco adopts an ordinance prohibiting the smoking of opium, apparently the first law in the United States to deal with the practice.

1884 Largely through the influence of the Women's Christian Temperance Union, the New York state legislature passes a bill requiring the inclusion of an anti-alcohol curriculum in all schools in the state. Pennsylvania follows suit the next year, as do many other states in succeeding years.

1887 Romanian chemist Lazăr Edeleanu first synthesizes amphetamine in an effort to make ephedrine synthetically. With no known use, the compound is essentially forgotten for about 40 years.

1893 Japanese chemist Nagayoshi Nagai synthesizes methamphetamine.

1902 Physician C. B. Burr writes in the *Journal of the American Medical Association* about the problems of morphine addiction and its treatment. This article is one of the earliest commentaries on the addictive properties of morphine and heroin and their potential medical implications.

1906 The U.S. Congress passes the Pure Food and Drug Law, among whose provision is a requirement that all products containing alcohol be labeled to indicate that fact.

1909   The U.S. Congress passes the Smoking Opium Exclusion Act, the first federal regulation of the nonmedical use of a substance. The law bans the importation, possession, and smoking of opium.

1910   New York becomes the first state to adopt a drunk driving law.

1912   The International Opium Convention is signed at The Hague, the Netherlands, signed by China, France, Germany, Italy, Japan, the Netherlands, Persia, Portugal, Russia, Siam, the United States, and the United Kingdom. The convention called on all signatories to make every effort to control "all persons manufacturing, importing, selling, distributing, and exporting morphine, cocaine, and their respective salts, as well as the buildings in which these persons carry such an industry or trade." The convention is the first effort at reaching an international agreement on the control of illicit drugs.

1914   The Harrison Act requires importers, exporters, manufacturers, and distributors of all opiate products to register with the U.S. government and pay taxes on their sales. The act does not make the use of opiates illegal.

1916   In the case of *United States v. Jin Fuey Moy* (241 U.S. 394 [1916]), the U.S. Supreme Court severely restricts implementation of the Harrison Act, passed two years earlier.

1919   Secretary of State Francis Polk certifies the ratification of the Eighteenth Amendment to the U.S. Constitution, placing severe restrictions on the manufacture, sale, and transportation of "intoxicating liquors" within the United States. The amendment was eventually ratified by every state in the union except for Connecticut and Rhode Island.

The International Opium Convention is incorporated into the conditions of the Versailles Peace Treaty signed at the end of World War I. This action obligated all signatories to the peace treaty to become signatories to the opium treaty also.

1922   The Narcotic Import and Export Act restricts the importation of crude opium into the United States except for medical use.

1924   The Heroin Act makes the manufacture and possession of heroin illegal.

1927   The Bureau of Prohibition in the Bureau of Internal Revenue is established as the enforcement arm of the Eighteenth Amendment to the Constitution, which had been adopted in 1919.

1928   Great Britain bans the use of cannabis for nonmedical purposes.

1930   The Federal Bureau of Narcotics is established to enforce provisions of the Harrison Narcotic Act of 1914 and the Narcotic Drugs Import and Export Act of 1922.

1931   At a meeting held in Geneva, a group of nations adopt the Convention for Limiting the Manufacture and Regulating the Distribution of Narcotic Drugs in an effort to bring under control the manufacture, distribution, and use of a number of narcotic drugs. The convention enters into force in 1933.

1932   The U.S. Congress passes the Uniform State Narcotics Act, which encourages all states to adopt model legislation described in the act so that the same penalties for drug use will be applied throughout the nation. By the mid-1930s, all states have adopted the model legislation, essentially establishing a national drug policy.

The pharmaceutical firm of Smith, Kline, and French markets amphetamine as Benzedrine, an over-the-counter inhalant for respiratory congestion.

1933   Secretary of State Cordell Hull certifies the ratification of the Twenty-First Amendment to the United States, nullifying the Eighteenth Amendment and ending national laws against the manufacture, sale, and transportation of alcoholic beverages in the United States.

1935   Two American alcoholics—William Griffith ("Bill") Wilson and Robert Holbrook ("Bob") Smith—found Alcoholics Anonymous.

1936   A film entitled *Reefer Madness* about the dangers of smoking marijuana is released to the general public. The film is reputedly produced originally by a small church group aimed at frightening their youth members about the risks of substance abuse. Although produced at little cost with a cast of essentially unknown actors, the film has come to be a cult classic and, in 2001, premiers as an off-Broadway musical show.

Representatives of a number of nations meet in Geneva to adopt the Convention for the Suppression of the Illicit Traffic in Dangerous Drugs, an effort to criminalize trafficking in illegal drugs. When the United States finds itself unable to support the final document, it loses any chance of being a strong step in preventing the worldwide distribution of illegal drugs.

1937   The American Medical Association endorses the sale of amphetamine tablets for the treatment of narcolepsy and attention deficit hyperactivity disorder.

The Marijuana Tax Act imposes a tax on anyone who deals in any form of cannabis, hemp, or marijuana. The act does not criminalize the use of marijuana, but it does provide for severe penalties for anyone who fails to pay the tax associated with cannabis use.

1941–1945   The U.S. government distributes both amphetamine and methamphetamine to military personnel to improve their performance in battle.

1948   The United Nations sponsors an international conference to update a treaty for the control of narcotic drugs signed in 1931. The document signed at the meeting is called the Protocol Bringing under International Control Drugs outside the Scope of the Convention of 13 July 1931 for Limiting the Manufacture and Regulating the Distribution of Narcotic Drugs. It takes an important step in recognizing that a number of substances not previously defined formally as illegal substances—including a number of synthetic products—have effects similar to those of marijuana, cocaine, heroin, morphine, and other "traditional" drugs.

1951   The Boggs Act increases federal penalties for violations of federal drug laws. The act is the first piece of legislation in which marijuana and other illegal drugs are given equal treatment.

Lois W., wife of Bill W., cofounder of Alcoholics Anonymous, and Anne B. found Al-Anon, a support group for family members of alcoholics.

1956 The Narcotics Control Act further increases federal penalties for violations of federal drug laws.

1957 The teenage son of alcoholic parents and members of Alcoholics Anonymous in California form Alateen, an organization designed to provide support for the children of one or more alcoholic parents. A year later, the organization is adopted by Al-Anon as a special committee of the organization.

1961 A conference sponsored by the United Nations adopts the Single Convention on Narcotic Drugs, an effort to update and consolidate a number of previously adopted conventions, protocols, and agreements on the manufacture, distribution, and sale of illegal drugs, including the International Opium Convention of 1912; the Agreement Concerning the Manufacture of, Internal Trade in and Use of Prepared Opium of 1925; the International Opium Convention of 1925; the Convention for Limiting the Manufacture and Regulating the Distribution of Narcotic Drugs of 1931; the Agreement for the Control of Opium Smoking in the Far East of 1931; the Protocol Amending the Agreements, Conventions and Protocols on Narcotic Drugs of 1912; 1925, 1931, 1936, and 1946; the Protocol Bringing under International Control Drugs Outside the Scope of the Convention of 1931; and the Protocol for Limiting and Regulating the Cultivation of the Poppy Plant, the Production of, International and Wholesale Trade in, and Use of Opium of 1953.

1964 In the largest and most definitive study of its kind, the so-called Grand Rapids Study finds that the risk of a driver being involved in an accident rises sharply with his or her blood alcohol concentration. These findings are replicated a number of times in the future with a variety of modifications in variables studied.

1965 The Drug Abuse Control Amendments Act is passed for the purpose of dealing with problems caused by the use of stimulants, depressants, and hallucinogens. It authorizes the Food and Drug Administration to designate such drugs as controlled substances and to require that a federal license be obtained for their distribution and sale. The possession of small amounts of such drugs for personal use is allowed.

An advisory committee to the surgeon general issues a report, "Smoking and Health," that represents the first significant review of the health effects of smoking. The report is instrumental in the passage in the same year of the Federal Cigarette Labeling and Advertising Act, which, among other provisions, requires that all cigarette packages carry the warning label: "Caution: Cigarette Smoking May Be Hazardous to Your Health."

1968   The Bureau of Narcotics and Dangerous Drugs is formed as an agency within the U.S. Department of Justice. It combines the preexisting Bureau of Narcotics and Bureau of Drug Abuse Control.

1970   The U.S. Congress passes the Comprehensive Drug Abuse Prevention and Control Act in an effort to consolidate a number of earlier laws regulating the manufacture and distribution of narcotics, stimulants, depressants, hallucinogens, anabolic steroids, and chemicals used in the production of controlled substances. Title II of the act is called the Controlled Substances Act, which establishes a five-tier system of categorizing drugs that is still used today.

The U.S. Congress passes legislation banning cigarette advertising on television and radio. The ban takes effect in 1971. The cigarette industry voluntarily agrees to list tar and nicotine content on all cigarette packages.

The U.S. Congress passes the Comprehensive Alcohol Abuse and Alcoholism Prevention, Treatment, and Rehabilitation Act of 1970. One provision of the act establishes the National Institute on Alcoholism and Alcohol Abuse (NIAAA), with the responsibility of conducting intramural research and supporting extramural research on issues of alcoholism and alcohol abuse.

1971   President Richard M. Nixon declares a "war on drugs," calling for an aggressive anti-drug policy at both federal and state levels. He calls drug abuse "Public Enemy #1" in the United States.

The United Nations Protocol on Psychotropic Substances is adopted in Vienna. The purpose of the protocol is to expand coverage of the 1961 Single Convention on Narcotic Drugs (which covered natural substances and their derivatives exclusively) to a host of synthetic psychotropic substances, such as ketamine, ephedrine, 3,4-methylenedioxymethamphetamine (MDMA), and tetrahydrocannabinol not covered by the 1931 agreement.

1972   The National Commission on Marihuana and Drug Abuse (also known as the Shafer Commission, after its chairman) issues its report, recommending, among other things, that simple possession of marijuana be decriminalized and that all distinctions between legal and illegal drugs be dropped. The commission has been created by the U.S. Congress by Public Law 91–513 to study the problem of substance abuse in the United States. President Richard M. Nixon declines to implement any of the commission's recommendations.

1973   As part of the Reorganization Plan No. 2 of 1973, President Richard M. Nixon establishes the Drug Enforcement Administration to replace the Bureau of Narcotics and Dangerous Drugs, the Office of Drug Abuse Law Enforcement, and a handful of other federal agencies with drug control responsibilities.

The Methadone Control Act provides funding for the establishment of clinics through which recovering heroin addicts can receive methadone therapy.

1974   The National Institute on Drug Abuse is created to conduct research on drug abuse and drug addiction.

1976   The Democratic Party national platform calls for decriminalization of marijuana, with the abolishment of all penalties for possession of one ounce or less of the drug.

1978   The U.S. Food and Drug Administration introduces the Compassionate Investigational New Drug program, allowing a small number of patients to use marijuana grown at a federal facility at the University of Mississippi to relieve symptoms of medical conditions. Currently four individuals remain in that program.

The U.S. Congress passes the American Indian Religious Freedom Act that acknowledges the elements of traditional Native American religious ceremonies and the conflicts that may arise between those ceremonies and some U.S. laws. It declares that Native Americans do have the right to practice their traditional religious customs. The use of peyote is implicitly, but not explicitly, guaranteed by this act.

1984   The 1965 Federal Cigarette Labeling and Advertising Act is amended to require that one of four warning labels appear in a specific format on cigarette packages and in most related advertising: "SURGEON GENERAL'S WARNING: Smoking Causes Lung Cancer, Heart Disease, Emphysema, and May Complicate Pregnancy," "SURGEON GENERAL'S WARNING: Quitting Smoking Now Greatly Reduces Serious Risks to Your Health," "SURGEON GENERAL'S WARNING: Smoking by Pregnant Women May Result in Fetal Injury, Premature Birth, and Low Birth Weight," or "SURGEON GENERAL'S WARNING: Cigarette Smoke Contains Carbon Monoxide."

The U.S. Congress passes the National Minimum Drinking Age Act (also known as the Uniform Drinking Age Act) requiring all states to raise the minimum age for drinking to 21. Any state that refuses to adopt this standard is subject to loss of 10 percent of the funds due it annually under the Federal Aid Highway Act.

1985   Minnesota becomes the first state to enact legislation setting aside a portion of the state tobacco tax for smoking prevention programs.

1986   The U.S. Congress passes the Anti-Drug Abuse Act of 1986. The act consists of two major titles, one dealing with

Anti-Drug Enforcement, and the other with International Narcotics Control. The first title is divided into 21 subtitles dealing with a host of issues, perhaps the most important of which is Subtitle E: Controlled Substances Analogue Enforcement Act of 1986, which states that substances that are chemically and pharmacologically similar to substances listed in Schedule I or Schedule II of the Controlled Substances Act of 1970 (known as analogues of the listed drugs) are also classified as Schedule I drugs. Perhaps the most controversial section is Subtitle B: Drug Possession Penalty Act of 1986, which establishes the so-called 100-to-1 rule, in which possession of 100 grams of powder cocaine (the drug of choice among wealthy white Americans) is considered to be legally equivalent to 1 gram of crack cocaine (used most commonly by blacks).

President Ronald Reagan signs Executive Order 12564 requiring all federal agencies to establish drug-free workplace programs.

First Lady Nancy Reagan launches her "Just Say No" campaign against drug use.

1988 The Anti-Drug Abuse Act of 1988 for the first time imposes penalties on the users of illegal drugs. Prior to this time, penalties for illegal drug use were limited to the producers and distributors of such substances. One provision of the act establishes the Office of National Drug Control Policy, with responsibility for developing policies for control of the nation's drug abuse problems.

Francis L. Young, administrative law judge at the Drug Enforcement Administration (DEA), issues an opinion that marijuana has clear and unquestionable medical uses and should be reclassified as a Schedule II drug from its current status as a Schedule I drug. The DEA declines to act on that recommendation.

The U.S. Congress passes the Chemical Diversion and Trafficking Act, whose purpose it is to reduce the supply of precursor chemicals and manufacturing devices (such as pill machines) used in the manufacture of drugs. Prior to the law, the United States was the major supplier of these materials to (primarily) South American companies, where raw materials were converted to commercial-grade drugs.

The U.S. Congress passes the Drug Free Workplace Act, which extends President Ronald Reagan's 1986 executive order to require all contractors and grantees of the federal government to develop programs for a drug-free workplace.

1990   The U.S. Congress passes legislation banning smoking on all U.S. commercial airline flights.

1992   President George H. W. Bush discontinues the Food and Drug Administration's Compassionate Investigational New Drug program because it conflicts with his administration's drug use policies.

1993   The U.S. Congress passes the Native American Free Exercise of Religion Act, which confirms, clarifies, and expands the American Indian Religious Freedom Act of 1978. In particular, it specifically allows the use of peyote, a drug banned by the Controlled Substances Act of 1970.

1994   China passes the nation's first laws requiring health warnings on cigarette packages, limiting tobacco advertising, and initiating antismoking programs.

Mississippi becomes the first state to sue the tobacco industry to recover costs for tobacco-related illnesses.

The Omnibus Crime Bill, introduced by then-senator Joseph Biden (D–DE), introduces the death penalty for anyone convicted of operating large-scale drug distribution programs, one of the first times the death penalty is permitted for crimes in which a death is not involved.

1995   The U.S. Sentencing Commission issues a report to the U.S. Congress confirming that serious racial imbalances exist in sentencing for powder cocaine and "crack" cocaine and recommending Congress act to ameliorate these disparities. Congress declines to do so, one of the very few times in history it refuses to follow the commission's recommendations.

In the case of *Vernonia v. Acton*, the U.S. Supreme Court rules, in a vote of 6 to 3, that a school district may impose suspicionless drug tests on students who wish to engage in extracurricular activities.

1996   Arizona voters pass Proposition 200, otherwise known as the Drug, Medicalization, Prevention and Punishment Act, which requires that a person convicted of possession or use of an illegal drug receive drug treatment for the first and second offense, and a prison term only after the third such conviction. Physicians in the state are also authorized to write prescriptions for Schedule I drugs when federal law permits such actions.

The U.S. Congress passes the Drug-Induced Rape Prevention and Punishment Act, which provides for penalties of up to 20 years in prison for supplying a drug to another person with the intent of committing a crime, such as rape, against that person. The primary motivation for the act is the spread of so-called date rape, in which one person provides a second person with a psychoactive drug—most commonly ketamine, gamma hydroxybutyrate (GHB), gamma butyrolactone (GBL), or Rohypnol—without that second person's knowledge or approval.

California voters pass Proposition 215, the Compassionate Use Act of 1996, which allows individuals with a doctor's prescription to grow small amounts of marijuana for their own personal medical use.

The U.S. Congress passes the Comprehensive Methamphetamine Control Act, which further restricts the sale of precursors used in the production of methamphetamine, such as pseudoephedrine, iodine, red phosphorus, and hydrochloric acid.

1997   The tobacco industry reaches a settlement with 46 state attorneys general to pay $360 billion over a period of 25 years to fund antismoking campaigns, to add health warnings to cigarette packages, and to pay substantial fines if the number of teenage smokers is not reduced.

For the first time in history, a major tobacco executive, Bennett LeBow, CEO of Liggett, admits during public testimony that cigarette smoking causes cancer.

1998   The U.S. Congress passes the Controlled Substances Trafficking Prohibition Act, which limits the amount of certain controlled substances that a person can bring into the United States for personal use to 50 pills or less or a two-week supply. The law is designed to remove a loophole that previously allowed individuals to bring back unlimited quantities of Schedule II drugs, supposedly for their own personal medical needs but, in reality, for resale in the United States.

2000   The U.S. Supreme Court rules that the Food and Drug Administration does not have the authority to regulate tobacco products.

The Drug Addiction Treatment Act of 2000 allows certain qualifying physicians to treat patients with opioid addictions using substances on Schedules III, IV, and V of the Controlled Substances Act. The only drug that meets this specification is buprenorphine.

President Bill Clinton signs a new federal law requiring all states to pass a law setting a blood alcohol concentration (BAC) of 0.08 percent as the legal limit. States that do not adopt this standard are to be denied a portion of the federal highway funding normally due them. Eventually 49 states do adopt such laws, the only exception being Massachusetts, where a BAC of 0.08 percent is considered legal proof of impairment, but is not illegal in and out itself.

The U.S. government gives $1.3 billion to Colombia for the purpose of improving its anti-drug campaign. The money is designated to be used for aerial spraying of coca and other drug crops, for training of Colombian troops in anti-drug programs, and for the purchase of equipment, such as helicopters, to be used against drug manufacturers and distributors.

2001   In the case of *United States v. Oakland Cannabis Buyers' Cooperative,* the U.S. Supreme Court unanimously rules that marijuana has no medical value and that its sale by the Oakland Cannabis Buyers' Cooperative (and similar organizations) is illegal.

2002 The British government changes its policies on the use of cannabis products, downgrading the drug from Class B to Class C. That change leaves the drug as an illegal substance, although an arrest for possession is likely to result in confiscation of the drug and a warning, but no prosecution, prison time, or fine.

2003 All forms of advertising for tobacco products in the United Kingdom is banned.

A ban by the European Union on the use of the terms "light" or "mild" on cigarette packages takes effect.

Concerned about the estimated 30,000 deaths annually caused by smoking, French president Jacques Chirac announces a "war on smoking" that includes an investment of more than $500 million for antismoking campaigns, a near-doubling of cigarette taxes, and greater limitations on places that people may smoke.

2004 All forms of advertising and promotions for tobacco products are banned in India.

2005 The U.S. Congress passes and President George W. Bush signs the USA PATRIOT Improvement and Reauthorization Act, which includes, as an unrelated amendment, a version of the Combat Meth Act, originally proposed by Sen. James Talent (R–MO). One of the primary features of the act is the imposition of severe restrictions on the sale of cough and cold products whose ingredients can be used in the manufacture of methamphetamine.

In the case of *Gonzales v. Raich,* the U.S. Supreme Court rules, by a vote of 6 to 3, that it is illegal for medical doctors to write prescriptions for their patients to use marijuana for medical purposes.

2006 In the case of *United States of America v. Philip Morris*, Judge Gladys Kessler finds that U.S. tobacco companies have engaged in a "massive 50-year scheme to defraud the public, including consumers of cigarettes, in violation of RICO [Racketeer Influenced and Corrupt Organizations Act of 1970]." She imposes a fine of $280 billion on the tobacco companies.

2009   Congress approves the largest-ever increase in the federal cigarette tax, boosting it 62 cents, to $1.01 a pack.

The U.S. Congress passes and President Barack Obama signs the Family Smoking Prevention and Tobacco Control and Federal Retirement Reform act, which authorizes the Food and Drug Administration to regulate cigarettes and other tobacco products.

For the first time in history, the number of fatalities due to prescription drugs exceeds the number of deaths from vehicle accidents in the United States.

2010   The U.S. Congress adopts the Secure and Responsible Drug Disposal Act of 2010, which outlines the circumstances under which a person "who has lawfully obtained a controlled substance in accordance with this title may, without being registered, deliver the controlled substance to another person for the purpose of disposal of the controlled substance."

The state of Florida passes the nation's first pill-mill-type bill, setting standards for doctors who prescribe narcotics.

2011   Representative Barney Frank (D–MA) introduces legislation that would remove marijuana from the list of controlled substances (i.e., decriminalize marijuana in the United States). He introduces a second bill that would require the secretary of health and human services to recommend a relisting of marijuana under some category other than Schedules I or II and declares that federal regulations shall not be construed to conflict with the decisions of individual states to permit the medical use of marijuana. Neither bill is acted upon.

2012   Voters in the state of Colorado approve Amendment 64, which permits the personal use of marijuana in the state. "Personal use" includes the cultivation of three immature and three mature cannabis plants and possession of one ounce of marijuana by individuals over the age of 21. Voters in Washington adopt a similar law that permits possession, but not growing, of marijuana.

2014   The U.S. House of Representatives passes a bill prohibiting the Drug Enforcement Administration from using funds to arrest medical cannabis patients in states with medical cannabis laws.

2015   An outbreak of HIV infections in rural Scott County, Indiana, is attributed to sharing of needles by individuals addicted to the opioid analgesic Opana (oxymorphone). As of mid-May 2015, more than 150 new cases of HIV had been diagnosed that could be traced to this nonmedical use of Opana. Indiana governor Mike Pence (Republican) reluctantly agrees to a needle exchange program to which he had previously been opposed as a possible way for ending the spread of the epidemic.

DEA agents carry out raids in Alabama, Arkansas, Louisiana, and Mississippi targeting pharmacists, physicians, and street-dealers who are selling prescription drugs for nonmedical purposes. More than 200 individuals are arrested as a result of the raids, which DEA officials called the "largest operation against illegal trafficking of prescription drugs" in U.S. history.

As of the end of 2015, 34 states have adopted one or more laws dealing with prescription drug abuse. No federal legislation has yet been adopted on the issue.

2016   A review of the impact of new marijuana laws published in the *Journal of Addiction Medicine* finds an increase in the number of adults using marijuana over the past decade, no change in the number of adolescents using the substance, a decrease in marijuana-related arrests, and an increase in the number of treatment admissions for the drug.

The state legislatures of Ohio and Pennsylvania approve the use of marijuana for medical purposes, bringing to 25 the number of states (and the District of Columbia) that have taken such actions by one means or another.

Congress passes a bill providing funding for opioid and heroin addiction programs. The three main components of the bill are new programs for diverting people stopped for minor opioid infractions from the criminal justice system into treatment programs; extended use of medications such as methadone and buprenorphine for the treatment of opioid addiction; and expanded use of naloxone by first responders in the treatment of opioid overdoses.

2017   Surgeon General Vivek H. Murthy issues the first ever national report on substance abuse in a document entitled "Facing Addiction in America: The Surgeon General's Report on Alcohol, Drugs, and Health."

Discussions of substance abuse often involve terminology that is unfamiliar to the average person. In some cases, the terms used are scientific or medical expressions used most commonly by professionals in the field. In other cases, the terms may be part of the so-called street slang that users themselves employ in talking about the drugs they consume, the paraphernalia associated with drugs, or the kind of experiences that accompany drug use. This glossary lists and defines some of the most common terms from each group.

addiction   A long-lasting and typically recurring psychological and/or physiological need for one or more substances, such as alcohol or tobacco, that generally results in permanent or long-lasting changes in the neurochemistry of the brain.

alcohol   In discussions of substance abuse, a term that refers to the chemical's correct chemical name, ethanol or ethyl alcohol. In chemistry, the term has a different and more general meaning, referring to a class of organic compounds that contains the hydroxyl functional group, —OH.

alcoholism   Physical dependence on alcohol such that discontinuing the use of alcohol results in withdrawal symptoms. Alcoholism is typically accompanied by the development of social and/or health problems serious enough to require professional help.

analgesic   A drug capable of relieving pain.

analog (also **analogue**) A chemical compound similar in structure to some other chemical compound.

antidepressant A drug that reduces or moderates depression, resulting in an elevation in one's mood.

ataxia Loss of control of muscular movement, manifested in an unsteady gait, unsteady movements, and clumsiness; a common symptom of mild drug overdose.

BAC Acronym for *blood alcohol content* or *blood alcohol concentration*, a measure of the amount of alcohol present in a person's body, usually represented as percent content or percent concentration, as 0.08 (i.e., 0.08%).

barbiturate A substance derived from the chemical barbituric acid ($C_4H_4N_2O_3$). Some examples of barbiturates are barbital (Veronal), phenobarbital (Luminal), pentobarbital (Nembutal), and sodium pentothal.

bhang A concoction or infusion made with leaves and flowers from the hemp plant, widely used on the Indian subcontinent as a recreational drug and as a drug for religious and ceremonial purposes.

binge drinking Excessive consumption of alcohol over a relatively brief period of time, which typically results in nausea, vomiting, loss of control over one's bodily functions and, in extreme cases, more serious symptoms, such as coma and death.

blackout Loss of memory about a particular event, such as the taking of a drug or overconsumption of alcohol.

bronchodilator A drug that relaxes and dilates the bronchial passages, allowing for easier breathing.

caffeine A mildly addictive alkaloid stimulant found in coffee, tea, kola nuts, and many synthetic beverages, such as soda drinks.

cannabinoid Any one of the substances found in the cannabis plant, *Cannabis sativa*, or, more generally, that has a chemical structure similar to that of tetrahydrocannabinol (THC) or that binds to cannabinoid receptors in the body.

cannabis The botanical name for the plant from which marijuana comes. Its correct botanical name is *Cannabis sativa*.

chemical dependence A condition that develops when one's body undergoes changes that result in a continual physiological need for a particular drug or other substance.

club drug *See* **designer drug**.

cocaine A powerful stimulant extracted from the leaves of the coca plant (*Erythroxylon coca*).

codeine An addictive alkaloid narcotic derived from opium, used as an antitussive and analgesic, and also abused as a recreational drug.

controlled substance analog *See* **designer drug**.

crack A highly addictive form of cocaine, made by mixing cocaine with baking soda and water.

cross-addiction Addiction to two substances belonging to different classes, such as alcohol and cocaine.

dependence A condition in which an individual develops a fixation on or craving for a drug that is not necessarily so severe as to be classified as an addiction but that may, nonetheless, require professional help to overcome.

designer drug (1) A synthetic chemical compound developed for the treatment of a specific disease or group of diseases; (2) A psychoactive chemical deliberately synthesized to avoid antidrug laws that mimics the effects of a banned drug. Also known as a controlled substance analog, club drug, or rave drug.

dissociative drug A substance that produces feelings of analgesia, disconnection, and alienation.

drug A chemical used in the diagnosis, cure, mitigation, treatment, or prevention of disease or to bring about an alternation in one's mental or emotional state.

dysphoria   A condition of unusually severe depression and/or anxiety, mental and/or physical discomfort, and general malaise.

ecstasy   A street name for 3-4 methylenedioxymethamphetamine (MDMA).

empathogen   A drug capable of producing strong emotional responses, such as emotional closeness, love, and affection. The term **entactogen** has been suggested as a synonym for the word.

enabling   The act of supporting or contributing to the destructive behavior of a substance abuser, sometimes based on the enabler's best intentions of helping that person.

endogenous   Produced naturally within the body.

entactogen   *See* **empathogen**.

flashback   Recurring emotional or sensory experiences that take place independently, and often at much later times, than an initial experience that, in the case of drugs, was the occasion of having consumed those drugs.

freebasing   A method of consuming cocaine by mixing it with ether so that it can be smoked.

hallucinogen   A substance that causes profound distortions in a person's perceptions of reality, causing an individual to see images, hear sounds, and feel sensations that seem real but do not exist.

inhalant   A substance of low volatility, such that it can be easily absorbed through the respiratory system.

laudanum   A tincture of opium, that is, opium powder dissolved in alcohol.

LSD   *See* **lysergic acid diethylamide**.

lysergic acid diethylamide   A semisynthetic chemical compound with very strong hallucinogenic effects, often known by its common names of LSD or acid.

mainlining   Taking a drug by injection into a vein.

methamphetamine   A highly addictive psychoactive drug belonging to the family of phenylethylamines, easily made by amateur chemists, and known by a variety of common names, depending in part on the form in which it is consumed, as "chalk," "crank," "crystal," "ice," glass," "meth," and "speed."

narcotic Any drug that, in small doses, produces insensitivity to pain, dulls the senses, and induces deep sleep, but in larger doses may result in numbness, convulsions, and coma.

neuron A nerve cell.

neurotransmitter A chemical that carries a nerve impulse between two neurons.

nicotine A very addictive alkaloid compound that occurs naturally in plants belonging to the genus Solanaceae, which includes the tobacco plant, of which it constitutes about 0.6–3.0 percent by dry weight.

opiate Any drug or other substance derived from or chemically related to opium.

opiate receptor A specialized receptor cell in neurons that bind to natural analgesic molecules present in the body.

opium An addictive narcotic extracted from the seeds of the opium poppy, *Papaver somniferum*.

OTC drug *See* **over-the-counter drug**.

overdose (verb) To take an excessive, risky, and potentially fatal quantity of a harmful substance.

over-the-counter drug A drug that can be purchased without a prescription.

paranoia A psychological disorder characterized by delusions of persecution or grandeur.

pharmacopoeia A catalog of drugs, chemicals, and medicinal preparations.

phenylethylamines A class of drugs whose members contain three functional groups—the phenyl group ($-C_6H_5$), ethyl group ($-C_2H_5$), and amine group ($-NH_2$)—that form the basis of a large number of natural and synthetic compounds with a variety of psychotropic effects. Drugs in this class may act as anorectics, antidepressants, bronchodilators, entactogens, hallucinogens, or stimulants.

precursor chemical   A chemical used to make some other substance, for example, the raw materials used to make illicit drugs.

prescription drug   A drug that can be purchased only with a medical prescription provided by a registered medical provider, such as a physician or a physician's assistant.

psychedelic   A substance capable of producing perceptual changes, such as vivid colors and weird shapes, as well as altered awareness of one's mind and body.

psychoactive   *See* **psychotropic**.

psychotropic   Having an effect on the mind.

rave drug   *See* **designer drug**.

relapse   The return of a condition, such as addiction to or dependency on a drug, which had formerly been successfully overcome.

schedule   (drug) A category into which the federal government classifies certain drugs based on their potential medical use and their possibility of illicit recreational applications.

secondhand smoke   Cigarette smoke inhaled involuntarily by nonsmoking individuals in a closed environment.

serotonin   A neurotransmitter associated with a number of mental and emotional functions, including appetite, learning, memory, mood, muscular contraction, and sleep. A number of drugs reduce or increase the amount of serotonin available in the brain, thereby moderating one or more of these actions.

smokeless tobacco   Tobacco that is consumed by some method other than smoking, for example, chewing tobacco or snuff.

snuff   Finely ground tobacco that is inhaled rather than smoked.

stimulant   When used in connection with drugs, a substance that temporarily increases physiological activity in the body, with a number of associated effects, such as increased awareness, interest, physical activity, wakefulness, endurance, and productivity. Physiological changes include increased heart rate and blood pressure.

synaptic gap The space between two neurons.

tetrahydrocannabinol A primary component of the cannabis plant, often represented simply as THC.

THC *See* **tetrahydrocannabinol**.

tolerance Immunity to the effects caused by a substance such that one requires a larger amount of the substance over time to achieve the same results obtained from smaller amounts earlier on in its use.

twelve-step program A program for recovery from alcoholism, drug addiction, and other behavioral problems originally proposed by Alcoholics Anonymous in its 1939 book *Alcoholics Anonymous: The Story of How More Than One Hundred Men Have Recovered from Alcoholism*.

withdrawal symptoms The physical, mental, and emotional effects that an individual experiences when he or she discontinues use of a substance to which he or she has become addicted or dependent.

About the Author

David E. Newton holds an associate's degree in science from Grand Rapids (Michigan) Junior College, a BA in chemistry (with high distinction), an MA in education from the University of Michigan, and an EdD in science education from Harvard University. He is the author of more than 400 textbooks, encyclopedias, resource books, research manuals, laboratory manuals, trade books, and other educational materials. He taught mathematics, chemistry, and physical science in Grand Rapids, Michigan, for 13 years; was professor of chemistry and physics at Salem State College in Massachusetts for 15 years; and was adjunct professor in the College of Professional Studies at the University of San Francisco for ten years.

The author's previous books for ABC-CLIO include *Global Warming* (1993), *Gay and Lesbian Rights* (1994, 2009), *The Ozone Dilemma* (1995), *Violence and the Mass Media* (1996), *Environmental Justice* (1996, 2009), *Encyclopedia of Cryptology* (1997), *Social Issues in Science and Technology: An Encyclopedia* (1999), *DNA Technology* (2009), *Sexual Health* (2010), *The Animal Experimentation Debate* (2013), *Marijuana* (2013), *World Energy Crisis* (2013), *Steroids and Doping in Sports* (2014), *GMO Food* (2014), *Science and Political Controversy* (2014), *Wind Energy* (2015), *Fracking* (2015), *Solar Energy* (2015), *Youth Substance Abuse* (2016), and *Global Water Crisis* (2016). His other recent books include *Physics: Oryx Frontiers of Science Series* (2000), *Sick!* (4 volumes) (2000), *Science, Technology, and Society: The Impact of Science in the 19th Century* (2 volumes; 2001), *Encyclopedia of Fire* (2002), *Molecular*

Nanotechnology: Oryx Frontiers of Science Series (2002), *Encyclopedia of Water* (2003), *Encyclopedia of Air* (2004), *The New Chemistry* (6 volumes; 2007), *Nuclear Power* (2005), *Stem Cell Research* (2006), *Latinos in the Sciences, Math, and Professions* (2007), and *DNA Evidence and Forensic Science* (2008). He has also been an updating and consulting editor on a number of books and reference works, including *Chemical Compounds* (2005), *Chemical Elements* (2006), *Encyclopedia of Endangered Species* (2006), *World of Mathematics* (2006), *World of Chemistry* (2006), *World of Health* (2006), *UXL Encyclopedia of Science* (2007), *Alternative Medicine* (2008), *Grzimek's Animal Life Encyclopedia* (2009), *Community Health* (2009), *Genetic Medicine* (2009), *The Gale Encyclopedia of Medicine* (2010–2011), *The Gale Encyclopedia of Alternative Medicine* (2013), *Discoveries in Modern Science: Exploration, Invention, and Technology* (2013–2014), and *Science in Context* (2013–2014).